T0263781

Plaque Imaging

Editor

J. KEVIN DEMARCO

NEUROIMAGING CLINICS OF NORTH AMERICA

www.neuroimaging.theclinics.com

Consulting Editor
SURESH K. MUKHERJI

February 2016 • Volume 26 • Number 1

ELSEVIER

1600 John F. Kennedy Boulevard • Suite 1800 • Philadelphia, Pennsylvania, 19103-2899

http://www.neuroimaging.theclinics.com

NEUROIMAGING CLINICS OF NORTH AMERICA Volume 26, Number 1
February 2016 ISSN 1052-5149, ISBN 13: 978-0-323-41700-6

Editor: John Vassallo (j.vassallo@elsevier.com)
Developmental Editor: Casey Jackson

© **2016 Elsevier Inc. All rights reserved.**

This publication and the individual contributions contained in it are protected under copyright by Elsevier, and the following terms and conditions apply to their use:

Photocopying
Single photocopies of single articles may be made for personal use as allowed by national copyright laws. Permission of the Publisher and payment of a fee is required for all other photocopying, including multiple or systematic copying, copying for advertising or promotional purposes, resale, and all forms of document delivery. Special rates are available for educational institutions that wish to make photocopies for non-profit educational classroom use. For information on how to seek permission visit www.elsevier.com/permissions or call: (+44) 1865 843830 (UK)/(+1) 215 239 3804 (USA).

Derivative Works
Subscribers may reproduce tables of contents or prepare lists of articles including abstracts for internal circulation within their institutions. Permission of the Publisher is required for resale or distribution outside the institution. Permission of the Publisher is required for all other derivative works, including compilations and translations (please consult www.elsevier. com/permissions).

Electronic Storage or Usage
Permission of the Publisher is required to store or use electronically any material contained in this periodical, including any article or part of an article (please consult www.elsevier.com/permissions). Except as outlined above, no part of this publication may be reproduced, stored in a retrieval system or transmitted in any form or by any means, electronic, mechanical, photocopying, recording or otherwise, without prior written permission of the Publisher.

Notice
No responsibility is assumed by the Publisher for any injury and/or damage to persons or property as a matter of products liability, negligence or otherwise, or from any use or operation of any methods, products, instructions or ideas contained in the material herein. Because of rapid advances in the medical sciences, in particular, independent verification of diagnoses and drug dosages should be made.

Although all advertising material is expected to conform to ethical (medical) standards, inclusion in this publication does not constitute a guarantee or endorsement of the quality or value of such product or of the claims made of it by its manufacturer.

Neuroimaging Clinics of North America (ISSN 1052-5149) is published quarterly by Elsevier Inc., 360 Park Avenue South, New York, NY 10010-1710. Months of issue are February, May, August, and November. Business and editorial offices: 1600 John F. Kennedy Blvd., Suite 1800, Philadelphia, PA 19103-2899. Business and editorial offices: 6277 Sea Harbor Drive, Orlando, FL 32887-4800. Periodicals postage paid at New York, NY, and additional mailing offices. Subscription prices are USD 365 per year for US individuals, USD 564 per year for US institutions, USD 100 per year for US students and residents, USD 415 per year for Canadian individuals, USD 718 per year for Canadian institutions, USD 525 per year for international individuals, USD 718 per year for international institutions and USD 260 per year for Canadian and foreign students and residents. To receive student/resident rate, orders must be accompanied by name of affiliated institution, date of term, and the *signature* of program/residency coordinator on institution letterhead. Orders will be billed at individual rate until proof of status is received. Foreign air speed delivery is included in all *Clinics* subscription prices. All prices are subject to change without notice. POSTMASTER: Send address changes to *Neuroimaging Clinics of North America*, Elsevier Health Sciences Division, Subscription **Customer Service, 3251 Riverport Lane, Maryland Heights, MO 63043. Telephone: 1-800-654-2452 (U.S. and Canada); 314-447-8871 (outside U.S. and Canada). Fax: 314-447-8029. E-mail:** journalscustomer service-usa@elsevier.com **(for print support);** journalsonlinesupport-usa@elsevier.com **(for online support)**.

Reprints. For copies of 100 or more of articles in this publication, please contact the Commercial Reprints Department, Elsevier Inc., 360 Park Avenue South, New York, NY 10010-1710. Tel.: 212-633-3874; Fax: 212-633-3820; E-mail: reprints@ elsevier.com.

Neuroimaging Clinics of North America is covered by *Excerpta Medical/EMBASE,* the RSNA Index of Imaging Literature, *MEDLINE/PubMed (Index Medicus),* MEDLINE/MEDLARS, SciSearch, Research Alert, and Neuroscience Citation Index.

PROGRAM OBJECTIVE

The goal of *Neuroimaging Clinics of North America* is to keep practicing radiologists and radiology residents up to date with current clinical practice in radiology by providing timely articles reviewing the state of the art in patient care.

TARGET AUDIENCE

Practicing radiologists, radiology residents, and other healthcare professionals who utilize neuroimaging findings to provide patient care.

LEARNING OBJECTIVES

Upon completion of this activity, participants will be able to:

1. Review and evaluate different methods of carotid plaque imaging, such as 3D MR imaging, PET imaging, and contrast-enhanced ultrasound imaging.
2. Discuss plaque assessment in the management of patients with cryptogenic stroke and asymptomatic carotid stenosis.
3. Recognize the use of multi-contrast magnetic resonance in the imaging of carotid plaque.

ACCREDITATION

The Elsevier Office of Continuing Medical Education (EOCME) is accredited by the Accreditation Council for Continuing Medical Education (ACCME) to provide continuing medical education for physicians.

The EOCME designates this enduring material for a maximum of 15 *AMA PRA Category 1 Credit*(s)™. Physicians should claim only the credit commensurate with the extent of their participation in the activity.

All other health care professionals requesting continuing education credit for this enduring material will be issued a certificate of participation.

DISCLOSURE OF CONFLICTS OF INTEREST

The EOCME assesses conflict of interest with its instructors, faculty, planners, and other individuals who are in a position to control the content of CME activities. All relevant conflicts of interest that are identified are thoroughly vetted by EOCME for fair balance, scientific objectivity, and patient care recommendations. EOCME is committed to providing its learners with CME activities that promote improvements or quality in healthcare and not a specific proprietary business or a commercial interest.

The planning committee, staff, authors and editors listed below have identified no financial relationships or relationships to products or devices they or their spouse/life partner have with commercial interest related to the content of this CME activity:

Abdelrahman Ali, MD; Anna Bayer-Karpinska, MD; Leo H. Bonati, MD; Mauricio Castillo, MD; Huijun Chen, PhD; J. Kevin DeMarco, MD; Marc R. Dweck, MD, PhD; Zahi A. Fayad, PhD; Anjali Fortna; Venu Gourineni, MD; William Kerwin, PhD; Alan Moody, FRCR, FRCP; Mahmud Mossa-Bassa, MD; Suresh K. Mukherji, MD, MBA, FACR; Paul J. Nederkoorn, MD, PhD; Dennis L. Parker, PhD; Grace Parraga, PhD; Tobias Saam, MD; Sandeep A. Saha, MD, FACP; Erin Scheckenbach; Andreas Schindler, MD; N. Singh, MD; Karthik Subramaniam; Jie Sun, MD; Carlos Torres, MD, FRCPC; John Vassallo; Alex T. Vesey, MD; Bruce Wasserman, MD; Nader Zakhari, MD, FRCPC; Qiang Zhang, MS.

The planning committee, staff, authors and editors listed below have identified financial relationships or relationships to products or devices they or their spouse/life partner have with commercial interest related to the content of this CME activity:

Steven B. Feinstein, MD, FACC, FESC is a consultant/advisor for General Electric.

Thomas S. Hatsukami, MD receives research support from Koninklijke Philips N.V.

J. David Spence, MD, FRCPC, FAHA is a consultant/advisor for, with stock ownership in, Vascularis Inc.

Ahmed Tawakol, MD is a consultant/advisor for Takeda Pharmaceutical Company Limited; Actelion Pharmaceuticals US, Inc; and Amgen Inc, and has research support from Takeda Pharmaceutical Company Limited; Actelion Pharmaceuticals US, Inc; and Genentech, Inc.

Chun Yuan, PhD is a consultant/advisor for, with research support from, Koninklijke Philips N.V.

UNAPPROVED/OFF-LABEL USE DISCLOSURE

The EOCME requires CME faculty to disclose to the participants:

1. When products or procedures being discussed are off-label, unlabelled, experimental, and/or investigational (not US Food and Drug Administration [FDA] approved); and
2. Any limitations on the information presented, such as data that are preliminary or that represent ongoing research, interim analyses, and/or unsupported opinions. Faculty may discuss information about pharmaceutical agents that is outside of FDA-approved labelling. This information is intended solely for CME and is not intended to promote off-label use of these medications. If you have any questions, contact the medical affairs department of the manufacturer for the most recent prescribing information.

TO ENROLL

To enroll in the *Neuroimaging Clinics of North America* Continuing Medical Education program, call customer service at 1-800-654-2452 or sign up online at http://www.theclinics.com/home/cme. The CME program is available to subscribers for an additional annual fee of USD 235.

METHOD OF PARTICIPATION

In order to claim credit, participants must complete the following:

1. Complete enrolment as indicated above.
2. Read the activity.
3. Complete the CME Test and Evaluation. Participants must achieve a score of 70% on the test. All CME Tests and Evaluations must be completed online.

CME INQUIRIES/SPECIAL NEEDS

For all CME inquiries or special needs, please contact elsevierCME@elsevier.com.

NEUROIMAGING CLINICS OF NORTH AMERICA

THE CLINICS ARE AVAILABLE ONLINE!
Access your subscription at:
www.theclinics.com

NEUROIMAGING CLINICS OF NORTH AMERICA

Contributors

CONSULTING EDITOR

SURESH K. MUKHERJI, MD, MBA, FACR
Professor and Chairman, Walter F. Patenge
Endowed Chair, Department of Radiology,
Michigan State University; Chief Medical
Officer and Director of Health Care Delivery,
Michigan State University Health Team, East
Lansing, Michigan

EDITOR

J. KEVIN DeMARCO, MD
Professor, Director of MRI, Department of
Radiology, Michigan State University, East
Lansing, Michigan

AUTHORS

ABDELRAHMAN ALI, MD
Cardiac MR PET CT Program, Massachusetts
General Hospital, Harvard Medical School,
Boston, Massachusetts

ANNA BAYER-KARPINSKA, MD
Institute for Stroke and Dementia Research,
Ludwig-Maximilians-University Hospital
Munich, Munich, Germany

LEO H. BONATI, MD
Stroke Center, Departments of Neurology and
Clinical Research, University Hospital Basel,
Basel, Switzerland

MAURICIO CASTILLO, MD, FACR
Professor of Radiology, Chief, Division of
Neuroradiology, Department of Radiology,
University of North Carolina School of
Medicine, Chapel Hill, Chapel Hill, North
Carolina

HUIJUN CHEN, PhD
Department of Biomedical Engineering, Tenure
Track Assistant Professor, Center for
Biomedical Imaging Research, School of
Medicine, Tsinghua University, Beijing, China

J. KEVIN DeMARCO, MD
Professor, Director of MRI, Department of
Radiology, Michigan State University, East
Lansing, Michigan

MARC R. DWECK, MD, PhD
British Heart Foundation Centre for
Cardiovascular Science, College of Medicine
and Veterinary Medicine, University of
Edinburgh, Edinburgh, United Kingdom;
Imaging Science Laboratories, Departments of
Radiology and Medicine, Translational and
Molecular Imaging Institute, Mount Sinai
School of Medicine, New York, New York

ZAHI A. FAYAD, PhD
Imaging Science Laboratories, Departments
of Radiology and Medicine, Translational
and Molecular Imaging Institute, Mount
Sinai School of Medicine, New York,
New York

STEVEN B. FEINSTEIN, MD, FACC, FESC
Division of Cardiology, Department of
Medicine, Rush University Medical Center,
Chicago, Illinois

VENU GOURINENI, MD
Division of Cardiology, Department of
Medicine, Rush University Medical Center,
Chicago, Illinois

THOMAS S. HATSUKAMI, MD
Professor, Department of Surgery;
Co-Director, Vascular Imaging Laboratory,
University of Washington, Seattle, Washington

WILLIAM KERWIN, PhD
Associate Professor, Department of Radiology,
School of Medicine, University of Washington,
Seattle, Washington

ALAN R. MOODY, FRCR, FRCP
Department of Medical Imaging, University of
Toronto, Toronto, Ontario, Canada

MAHMUD MOSSA-BASHA, MD
Assistant Professor of Radiology, Division of
Neuroradiology, University of Washington
Medical Center; Director of Cross-Sectional
Neurovascular Imaging, University of
Washington School of Medicine, Seattle,
Washington

PAUL J. NEDERKOORN, MD, PhD
Neurologist, Clinical Epidemiologist,
Department of Neurology, Academic Medical
Center Amsterdam, Amsterdam, The
Netherlands

DENNIS L. PARKER, PhD
Professor, Department of Radiology, Imaging
and Neurosciences Center; Director, Utah
Center for Advanced Imaging Research
(UCAIR), University of Utah, Salt Lake City,
Utah

GRACE PARRAGA, PhD
Imaging Research Laboratories, Department of
Medical Biophysics, Robarts Research
Institute, Western University, London, Ontario,
Canada

TOBIAS SAAM, MD
Institute for Clinical Radiology,
Ludwig-Maximilians-University Hospital
Munich, Munich, Germany

SANDEEP A. SAHA, MD, FACP
Division of Cardiology, Department of
Medicine, Rush University Medical Center,
Chicago, Illinois

ANDREAS SCHINDLER, MD
Institute for Clinical Radiology,
Ludwig-Maximilians-University Hospital
Munich, Munich, Germany

NAVNEET SINGH, MD
Department of Medical Imaging,
University of Toronto, Toronto, Ontario,
Canada

J. DAVID SPENCE, MD, FRCPC, FAHA
Director, Departments of Neurology and
Clinical Pharmacology, Stroke Prevention and
Atherosclerosis Research Centre, Robarts
Research Institute, Western University,
London, Ontario, Canada

JIE SUN, MD
Acting Instructor, Department of
Radiology, University of Washington, Seattle,
Washington

AHMED TAWAKOL, MD
Cardiac MR PET CT Program, Division of
Cardiology, Massachusetts General Hospital,
Harvard Medical School, Boston,
Massachusetts

CARLOS TORRES, MD, FRCPC
Associate Professor of Radiology;
Program Director-Neuroradiology;
Department of Radiology, University
of Ottawa; Department of Medical
Imaging, The Ottawa Hospital, Ottawa,
Ontario, Canada

ALEX T. VESEY, MD
British Heart Foundation Centre for
Cardiovascular Science, College of
Medicine and Veterinary Medicine,
University of Edinburgh, Edinburgh,
United Kingdom

BRUCE A. WASSERMAN, MD
Professor of Radiology, Director of
Diagnostic Neurovascular Imaging,
Director of Translational Neuroradiology,
Russell H. Morgan Department of Radiology
and Radiological Sciences, Johns Hopkins
School of Medicine, Baltimore, Maryland

CHUN YUAN, PhD
Co-Director, Vascular Imaging Lab; Professor,
Department of Radiology; Director,
Bio-Molecular Imaging Center, University of
Washington, Seattle, Washington

NADER ZAKHARI, MD, FRCPC
Neuroradiology Fellow, Department of
Radiology, University of Ottawa; Department of
Medical Imaging, The Ottawa Hospital,
Ottawa, Ontario, Canada

QIANG ZHANG, MS
Department of Biomedical Engineering,
Center for Biomedical Imaging Research,
School of Medicine, Tsinghua University,
Beijing, China

Contents

There has been significant progress made in 3-dimensional (3D) carotid plaque MR imaging techniques in recent years. Three-dimensional plaque imaging clearly represents the future in clinical use. With effective flow-suppression techniques, choices of different contrast weighting acquisitions, and time-efficient imaging approaches, 3D plaque imaging offers flexible imaging plane and view angle analysis, large coverage, multivascular beds capability, and can even be used in fast screening.

Plaque imaging by MR imaging provides a wealth of information on the characteristics of individual plaque that may reveal vulnerability to rupture, likelihood of progression, or optimal treatment strategy. T1-weighted and T2-weighted images among other options reveal plaque morphology and composition. Dynamic contrast-enhanced–MR imaging reveals plaque activity. To extract this information, image processing tools are needed. Numerous approaches for analyzing such images have been developed, validated against histologic gold standards, and used in clinical studies. These efforts are summarized in this article.

The incorporation of a short, easy-to-acquire and simple to read sequence to visualize the vessel wall and detect intraplaque hemorrhage (IPH) is achievable now. Demonstration of IPH may be helpful in primary or secondary prevention of neuro-ischemic events, assessment prior to carotid intervention and the general definition of an individual's vascular phenotype. The addition of an IPH-detecting vessel wall sequence only adds 5 to 6 minutes to a standard carotid MRI examination making clinical translation feasible and achievable.

Atherosclerosis is a complex inflammatory process and an integral component of myocardial infarction and stroke. Atherosclerotic plaques can be detected using ultrasonography, myocardial perfusion imaging, coronary angiography, multidetector computed tomography (CT), and MR imaging. These modalities assess the luminal encroachment of the plaques or the structural features. Imaging plaque biology in concert with plaque structure may provide important insights. PET scanning using 18F fluorodeoxyglucose. (^{18}F FDG-PET) is commonly combined with CT scanning to characterize oncological processes. This review examines the role of ^{18}F FDG-PET/CT imaging in the characterization of atherosclerotic plaque biology.

By harnessing the versatility and soft tissue imaging capabilities of MR imaging alongside the unmatched sensitivity and biomolecular flexibility of PET, the potential to provide detailed multiparametric plaque characterization in the carotid arteries is clear. The ability to acquire simultaneous, and dynamic multimodal data is perhaps PET/MR's greatest strength that will be of major interest to researchers investigating carotid and coronary atherosclerosis alike. This review summarizes the current status of dedicated hybrid PET/MR imaging, to crystallize the rationale for and advantages of this technique with respect to carotid atherosclerosis, and to discuss current limitations, challenges, and future directions.

Measurement of plaque burden is different from measurement of carotid intima-media thickness (IMT). Carotid total plaque area is a stronger predictor of cardiovascular risk than IMT, and in contrast to progression of IMT, which does not predict cardiovascular events, progression of total plaque area and total plaque volume strongly predict cardiovascular events. Measurement of plaque burden is useful in genetic research, and in evaluation of new therapies for atherosclerosis. Perhaps more importantly, it can be used for management of patients. A strategy called "treating arteries instead of treating risk factors" markedly reduces risk among patients with asymptomatic carotid stenosis.

Contrast-enhanced ultrasonography (CEUS) is a rapidly evolving modality for imaging carotid artery disease and systemic atherosclerosis. CEUS coupled with diagnostic ultrasonography predicts the degree of carotid artery stenosis and is comparable with computed tomography and magnetic resonance angiography. This article reviews the literature on the evolving role of CEUS for the identification and characterization of carotid plaques with an emphasis on detection of intraplaque neovascularization and related high-risk morphologic features notably present in symptomatic patients. CEUS carotid imaging may play a prominent additive role in risk stratifying patients and serve as a powerful tool for monitoring therapeutic interventions.

In up to 40% of ischemic stroke cases the etiology remains unknown. A substantial proportion of these patients has non- or only mildly stenosing carotid artery plaques not fulfilling common criteria for large artery stroke, but beeing suspicious for arterio-arteriell embolism. Several imaging techniques allow the non-invasive analysis of plaque features. Nevertheless, carotid MRI might be best suited to assess the key features of vulnerable plaques. This review article discusses potential causes of cryptogenic stroke, the role of plaque imaging in non-stenosing plaques and the association of vulnerable plaques and specific plaque features with stroke risk and stroke recurrence.

The continued occurrence of stroke despite advances in medical therapy for asymptomatic carotid stenosis (ACS) strongly indicates that individual response to medical therapy may vary widely. This article reviews the literature that identifies MR imaging and ultrasound plaque features which are seen in patients at increased risk of future cardiovascular events. Imaging can identify plaque phenotype that is the most amendable to intensive medical therapy. There is also good evidence that plaque imaging can measure the individual response to medical therapy and the lack of response identifies a high-risk group of ACS patients.

Although treatment guidelines are well established for symptomatic patients with greater than 69% carotid stenosis on catheter angiography, optimal management of lower degrees of stenosis remain unclear. Vessel wall MR imaging of the carotid arteries has proved helpful in the evaluation of plaque burden and vulnerable plaque characteristics, and in stratifying risk in low-grade carotid stenosis. This article discusses the pathophysiology and imaging of atherosclerotic plaques resulting in low-grade carotid stenosis, and the corresponding stroke risk and association with plaque elsewhere in the cardiovascular system.

The heart and the carotid arteries are the most common sites of origin of embolic disease to the brain. Clots arising from these locations are the most common types of brain emboli. Less common cerebral emboli include air, fat, calcium, infected vegetations, and tumor cells as well as emboli originating in the venous system. Although infarcts can be the final result of any type of embolism, described herein are the ancillary and sometimes unique imaging features of less common types of cerebral emboli that may allow for a specific diagnosis to be made or at least suspected in many patients.

Many of the current guidelines for the management of carotid atherosclerosis are based on clinical trial findings published more than 2 decades ago. The lack of plaque information in clinical decision making represents a major shortcoming and highlights the need for contemporary trials based on characteristics of the athero-sclerotic lesion itself, rather than luminal stenosis alone. This article summarizes the major dilemmas clinicians face in current practice, and discusses the rationale and evidence that plaque imaging may help to address these challenges and optimize the clinical management of carotid artery disease in the future.

At present, patients with carotid disease are selected for invasive recanalization therapies mainly based on the degree of luminal narrowing and the presence or absence of recent ischemic symptoms. A more sophisticated risk model takes into account other clinical variables, such as age, sex, and the type of recent symptoms, as well as presence of ulcerated plaque. A growing body of evidence shows that noninvasive imaging of the carotid plaque by various methods reliably identifies structural correlates of plaque vulnerability, which are associated with an increased risk of cerebrovascular events.

Foreword
Plaque Imaging

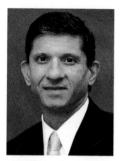

Suresh K. Mukherji, MD, MBA, FACR
Consulting Editor

I wish to thank Dr Kevin DeMarco for guest-editing this issue on carotid plaque imaging. This topic is obviously very important and constantly evolving. The focus of this issue is the clinical applications of modern plaque imaging. Dr DeMarco has assembled a talented group of international experts to author these excellent reviews on the "current state" of carotid plaque imaging. There are articles dedicated to 3D MR imaging of carotid plaque, computer-assisted analysis of multicontrast carotid plaque MR imaging, ultrasound (3D and contrast-enhanced techniques), and PET-CT and PET-MR imaging of carotid plaque. The issue also includes an essential article on the clinical impact of plaque imaging that underscores the importance of what we do and also why further investments in this field are clearly needed. The authors have done an amazing job with their contributions, and I want to thank all of them for their efforts and commitment to this wonderful issue.

On a personal note, I have had the pleasure of working with Kevin for the past three years in the Department of Radiology at Michigan State University. Kevin is really an extraordinary individual whose unbridled passion for carotid plaque imaging is only superseded by his devotion to his family. I was delighted when Kevin accepted this invitation but am even happier to call him a friend. Thank you, Kevin!

Suresh K. Mukherji, MD, MBA, FACR
Department of Radiology
Michigan State University Health Team
Michigan State University
846 Service Road
East Lansing, MI 48824, USA

E-mail address:
mukherji@rad.msu.edu

Neuroimag Clin N Am 26 (2016) xv
http://dx.doi.org/10.1016/j.nic.2015.10.002
1052-5149/16/$ – see front matter © 2016 Published by Elsevier Inc.

Preface
Carotid Plaque Imaging Comes of Age

 CrossMark

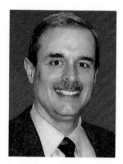

J. Kevin DeMarco, MD
Editor

I hope you have as much fun reading this issue of *Neuroimaging Clinics* as I had putting it together. As you can tell, all the world experts in carotid plaque imaging that contributed to this issue have a deep passion for improving our patients' health and well-being. Simply measuring carotid stenosis is so last millennium. We have so many tools to help clinicians better gauge the future cardiovascular risk of their patients. The challenge is translating their excellent research on carotid plaque imaging into useful clinical imaging strategies.

The focus of this issue is the clinical application of this excellent carotid plaque research. A talented group of international experts reviews the current state-of-the-art MR imaging of carotid plaque with recent efforts to utilize all 3D MR imaging of carotid plaque and computer-assisted analysis of multicontrast carotid plaque MR imaging and to incorporate carotid plaque imaging into routine clinical carotid MR angiography. Another distinguished group of experts share with us current state-of-the-art PET-CT and PET-MR imaging of carotid plaque. Last, but certainly not least, we read about the exciting developments of 3D carotid plaque ultrasound and contrast-enhanced carotid plaque ultrasound.

After reviewing the best that MR imaging, PET, and ultrasound has to offer, we hear from radiologists on their efforts to better assess risk through the detection of vulnerable plaque in patients with "cryptogenic" stroke, use of plaque imaging in asymptomatic carotid stenosis patients, as well as implications of MR imaging in patients with low-grade carotid stenosis. We also read about unusual causes of cerebral embolism and how the radiologist can suggest the correct diagnosis that will significantly impact patient management.

We end this issue with what I hope will be a terrific resource for you to begin a discussion with your referring clinicians about using carotid plaque imaging. A world-renowned vascular surgeon and a stroke neurologist give us their clinical perspective of using carotid plaque imaging to decide on optimal treatment of patients with carotid stenosis.

I would like to thank all the authors for their excellent work and hope that, you, the readers, can take advantage of their efforts to improve the care of your patients with carotid stenosis.

J. Kevin DeMarco, MD
Department of Radiology
Michigan State University Health Team
Michigan State University
846 Service Road
East Lansing, MI 48824, USA

E-mail address:
jkd@rad.msu.edu

Neuroimag Clin N Am 26 (2016) xvii
http://dx.doi.org/10.1016/j.nic.2015.10.001
1052-5149/16/$ – see front matter © 2016 Published by Elsevier Inc.

Three-Dimensional Carotid Plaque MR Imaging

Chun Yuan, PhD[a],*, Dennis L. Parker, PhD[b]

KEYWORDS

- 3D MR imaging • Vessel wall imaging • Vulnerable plaque • Atherosclerosis imaging • 3D MRA
- 3D vessel wall imaging

KEY POINTS

- Significant progress has been made in 3-dimensional (3D) carotid plaque imaging techniques in recent years.
- Due to fast imaging times and results comparable to many clinical techniques, 3D vessel wall imaging by MR imaging may be able to improve on current clinical assessments.
- Our ability to predict clinical outcomes is limited by our knowledge of atherosclerosis etiology and progression; 3D techniques may enable us to study understand the origin and outcomes of carotid atherosclerosis.
- Information on the condition of carotid atherosclerosis may provide a useful window to understanding system-wide disease burden and assess overall cardiovascular risk.

INTRODUCTION

Carotid atherosclerosis, especially atherosclerotic plaques at the carotid bifurcation, is a significant cause of ischemic stroke, a leading cause of death and disability worldwide. A primary goal of imaging of carotid atherosclerosis is, therefore, to identify lesions that will lead to ischemic stroke. Carotid plaques typically become flow-limiting as they progress. The simple assessment of luminal narrowing (stenosis), however, has proven to be of limited value in predicting the risk of ischemic stroke. Furthermore, atherosclerosis is a systemic condition that affects large and medium-sized arteries, especially the coronary artery, so information on the condition of carotid atherosclerosis may provide a useful window to understanding system-wide disease burden and assess overall cardiovascular risk. Thus, carotid plaque imaging has 2 primary goals: one is to identify high-risk plaques that can cause stroke or other ischemic events, the other is to screen for the presence of plaques for overall cardiovascular evaluation.

High-risk plaques are defined as plaques that are likely to rupture, leading to thrombosis in situ and/or downstream and potentially ischemic events. Based on histologic examination of coronary atherosclerosis, key features of high-risk plaques include a large lipid-rich necrotic core (LRNC) with an overlying thin (or ruptured) fibrous cap (FC), active inflammation, plaque fissures,

Disclosure Statement: Dr C. Yuan holds grants from the National Institutes of Health and (R21EB017514 & R01HL103609) Philips Medical. He also serves as a Member of Radiology Advisory Network, Philips. Dr D.L. Parker has nothing to disclose.
[a] Vascular Imaging Lab, Department of Radiology, Bio-Molecular Imaging Center, University of Washington, Box 358050, 850 Republican Street, Seattle, WA 98109-4714, USA; [b] Department of Radiology, Imaging & Neurosciences Center, Utah Center for Advanced Imaging Research (UCAIR), University of Utah, 729 Arapeen Drive, Salt Lake City, UT 84108, USA
* Corresponding author.
E-mail address: cyuan@uw.edu

1052-5149/16/$ – see front matter © 2016 Elsevier Inc. All rights reserved.

calcium nodules on the luminal surface, and the presence of intraplaque hemorrhage (IPH).[1] These are mainly plaque compositional features. There have been few histologic definitions of high-risk plaques of the carotid arteries, perhaps due to limited access to intact carotid atherosclerosis specimens.[1] Interestingly, recent literature has pointed to features that can be identified by MR carotid plaque imaging in prospective studies, such as the presence of LRNC, IPH, and luminal surface disruption, as those at high risk for rupture or subsequent events.[2,3]

Ultrasound, especially intima media thickness (IMT) measurement, has been used extensively as a screening tool to use carotid artery condition to assess cardiovascular risk.[4] Recent development in ultrasound, however, suggest that 2-dimensional (2D) and 3D B-mode ultrasound capable of visualizing the presence of plaques at the carotid region may provide improved predictive power of future cardiovascular risk[5,6] over IMT. This leads to an interesting question on whether MR imaging can also play a role in screening, with its apparent advantages in soft tissue contrast and 3D capabilities.

This article is focused on MR imaging techniques for carotid arteries, with a major emphasis on 3D techniques, which are considered the future of carotid plaque imaging applications.

TECHNICAL CONSIDERATIONS AND EXISTING 2D IMAGING TECHNIQUES

Essential technical considerations for carotid plaque imaging includes the following: hardware considerations, such as field strength and specialized radiofrequency (RF) coils, imaging factors, such as spatial resolution and signal-to-noise ratio (SNR), and scan time, and tissue-specific factors, including tissue contrast, contrast-to-noise (CNR) for specific vessel wall and atherosclerotic plaque tissue identification, and motion artifact suppression. Most of all, vessel wall visualization and the identification of components of atherosclerosis require effective suppression of signals from circulating blood. The carotid bifurcation, the most frequent site of carotid atherosclerosis, exhibits complex flow pattern that includes flow recirculation. Thus, complete flow suppression requires special consideration of the flow conditions at the carotid bifurcation.

Over the years, there have been extensive technical developments and validation for 2D-based carotid plaque imaging. The developments can be summarized as follows. (1) Initial development of carotid imaging was on 1.5-T scanners with extensive validation conducted using histology of carotid plaque specimens as the gold standard.[7,8]

Studies then showed 3-T clinical scanners offer clear SNR advantages[9] for carotid imaging. With application of specific RF coils and optimization of sequences, plaque composition can be identified with similar repeatability at 3.0 T and 1.5 T.[10] However, quantification of some components, such as calcification and IPH, may differ due to higher susceptibility effects at 3 T.[11] Additionally, the specific absorption rate is higher at 3 T and should be accounted for in protocol optimization. (2) Phased array surface coils with a small diameter and applied close to the neck provide improved SNR and are often used for vessel wall MR imaging.[12,13] In general, a spatial resolution of 0.5 to 0.6 mm in plane and 2-mm slice thickness has been used in many studies within clinically acceptable imaging time.[8] Most commonly reported longitudinal coverage has been approximately 3 cm centered at the carotid bifurcation. (3) There are many options for flow suppression with double inversion recovery[14] and motion sensitization[13,14] as the 2 most popular and effective techniques. (4) For full characterization of carotid plaque, from lesion burden to tissue composition to luminal surface condition, a multicontrast-imaging approach is highly desired, which includes both bright and black blood techniques, T1 and T2 or the application of contrast enhancement.[15]

This 2D multicontrast approach, although well accepted, has a number of shortcomings. It can be complicated to acquire multiple sequences with registered slice locations, the scan time tends to be long, the voxel size is not isotropic such that spatial information about plaque composition may be missed, and the longitudinal coverage is rather limited.

THREE-DIMENSIONAL CAROTID PLAQUE MR IMAGING: ESTABLISHED TECHNIQUES

Three-dimensional MR imaging acquisition, in general, enjoys improved spatial resolution and SNR compared with 2D imaging and can provide increased resolution in the slice-select direction. Isotropic voxels can potentially improve measurement accuracy and reproducibility of carotid MR imaging by minimizing slice-positioning error, allowing registration of images in serial studies.[16–18] But 3D imaging also faces several challenges, including relatively long scan time in which any motion may corrupt the entire data set as opposed to a subset of data in 2D acquisition. Furthermore, the in-flow–based flow-suppression techniques used widely in 2D acquisition maybe less effective, as the acquisition volume in 3D tends to be much larger. A desirable 3D sequence should have the following features: time-efficient acquisition, effective flow suppression, large coverage and isotropic voxel acquisition, and desirable contrast weighting.

Three-Dimensional Motion-Sensitized Driven Equilibrium Prepared Rapid Gradient Echo

Dr Balu and colleagues[19] introduced the 3D motion-sensitized driven equilibrium prepared rapid gradient echo (MERGE) technique in 2011. It is a combination of low flip angle gradient echo acquisition with a flow-suppression preparation module named motion-sensitized driven equilibrium (MSDE).[20] This motion-suppression technique is based on dephasing flowing blood signals and is relatively independent of imaging acquisition plane. With 3D MERGE, it allows isotropic acquisition (examples of $0.7 \times 0.7 \times 0.7$ mm^3) with much larger longitudinal coverage than 3 cm, and effective flow suppression with an acquisition time of 2 minutes. As a gradient echo–based acquisition, this technique offered a mixed T1 and T2 contrast weighting

and has been shown to be able to identify the presence of vessel wall lesions and quantify plaque burdens.

In a recently published clinical validation study, Zhao and colleagues[21] assessed 3D MERGE's ability to measure stenosis using digital subtraction angiography (DSA) as a gold standard (Fig. 1). In this study, an improved MSDE 3D sequence[22] was used with 0.8-mm isotropic resolution and 25-cm longitudinal coverage in 2 minutes 42 seconds acquisition time. The researchers showed, by comparing results of 52 patients, that 3D MERGE is accurate to quantify moderate to severe carotid stenosis (see Fig. 1). As demonstrated in this figure, one can appreciate both the stenotic site and the complex lesion that caused the narrowing and its distribution. Interestingly, because of the coverage, effective flow suppression, and the ability to visualize a large segment of the vessel wall, their study demonstrated the presence of lesions there were undetected by DSA. With the short 2-minute to 3-minute acquisition time for bilateral carotid

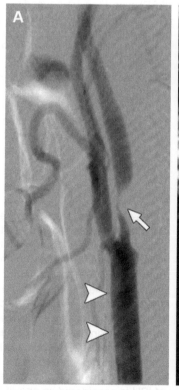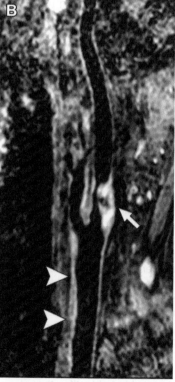

Fig. 1. Both (A) lateral projection DSA image and (B) oblique 3D BB MR image show advanced atherosclerotic disease (arrows), which caused severe internal carotid artery stenosis. The common carotid artery wall thickening (arrowheads) was visualized on (B), the 3D black blood (BB) MR image, but presented as normal on (A), the DSA image. (From Zhao H, Wang J, Liu X, et al. Assessment of carotid artery atherosclerotic disease by using three-dimensional fast black-blood MR imaging: comparison with DSA. Radiology 2015;274(2):510; with permission.)

artery imaging, 3D MERGE may be a powerful screening tool for high-risk populations and the application of 3D MERGE may extend beyond the carotid artery. In a separate study, Makhijani and colleagues[23] used compressed sensing with a hidden Markov tree model to accelerate 3D MERGE acquisition and showed that a factor of 4.5 acceleration was possible without visible degradation of diagnostic quality and quantitative measurements.

This technique, however, can lead to signal loss due to tissue water diffusion during the flow dephasing gradients and the effects of eddy currents caused by the rapid gradient switching. Since the original introduction, several techniques were introduced to reduce this signal loss and explore its use in multiple contrast weighting and in other vascular applications.[22,24–26] Zhu and colleagues[23] recently published a study focused on the optimization of improved MSDE (iMSDE) module for both 2D and 3D blood suppression in T1-weighted (T1W) and T2-weighted (T2W) spin echo acquisition and demonstrated the feasibility. This study showed iMSDE achieved better flow suppression than double-inversion recovery but with reduced vessel wall CNR efficiency in both T1W and T2W images.

Three-Dimensional Magnetization Prepared Rapid Acquisition Gradient Echo

Moody and colleagues[27] was the first to introduce the use of heavily T1W 3D imaging technique to identify a marker of complicated plaque. They named this approach direct thrombus imaging initially and the technique was based on 3D magnetization prepared rapid acquisition gradient echo (MPRAGE). With a 3.5-minute acquisition time and a spatial resolution of roughly $1 \times 2 \times 1$ mm^3, Murphy and colleagues[28] showed that detection of high signals within plaques is prevalent in the ipsilateral carotid arteries of patients with recent cerebral ischemic events. This high signal feature was later shown to be from IPH. MPRAGE offers a simple, straightforward approach to identify IPH in plaques and was later shown to have higher diagnostic capability for the detection and quantification of IPH compared with standard T1W and time of flight (TOF) approaches.[11]

Because of the heavy T1 weighting, MPRAGE was also found to be unable to identify other plaque tissues, especially coexisting calcification. Further, because MPRAGE is not a black blood technique, blood signals may sometimes be confused as IPH signals. It is worth noting, however, that since the introduction by Moody and colleagues[27] in 2003, this technique has been used in many studies that helped to establish the importance that detection of IPH as a high-risk feature of carotid plaque[2,3] (Fig. 2).

Three-Dimensional Fast (Turbo) Spin Echo–Based Approach

Three-dimensional fast spin echo (FSE) is an effective spin echo acquisition technique that is able to generate T1, proton density, and T2W images. Recently, a black blood version combined with variable flip angle acquisition to reduce acquisition time was developed, named 3D SPACE (variable-flip-angle 3D TSE T2w), for vessel wall imaging.[29] The advantage of this technique is its spin echo–based acquisition with better control over tissue contrast selection and it has natural flow suppression capability due to the application of series spin echo trains. The initial technique was used to generate T2W images to study femoral vessel wall with a spatial resolution of $0.72 \times 0.72 \times 0.72$ mm^3 and 11-minute acquisition. Carotid vessel wall imaging with improved flow suppression through flow phase dephasing (FSD) was then introduced.[30] In this study, Fan and colleagues demonstrated the effectiveness of the FSD magnetization preparation in improving blood signal suppression of SPACE for isotropic 3D acquisition at $0.63 \times 0.63 \times 0.63$ mm^3 and 6.4 minutes. The longitudinal coverage (Fig. 3) almost doubled the 3-cm coverage by the 2D technique. In another implementation of a 3D FSE technique, Zhu and colleagues[26] compared the performance of precontrast and postcontrast 3D CUBE to identify nonenhancing LRNC and showed good results.

Three-Dimensional Time of Flight

Three-dimensional TOF has been used for carotid imaging clinically for more than 20 years.[31] A commonly used approach to screen luminal stenosis is to evaluate the maximum intensity projection (MIP) from different angles. Recently Yim and colleagues[32] and Yoshimura and colleagues[33] found that MIP also can be used to identify IPH because IPH appears to have high-intensity signal (HIS). This is not surprising because most TOF techniques have T1 weighting and IPH is hyperintensive on T1W images.[34–36] But this is very interesting because the presence of IPH is considered as one of the important features of high-risk carotid plaques[2,37] and also because 3D TOF is routinely used in the clinical setting and is simple to implement. Gupta and colleagues[3] recently expanded this concept to

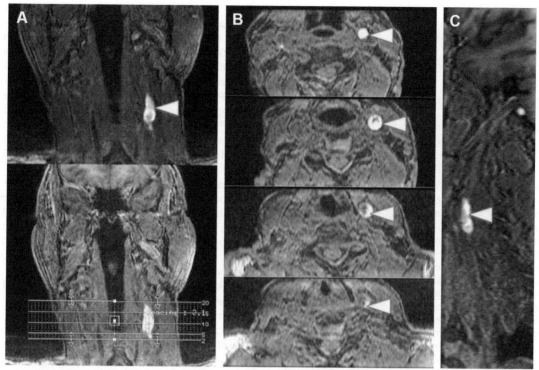

Fig. 2. Multiplanar images (*A* coronal, *B* axial, *C* sagittal) of carotid intraplaque hemorrhage (*arrowheads*) within the wall of the left carotid artery. Intraplaque hemorrhage is detected using a 3D T1W fat-suppressed fast field echo sequence by exploiting the T1 shortening effects of methemoglobin and the technique has been histologically validated. (*From* Singh N, Moody AR, Rochon-Terry G, et al. Identifying a high risk cardiovascular phenotype by carotid MR imaging-depicted intraplaque hemorrhage. Int J Cardiovasc Imaging 2013;29(7):1479; with permission.)

evaluate the association of HIS with symptomatic status (stroke and transient ischemic attack) and found that detection of HIS within carotid plaques is strongly associated with ipsilateral ischemic events. The study of Gupta and colleagues[3] further confirmed the usefulness of 3D TOF in plaque imaging and their results on IPH's relationship with prior symptomatic status is similar to previous reports based on more comprehensive and sensitive plaque-imaging techniques.[27,38]

A word of caution, however, was raised in another study led by Yamada, and colleagues.[39] In a study of 76 patients with a suspected carotid artery stenosis or carotid plaque by ultrasonography underwent multicontrast carotid cardiovascular magnetic resonance (CMR). HIS presence and volume were measured from 3D TOF-magnetic resonance angiography (MRA) MIP images, whereas IPH and LRNC volumes were separately measured from multicontrast CMR. The investigators found that HIS on MIP images are associated with an increased size of IPH and LRNC, particularly in those with moderate to severe stenosis.

But because IPH was frequently detected in arteries with low-grade stenosis, where TOF-MRA MIP images were found to have low sensitivity, methods with higher sensitivity for IPH while preserving the desirable capability of visualizing the lumen in 3D are needed to better evaluate this subpopulation.

In summary, 3D MERGE, MPRAGE, TOF, and FSE (with its various versions) are the main techniques for carotid plaque imaging: individually and combined, these sequences offer isotropic resolution, bright and black blood, large-coverage acquisition. Collectively, they can replace 2D multiple-contrast to fully characterize carotid plaques from burden, to composition, and to FC conditions.

THREE-DIMENSIONAL CAROTID PLAQUE IMAGING: NOVEL TECHNIQUES

Recently, some very exciting concepts and techniques have begun to emerge in 3D carotid plaque imaging. These methods are intended to streamline the image acquisition and improve

A   **B**

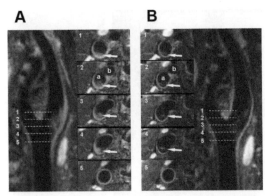

Fig. 3. Comparison of location-matched SPACE (*A*) and FSD-SPACE (*B*) images acquired from a healthy volunteer. Using multiplanar reconstruction (MPR), both longitudinal and cross-sectional views of the carotid artery can be visualized. The FSD preparation can dramatically suppress the residual blood signal (*arrows*) shown on SPACE images, thus resulting in larger apparent lumen and higher wall-lumen contrast. The locations of the 5 cross-sectional images (nos. 1–5) are indicated by the dashed line on the longitudinal images. [a] Internal carotid lumen; [b] external carotid lumen. (*From* Fan Z, Zhang Z, Chung YC, et al. Carotid arterial wall MR imaging at 3T using 3D variable-flip-angle turbo spin-echo (TSE) with flow-sensitive dephasing (FSD). J Magn Reson Imaging 2010;31(3):652; with permission.)

acquisition efficiency by obtaining multiple tissue contrasts in one single acquisition. With detecting IPH becoming a major interest, these techniques tend to all have an option to acquire heavily T1W black blood images and combined with other tissue or lumen contrasts. Another concept is to imbed carotid plaque imaging in an angiographic technique as such that it can be easily implemented in clinical setting when MRA is ordered.

Simultaneous Noncontrast Angiography and Intraplaque Hemorrhage Imaging

Wang and colleagues[40] introduced this exciting new technique in 2013. The simultaneous noncontrast angiography and intraplaque hemorrhage (SNAP) sequence used a phase-sensitive acquisition, and was designed to provide positive signals corresponding to IPH and negative signals corresponding to blood signal in the vessel lumen. The technique was designed to have better IPH contrast as compared with MPRAGE because it used phase-sensitive image reconstruction. For the same reason, flowing blood signals can be

either suppressed, as in black blood, or constructed as angiographic images. It takes 5 minutes to acquire an SNAP data set with $0.8 \times 0.8 \times 0.8$ mm^3 isotropic resolution and a longitudinal coverage of 16 cm. SNAP shows great promise for imaging both lumen size and carotid IPH with a single scan. With its large coverage, high resolution, and simultaneous MRA/IPH images, SNAP has the potential to become the first-line imaging method for patients with atherosclerosis in a clinical environment (Fig. 4).

Dr Balu and colleagues[41] later on introduced a dual-contrast vessel wall MR imaging concept based on the phase-sensitive polarity maps that are the core of SNAP technology. By adjusting the imaging parameters in SNAP sequence and adding new image reconstruction scheme to combine phase and magnitude signal together, they are able to acquire 4 sets of images from 1 single acquisition that provide information on plaque burden, luminal stenosis, IPH, and juxtaluminal calcification (Fig. 5). This concept expands the utility of SNAP to multiple-contrast.

Multicontrast Atherosclerosis Characterization of Carotid Plaque

Fan and colleagues[42] recently introduced another exciting 3D-based technique that is intended to generate multicontrast, coregistered images with hyper-T1W, gray blood, and T2W images. Multicontrast atherosclerosis characterization (MATCH), which is based on 3D spoiled segmented fast flow angle shot and flow-sensitive dephasing preparation for blood suppression, it is a gradient echo–based acquisition with in-plane resolution of 0.55×0.55 mm^2, 2-mm slice thickness, longitudinal coverage of approximately 3 cm, and acquisition time of 4 minutes and 45 seconds. In a pilot study, Fan and his coresearchers[42] found that MATCH was able to obtain a comparable ability to detect carotid plaque components such as LRNC, IPH, Calcium and loose matrix with no problems of misregistration compared with the conventional 2D multicontrast protocol. This technique, however, does not provide luminal narrowing information and the acquisition time will need to be further reduced to have larger longitudinal coverage (Fig. 6).

Three-Dimensional SHINE

Zhu and colleagues[43] in 2010 introduced one of the earliest multicontrast 3D acquisition techniques named 3D SHINE (Spoiled Gradient recalled echo pulse sequence for Hemorrhage

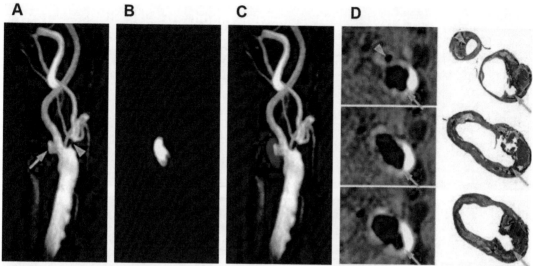

Fig. 4. SNAP with histology confirmation. Three-dimensional MIP images of the MRA portion (*A*), IPH portion (*B*), and color-coded joint view (*C*) of the SNAP images. Both IPH and luminal MRA were nicely delineated throughout the 160-mm coverage of bilateral carotid arteries. Even in small branches of the carotid artery, high-risk features like ulceration (*arrows*) and high-level stenosis (*arrowheads*) were visualized. On cross-sectional reformatted images (*D*), both IPH and luminal shapes were confirmed by the matched Mallory's trichrome histology slides. (*From* Wang J, Börnert P, Zhao H, et al. Simultaneous noncontrast angiography and intraplaque hemorrhage (SNAP) imaging for carotid atherosclerotic disease evaluation. Magn Reson Med 2013;69(2):341; with permission.)

assessment using INversion recovery and multiple Echoes). Similar to MATCH, this is also a 3D gradient echo–based approach (spoiled gradient recalled echo pulse) with multiple echo acquisition. This technique is intended to acquire black blood images with high-resolution volumetric coverage, multiple tissue contrasts, high SNR and CNR, and similar sensitivity and specificity in detecting whether IPH was present on an artery. The multiple echoes acquired with 3D SHINE allowed the estimation of IPH T_2^* and then the subsequent characterization of IPH (T_2^* for type I <14 ms, and for type II >14 ms) (**Fig. 7**).

Three-Dimensional Delay Alternating with Nutation for Tailored Excitation

Delay alternating with nutation for tailored excitation (DANTE) pulse trains have been used as frequency-selective excitation methods in Fourier transform MR imaging and for spatial tagging in MR imaging.[44] Recently, Li and colleagues[45] demonstrated that nonselective DANTE pulse trains can be used in combination with gradient pulses and short repetition times to eliminate signal from moving fluid and structures. Although the longitudinal magnetization of static tissue is mostly preserved, the magnetization from flowing spins fails to establish transverse steady state is almost completely attenuated due to the spoiling effect caused by flow along the applied gradient. The attenuation of flowing spins is effectively insensitive to spin velocity (above a very low threshold) and can be approximately quantified with a simple T1 longitudinal magnetization decay model. Based on this contrast mechanism, the

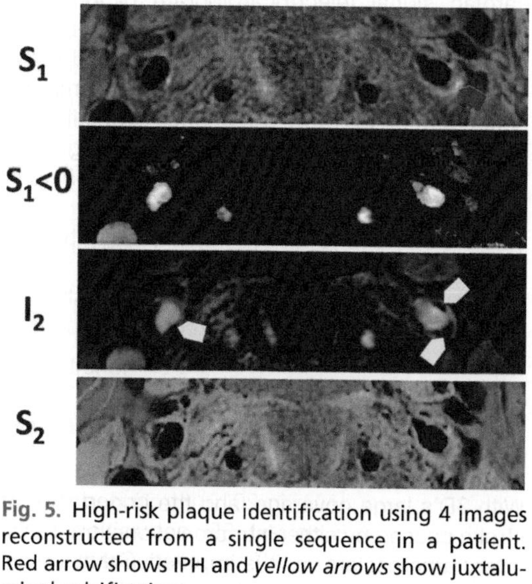

S_1

$S_1<0$

I_2

S_2

Fig. 5. High-risk plaque identification using 4 images reconstructed from a single sequence in a patient. Red arrow shows IPH and *yellow arrows* show juxtaluminal calcification.

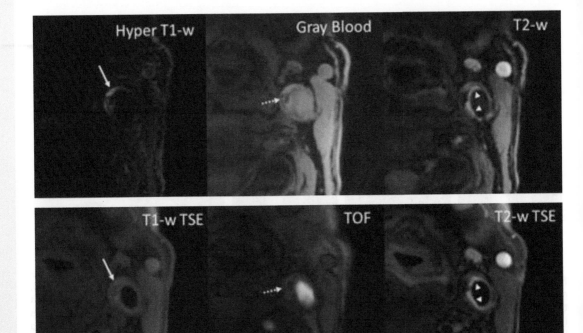

Fig. 6. A slice with coexistent plaque components including acute intraplaque hemorrhage (*solid arrows*), calcification (*dashed arrows*), and loose matrix (*arrowheads*). With the MATCH protocol, the unique contrast weightings and spatial coregistration facilitate easier identification of coexistent components and better appreciation of their spatial relations. The loose matrix is also hyperintense on T1W TSE, mimicking hemorrhage. However, it is not as hyperintense as hemorrhage on TOF. (*From* Fan Z, Yu W, Xie Y, et al. Multi-contrast atherosclerosis characterization (MATCH) of carotid plaque with a single 5-min scan: technical development and clinical feasibility. J Cardiovasc Magn Reson 2014;16:53; with permission.)

DANTE preparation was applied to black blood vessel imaging and demonstrated excellent blood signal suppression and static tissue signal preservation.

CINE Retrospective Ordering and Compressed Sensing (ciné-ROCS) Turbo Spin Echo, Motion-Sensitized Driven Equilibrium Prepared Rapid Gradient Echo, and Magnetization Prepared Rapid Acquisition Gradient Echo

Mendes and colleagues[46] investigated the effects of periodic motion in the neck on 2D and 3D carotid images. In conventional 2D and 3D turbo spin echo (TSE) acquisitions, periodic motion of blood, arterial wall, and surrounding tissue with the cardiac or respiratory cycle can cause image degradation. Mendes and colleagues[46] demonstrated that the measurement data acquired with conventional 2D and 3D TSE can be phase-ordered with the subject's cardiac signal (electrocardiogram or pressure pulse data) and the resulting sparse series of phase-ordered bins can be reconstructed using compressed sensing methods as a temporal sequence of 2D and 3D images. Despite the increased number of images (and resulting interpretation load), this technique appears to help in the discrimination of some artifacts. For TSE, ciné-ROCS reconstruction requires: (1) two or more measurement averages, and (2) a TR that spreads the measurements uniformly into the times of multiple selected cycle phases (**Fig. 8**).

Three-Dimensional for Joint Intracranial and Extracranial Vessel Wall Imaging

With 3D's large coverage, and the importance of stroke caused by either intracranial or extracranial artery atherosclerosis, it is imperative that vessel wall imaging be extended from carotid to

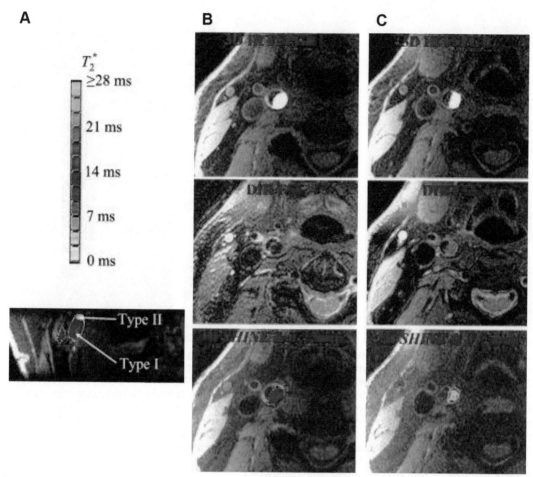

Fig. 7. An intraplaque hemorrhage with both type I and type II hemorrhagic regions is shown. The high-contrast hemorrhagic region is clearly depicted by 3D IR FSPGR or 3D SHINE. The $T*_2$ value is color coded with the bar at the upper-left corner. The type I hemorrhage tends to have a $T*_2$ value below 14 ms, and type II hemorrhage tends to have a $T*_2$ value above 14 ms. The 2 hemorrhage types are shown clearly in the reformatted coronal view (A). Consistent with the results from 3D SHINE, (B) type I hemorrhage (shown are axial slices at predominately type I region) appears to be hypointense in DIR FSE, and (C) type II hemorrhage (shown are axial slices at predominately type II region) appears to be iso-intense in DIR FSE. DIR, double inversion recovery; FSPGR, fast spoiled gradient recalled sequence; IR, inversion recovery. (*From* Zhu DC, Vu AT, Ota H, et al. An optimized 3D spoiled gradient recalled echo pulse sequence for hemorrhage assessment using inversion recovery and multiple echoes (3D SHINE) for carotid plaque imaging. Magn Reson Med 2010;64(5):1344; with permission.)

intracranial space. Zhou and colleagues[47] recently evaluated the performance of a novel 3D multicontrast approach for this purpose. Added with a custom-designed 36-channel neurovascular coil on a 3T scanner, they acquired images with 3D MERGE, SNAP, and volume isotropic turbo spin-echo acquisition (VISTA) (which is a different version of 3D FSE) sequences with T1, T2, and heavy T1 weighting covering the entire intracranial and extracranial vasculature. The 3D multicontrast images were acquired within 15 minutes, allowed the vessel wall visualization with 0.8 mm isotropic

spatial resolution covering intracranial and extracranial segments (25 cm head-to-toe direction). Quantitative wall and lumen SNR measurements for each sequence showed effective blood suppression at all selected locations ($P<.0001$). Although the wall-lumen CNR varied across measured locations, each sequence provided good or adequate image quality in both intracranial and extracranial segments (**Fig. 9**). This study shows the feasibility of a time-efficient complete workup of intracranial and extracranial vascular evaluation to identify high-risk plaques.

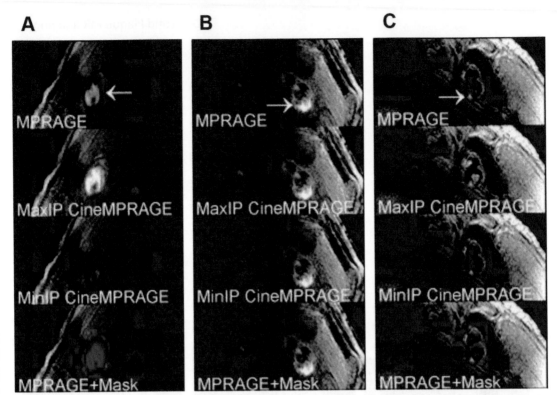

Fig. 8. Identification of potential hemorrhage and hemorrhage mimicking flow artifacts using CineMPRAGE image reconstruction. A patient with flow artifact is shown in (*A*), whereas patients with potential IPH are shown in (*B*) and (*C*). The top row is the MPRAGE images reconstructed using the standard MPRAGE technique. In all cases, there are pixels with signal intensities above 1.5 × sternocleidomastoid muscle. The maximum and minimum intensity projections (taken along the temporal direction) of the CineMPRAGE reconstruction are shown in the second and third rows, respectively. Although the potential hemorrhage signal is constant, the flow artifact varies across the cardiac cycle as evidenced by the difference in the maximum and minimum intensity projections. Color maps corresponding to the CineMPRAGE signal variation are overlaid on the conventional MPRAGE images on the bottom row. (*From* Mendes J, Parker DL, Kim SE, et al. Reduced blood flow artifact in intraplaque hemorrhage imaging using Cine MPRAGE. Magn Reson Med 2013;69(5):1282; with permission.)

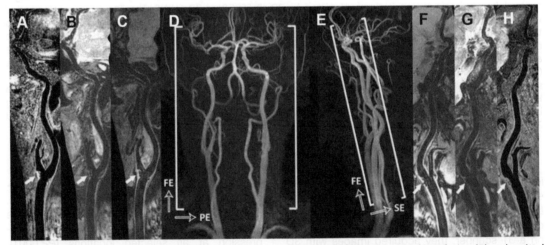

Fig. 9. Illustration of 3D multicontrast imaging coverage. Three stations of 3D TOF coronal MIP fusion (*D*) and sagittal MIP fusion (*E*) are illustrated here only for a clear definition of imaging field of view. The curved multiplanar reconstruction examples show the right (*A–C*) and left (*F–H*) side arteries ranging from CCA through ICA to MCA, where (*C*, *F*), (*B*, *G*), and (*A*, *H*) correspond to the results of 3D-MERGE, T2W VISTA, and SNAP, respectively. Note the plaques were detected at bilateral carotid bifurcations on all different contrast weighted images as shown by solid arrows. CCA, common carotid artery; ICA, internal carotid artery, MCA, middle cerebral artery. (*From* Zhou Z, Li R, Zhao X. Evaluation of 3D multi-contrast joint intra- and extracranial vessel wall cardiovascular magnetic resonance. J Cardiovasc Magn Reson 2015;17:41; with permission.)

SUMMARY

In summary, there has been significant progress made in 3D carotid plaque imaging techniques in recent years. Three-dimensional plaque imaging clearly represents the future in clinical use. With effective flow-suppression techniques, choices of different contrast weighting acquisitions, and time-efficient imaging approaches, 3D plaque imaging offers flexible imaging plane and view angle analysis, large coverage, multivascular beds capability, and even can be used in fast screening.

REFERENCES

1. Virmani R, Kolodgie FD, Burke AP, et al. Atherosclerotic plaque progression and vulnerability to rupture: angiogenesis as a source of intraplaque hemorrhage. Arterioscler Thromb Vasc Biol 2005;25(10):2054–61.

2. Saam T, Hetterich H, Hoffmann V, et al. Meta-analysis and systematic review of the predictive value of carotid plaque hemorrhage on cerebrovascular events by magnetic resonance imaging. J Am Coll Cardiol 2013;62(12):1081–91.

3. Gupta A, Baradaran H, Schweitzer AD, et al. Carotid plaque MRI and stroke risk: a systematic review and meta-analysis. Stroke 2013;44(11):3071–7.

4. O'Leary DH, Polak JF. Intima-media thickness: a tool for atherosclerosis imaging and event prediction. Am J Cardiol 2002;90(10C):18L–21L.

5. Sillesen H. Carotid intima-media thickness and/or carotid plaque: what is relevant? Eur J Vasc Endovasc Surg 2014;48(2):115–7.

6. Spence JD. Carotid plaque measurement is superior to IMT. Invited editorial comment on: carotid plaque, compared with carotid intima-media thickness, more accurately predicts coronary artery disease events: a meta-analysis-Yoichi Inaba, M.D., Jennifer A. Chen M.D., Steven R. Bergmann M.D., Ph.D. Atherosclerosis 2012;220(1):34–5.

7. Cai JM, Hatsukami TS, Ferguson MS, et al. Classification of human carotid atherosclerotic lesions with in vivo multicontrast magnetic resonance imaging. Circulation 2002;106(11):1368–73.

8. Yuan C, Kerwin WS. MRI of atherosclerosis. J Magn Reson Imaging 2004;19(6):710–9.

9. Yarnykh VL, Terashima M, Hayes CE, et al. Multicontrast black-blood MRI of carotid arteries: comparison between 1.5 and 3 tesla magnetic field strengths. J Magn Reson Imaging 2006;23(5):691–8.

10. Kerwin WS, Liu F, Yarnykh V, et al. Signal features of the atherosclerotic plaque at 3.0 Tesla versus 1.5 Tesla: impact on automatic classification. J Magn Reson Imaging 2008;28(4):987–95.

11. Ota H, Yarnykh VL, Ferguson MS, et al. Carotid intraplaque hemorrhage imaging at 3.0-T MR imaging: comparison of the diagnostic performance of three T1-weighted sequences. Radiology 2010;254(2):551–63.

12. Hayes CE, Mathis CM, Yuan C. Surface coil phased arrays for high-resolution imaging of the carotid arteries. J Magn Reson Imaging 1996;6(1):109–12.

13. Tate Q, Kim SE, Treiman G, et al. Increased vessel depiction of the carotid bifurcation with a specialized 16-channel phased array coil at 3T. Magn Reson Med 2013;69(5):1486–93.

14. Edelman RR, Chien D, Kim D. Fast selective black blood MR imaging. Radiology 1991;181(3):655–60.

15. Yuan C, Kerwin WS, Ferguson MS, et al. Contrast-enhanced high resolution MRI for atherosclerotic carotid artery tissue characterization. J Magn Reson Imaging 2002;15(1):62–7.

16. Antiga L, Wasserman BA, Steinman DA. On the overestimation of early wall thickening at the carotid bulb by black blood MRI, with implications for coronary and vulnerable plaque imaging. Magn Reson Med 2008;60(5):1020–8.

17. Balu N, Chu B, Hatsukami TS, et al. Comparison between 2D and 3D high-resolution black-blood techniques for carotid artery wall imaging in clinically significant atherosclerosis. J Magn Reson Imaging 2008;27(4):918–24.

18. Balu N, Kerwin WS, Chu B, et al. Serial MRI of carotid plaque burden: influence of subject repositioning on measurement precision. Magn Reson Med 2007;57(3):592–9.

19. Balu N, Yarnykh V, Chu B, et al, editors. Carotid plaque assessment using fast 3D isotropic-resolution black-blood MRI. International Society of Magnetic Resonance in Medicine; 2009.

20. Wang J, Yarnykh VL, Hatsukami T, et al. Improved suppression of plaque-mimicking artifacts in black-blood carotid atherosclerosis imaging using a multi-slice motion-sensitized driven-equilibrium (MSDE) turbo spin-echo (TSE) sequence. Magn Reson Med 2007;58(5):973–81.

21. Zhao H, Wang J, Liu X, et al. Assessment of carotid artery atherosclerotic disease by using three-dimensional fast black-blood MR imaging: comparison with DSA. Radiology 2015;274(2):508–16.

22. Wang J, Yarnykh VL, Yuan C. Enhanced image quality in black-blood MRI using the improved motion-sensitized driven-equilibrium (iMSDE) sequence. J Magn Reson Imaging 2010;31(5):1256–63.

23. Makhijani MK, Balu N, Yamada K, et al. Accelerated 3D MERGE carotid imaging using compressed sensing with a hidden Markov tree model. J Magn Reson Imaging 2012;36(5):1194–202.

24. Wang J, Gerretsen SC, Maki JH, et al. Time-efficient black blood RCA wall imaging at 3T using improved motion sensitized driven equilibrium (iMSDE): feasibility and reproducibility. PLoS One 2011;6(10):e26567.

25. Obara M, Kuroda K, Wang J, et al. Comparison between two types of improved motion-sensitized driven-equilibrium (iMSDE) for intracranial black-blood imaging at 3.0 tesla. J Magn Reson Imaging 2014;40(4):824–31.

26. Zhu C, Graves MJ, Yuan J, et al. Optimization of improved motion-sensitized driven-equilibrium (iMSDE) blood suppression for carotid artery wall imaging. J Cardiovasc Magn Reson 2014;16:61.

27. Moody AR, Murphy RE, Morgan PS, et al. Characterization of complicated carotid plaque with magnetic resonance direct thrombus imaging in patients with cerebral ischemia. Circulation 2003;107(24):3047–52.

28. Murphy RE, Moody AR, Morgan PS, et al. Prevalence of complicated carotid atheroma as detected by magnetic resonance direct thrombus imaging in patients with suspected carotid artery stenosis and previous acute cerebral ischemia. Circulation 2003;107(24):3053–8.

29. Zhang Z, Fan Z, Carroll TJ, et al. Three-dimensional T2-weighted MRI of the human femoral arterial vessel wall at 3.0 Tesla. Invest Radiol 2009;44(9):619–26.

30. Fan Z, Zhang Z, Chung YC, et al. Carotid arterial wall MRI at 3T using 3D variable-flip-angle turbo spin-echo (TSE) with flow-sensitive dephasing (FSD). J Magn Reson Imaging 2010;31(3):645–54.

31. Parker DL, Yuan C, Blatter DD. MR angiography by multiple thin slab 3D acquisition. Magn Reson Med 1991;17(2):434–51.

32. Yim YJ, Choe YH, Ko Y, et al. High signal intensity halo around the carotid artery on maximum intensity projection images of time-of-flight MR angiography: a new sign for intraplaque hemorrhage. J Magn Reson Imaging 2008;27(6):1341–6.

33. Yoshimura S, Yamada K, Kawasaki M, et al. High-intensity signal on time-of-flight magnetic resonance angiography indicates carotid plaques at high risk for cerebral embolism during stenting. Stroke 2011;42(11):3132–7.

34. Yuan C, Mitsumori LM, Ferguson MS, et al. In vivo accuracy of multispectral magnetic resonance imaging for identifying lipid-rich necrotic cores and intraplaque hemorrhage in advanced human carotid plaques. Circulation 2001;104(17):2051–6.

35. Chu B, Kampschulte A, Ferguson MS, et al. Hemorrhage in the atherosclerotic carotid plaque: a high-resolution MRI study. Stroke 2004;35(5):1079–84.

36. Kampschulte A, Ferguson MS, Kerwin WS, et al. Differentiation of intraplaque versus juxtaluminal hemorrhage/thrombus in advanced human carotid atherosclerotic lesions by in vivo magnetic resonance imaging. Circulation 2004;110(20):3239–44.

37. Takaya N, Yuan C, Chu BC, et al. Presence of intraplaque hemorrhage stimulates progression of carotid atherosclerotic plaques: a high-resolution MRI study. Circulation 2005;111:2768–75.

38. Yuan C, Zhang S, Polissar NL, et al. Identification of fibrous cap rupture with magnetic resonance imaging is highly associated with recent TIA or stroke. Circulation 2002;105(2):181–5.

39. Yamada K, Song Y, Hippe DS, et al. Quantitative evaluation of high intensity signal on MIP images of carotid atherosclerotic plaques from routine TOF-MRA reveals elevated volumes of intraplaque hemorrhage and lipid rich necrotic core. J Cardiovasc Magn Reson 2012;14:81.

40. Wang J, Börnert P, Zhao H, et al. Simultaneous non-contrast angiography and intraplaque hemorrhage (SNAP) imaging for carotid atherosclerotic disease evaluation. Magn Reson Med 2013;69(2):337–45.

41. Balu N, Liu H, Chen S, et al. Dual contrast vessel wall MRI using phase sensitive polarity maps, Proceedings of the 22st Scientific Meeting and Exhibition, International Society of Magnetic Resonance in Medicine. Milan (Italy), May 10–16, 2014.

42. Fan Z, Yu W, Xie Y, et al. Multi-contrast atherosclerosis characterization (MATCH) of carotid plaque with a single 5-min scan: technical development and clinical feasibility. J Cardiovasc Magn Reson 2014;16:53.

43. Zhu DC, Vu AT, Ota H, et al. An optimized 3D spoiled gradient recalled echo pulse sequence for hemorrhage assessment using inversion recovery and multiple echoes (3D SHINE) for carotid plaque imaging. Magn Reson Med 2010;64(5):1341–51.

44. Li L, Chai JT, Biasiolli L, et al. Black-blood multicontrast imaging of carotid arteries with DANTE-prepared 2D and 3D MR imaging. Radiology 2014;273(2):560–9.

45. Li L, Miller KL, Jezzard P. DANTE-prepared pulse trains: a novel approach to motion-sensitized and motion-suppressed quantitative magnetic resonance imaging. Magn Reson Med 2012;68(5):1423–38.

46. Mendes J, Parker DL, Kim SE, et al. Reduced blood flow artifact in intraplaque hemorrhage imaging using CineMPRAGE. Magn Reson Med 2013;69(5):1276–84.

47. Zhou Z, Li R, Zhao X, et al. Evaluation of 3D multi-contrast joint intra- and extracranial vessel wall cardiovascular magnetic resonance. J Cardiovasc Magn Reson 2015;17:41.

Analysis of Multicontrast Carotid Plaque MR Imaging

Huijun Chen, PhD[a], Qiang Zhang, MS[b],
William Kerwin, PhD[c],*

KEYWORDS

- MR imaging • Atherosclerosis • Morphology • Composition • Contrast enhancement
- Biomechanics • Image processing

KEY POINTS

- Quantitative analyses of atherosclerotic plaque are enabled by image processing.
- Analyses of traditional MR images (T1-weighted, T2-weighted, and so forth) yield measurements of plaque morphology and composition.
- Dynamic contrast-enhanced (DCE)–MR imaging and kinetic modeling can be used to assess plaque perfusion characteristics related to inflammation.
- Coupling these techniques with computational models reveals plaque biomechanical forces.

INTRODUCTION

In clinical practice, luminal stenosis measured from angiography is the most widely used parameter for risk prediction of atherosclerotic plaque.[1] Together with the development of high-resolution multicontrast vessel wall MR imaging techniques, vessel wall features have drawn more attention in addition to luminal stenosis,[2–6] including morphologic, compositional, physiologic, and hemodynamic features.

Morphologic features of atherosclerotic plaque usually quantified from multicontrast carotid MR imaging are mainly used to evaluate the plaque burden, including vessel wall thickness, area, volume, and some normalized indexes, such as the normalized wall index (NWI).[7–16] Segmentation of the lumen and outer-wall boundaries from black-blood carotid MR images is the key to acquiring those quantitative morphologic features. Some automatic lumen/outer-wall boundary segmentation algorithms and how to measure those plaque burden features from the lumen/outer-wall boundaries are discussed.

Atherosclerotic plaque has complex contents. Researchers have found that components have different signals in different weightings in multicontrast carotid MR images,[12] providing a unique opportunity to identify those components. Many studies have found that some compositional features detected by multicontrast MR imaging can be used for vulnerable plaque identification, such as the thin fibrous cap, large necrotic core, and intraplaque hemorrhage.[12,17–21] Methods of segmenting the plaque components, including multicontrast image registration and pattern recognition–based composition detection methods, are discussed.

Disclosure Statement: W. Kerwin is a former employee of VPDiagnostics, Inc (through 2013) and holds several patents related to the work. The remaining authors have nothing to disclose.
[a] Department of Biomedical Engineering, Center for Biomedical Imaging Research, School of Medicine, Tsinghua University, Room No. 109, Haidian District, Beijing, China; [b] Department of Biomedical Engineering, Center for Biomedical Imaging Research, School of Medicine, Tsinghua University, Room No. 120, Haidian District, Beijing, China; [c] Department of Radiology, School of Medicine, University of Washington, 850 Republican Street, Seattle, WA 98109, USA
* Corresponding author.
E-mail address: bkerwin98136@yahoo.com

1052-5149/16/$ – see front matter © 2016 Elsevier Inc. All rights reserved.

Recently, advances in carotid plaque MR imaging and analysis techniques have allowed researchers to evaluate atherosclerosis at the physiologic level. Physiologically, plaque vascularity and accumulations of macrophages are highly associated with plaque instability.[22,23] To quantify the plaque angiogenesis and inflammation, DCE, an MR imaging technique, has been proposed and successfully validated.[1,24,25] This article introduces the processing and modeling of DCE carotid plaque MR images.

Lastly, hemodynamic conditions are believed related to pathogenesis of atherosclerotic plaque.[26,27] Methods of extracting hemodynamic features from carotid plaque MR imaging, including the wall shear stress (WSS) and tensile stress, are discussed.[28–34]

PLAQUE BURDEN

Plaque burden is a measure of atherosclerotic plaque size. Based on the imaging and processing protocol, plaque burden metrics can be 2-D cross-sectional vessel wall thickness, area, 3-D volume, and other metrics. No matter which plaque burden metric is chosen, precise segmentation of the inner and outer boundaries of the vessel wall is an essential step. Black-blood carotid plaque MR imaging can show the vessel wall clearly, allowing automatic segmentation. Segmentation methods are in 2 categories: 2-D–based segmentation and 3-D–based segmentation. The 2-D segmentation methods detect the boundaries in cross-sectional images, whereas the 3-D segmentation techniques segment the surface directly. After lumen and outer-wall boundaries are detected, a range of morphology metrics can be calculated.

Imaging protocols

For plaque burden assessment, the protocol should include: T1-weighted, 2-D or 3-D acquisitions, black-blood preparation, fat saturation, in-plane resolution less than 1 mm, slice thickness 2 mm or less.

2-D Boundary Detection

Detection of the lumen and outer-wall boundaries has been accomplished most often by placing contours on stacks of 2-D cross-sectional images. Active contour methods, such as B-spline snakes, are available that deform an initial contour estimate to match the boundary apparent in the image.[35] For greater automation, techniques have been developed that propagate a contour from image to image. One such technique is the Markov shape model (**Fig. 1**), in which the expected shape in the subsequent image is estimated based on the shape in the current image.[36]

3-D Boundary Detection

As imaging methods have advanced to allow black-blood preparation in isotropic 3-D images, a new approach to boundary detection has emerged in which the entire lumen or outer-wall volume is segmented as a whole, rather than as a series of parallel contours. One such approach uses graph-cuts global optimization (**Fig. 2**) to simultaneously extract the lumen and vessel wall.[37] Constraints ensure that the lumen is contained within the larger vessel wall volume.

Plaque Burden Quantification

After the lumen and outer-wall boundaries have been identified, plaque burden metrics, such as thickness, area, and volume, can be calculated.

Vessel wall thickness calculation

Because of the various shapes of the diseased carotid artery, thickness measurement is a challenge. The key to calculating thickness is to find the matching lines connecting corresponding points between the lumen and outer-wall contours. Such correspondence, however, cannot be easily defined in carotid artery with severe plaque. The intuitive matching method of shortest distance may generate wrong matching lines, such as lines that cross the lumen (**Fig. 3**). Han and colleagues[38] propose using the Delaunay triangulation technique to find the corresponding points, which can produce a stable result for various plaque shapes. Once the Delaunay triangulation is completed, the matching lines can be defined by the triangular midlines of all triangles.

Vessel wall area and volume

In addition to thickness, vessel wall area is a commonly used burden metric. The vessel wall area can be calculated by measuring the area enclosed by the outer-wall boundary minus the area enclosed by the lumen boundary. With known area, the plaque volume is calculated using the Simpson rule, which sums the areas of all images times the separation between images.[39]

Normalized wall index

Although the absolute value of vessel wall area measurement can reflect the plaque burden, it does not account for the variance of carotid artery size in the population, which may introduce bias in clinical use. To solve this problem, a normalized metric has been proposed[35]: the NWI, which

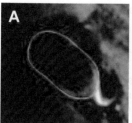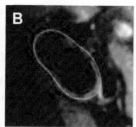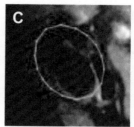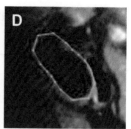

Fig. 1. Image (A) is proximal to image (B) and is used to refine the search space of the Markov shape model (B). (C, D) Examples of initializations obtained, respectively, without and with knowledge of the preceding shape. (*From* Underhill H, Kerwin W. Markov shape models: object boundary identification in serial magnetic resonance images, in proceedings 14th scientific meeting. International Society for Magnetic Resonance in Medicine. vol. 14. 2006. p. 829.)

normalized the plaque area by the vessel size. NWI is defined as the area of the vessel wall divided by the area of the lumen plus wall and ranges from approximately 0.4 for a normal artery to near 1.0 for a highly stenotic artery. In some cases, NWI is calculate in terms of wall and lumen volumes instead of areas.[14]

Validation, Reproducibility, and Clinical Studies of the Morphologic Metrics

Yuan and colleagues[11] have shown that the maximal wall area measurements from in vivo and ex vivo MR imaging strongly agree. In another study comparing in vivo and ex vivo plaque MR images, the correlation coefficients were found as high as 0.92 for wall volume measurement, 0.91 for maximum wall area measurement, and 0.90 for minimum lumen area measurement.[10] In a histology validated study,[12] the area measurements of wall can be correlated with histology ($r = 0.84$; $P<.001$).

The interscan, interobserver, and intraobserver reproducibilities of vessel wall morphology measurements have been investigated. The interscan reproducibility of the mean wall thickness is high (intraclass correlation coefficient [ICC] = 97% and coefficient of variation [CV] = 3.87%), the maximum wall thickness has lower interscan reproducibility (ICC = 87% and CV = 14.79%), the NWI has good interscan reproducibility (ICC = 98% and CV = 3.02%), and the interscan reproducibilities are also high for wall volume (ICC = 94% and CV = 4.2%), lumen volume (ICC = 99% and CV = 2.6%), and total vessel volume (ICC = 97% and CV = 2.25%).[8] In a study involving 4 scans,[14] the measurement error was as low as 5.8% for wall volume and 3.2% for a volume-based NWI. Intraobserver and interobserver variability of maximum wall area is also excellent (ICC ranging from 0.90 to 0.98).[11]

All the morphologic metrics of plaque have been widely used in clinical studies. Takaya and colleagues[9] found that maximum wall thickness is

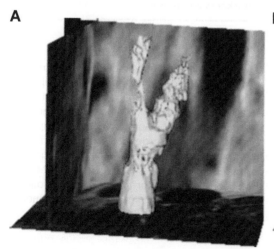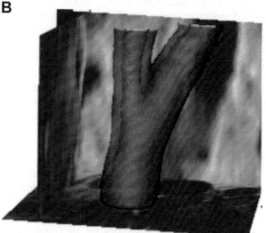

Fig. 2. The segmentation example: (A) the initial surface obtained by region growing and (B) the final lumen and outer-wall surface generated by the algorithm. (*From* Ukwatta E, Yuan J, Rajchl M, et al. 3-D carotid multi-region MRI segmentation by globally optimal evolution of coupled surfaces. IEEE Trans Med Imaging 2013;32(4):770–85; with permission.)

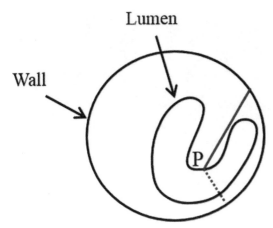

Lumen

Wall

P

Fig. 3. An example showing the possible failure in finding the matching lines between lumen and outer-wall contours. The red solid line gives the correct matching line at the point P, whereas the red dotted line shows the wrong matching line found by the shortest distance method.

associated with the subsequent cerebrovascular events (the hazard ratio for 1 mm increase is 1.6; $P = .008$) over a mean follow-up of 38.2 months. Saam and colleagues[13] has found that the lumen area of symptomatic plaque tends smaller compared with asymptomatic plaque ($P = .008$). Phan and colleagues[15] find that the patients with low high-density lipoprotein cholesterol ($\leq$35 mg/dL) have larger wall volume (97 ± 23 mm^3) than the patients whose high-density lipoprotein cholesterol levels are greater than 35 mg/dL (81 ± 19 mm^3). Morphologic metrics can also be used in longitudinal studies. Mean wall thickness and NWI have been used in therapeutic response study.[16] Zhao and colleagues[40] found that the treated patients had a smaller luminal area (55 mm^2 vs 44 mm^2) and plaque area (58 mm^2 vs 64 mm^2) compared with patients who did not receive the intensive lipid-lowering therapy. Takaya and colleagues[41] found that intraplaque hemorrhage can stimulate the plaque progression based on wall volume increase (wall volume change in subjects with and without intraplaque hemorrhage is 6.8% vs −0.15% [$P = .009$]).

What the Physician Needs to Know
- Several different measurements of plaque burden are used, including wall thickness, area, volume, and derived parameters, such as NWI.
- The key to all measurements of burden is accurate detection of lumen and outer-wall boundaries.
- Several tools are available to facilitate vessel boundary detection.

- Plaque burden measurements are accurate and reproducible.

PLAQUE COMPONENTS

In addition to plaque burden, the compositional characteristics of plaque are believed related the cerebral events.[19] The major plaque components identified by multicontrast carotid MR imaging include necrotic/lipid core,[19] intraplaque hemorrhage,[21] calcification,[14] loose matrix,[12] and fibrous cap.[17,18] The thin fibrous caps and large necrotic cores can cause plaque structural weakness.[1] Calcified nodule impinging into the lumen lead to fragile thrombus.[42] Strong correlations are found between intraplaque hemorrhage and cerebral events.[43,44] Thus, it is important to quantify not only the morphologic features but also the compositional characteristics.

The principle for multicontrast MR imaging–based plaque component identification is that the intensity features from multiple magnetic resonance (MR) weightings can differentiate plaque components, whereas different compositions may show similar signals in a single-contrast weighting.[12] Thus, the multiple MR weightings must be spatially aligned using registration technique before the component segmentation.[45]

Imaging protocols
For plaque component assessment, the protocol should include: multicontrast weighted imaging (T1, T2, contrast-enhanced T1, and time-of-flight), 2-D or 3-D acquisitions, black-blood and bright-blood preparation, fat saturation, in-plane resolution less than 1 mm, and slice thickness 2 mm or less.

Multicontrast Image Registration

The misalignment among multicontrast carotid MR images caused by patient motion is a major challenge in component identification. Patient motion must be corrected to well under 1 mm, given the fine image resolution and presence of components that may be on the order of 1 mm in size. To solve the misalignment caused by rigid motion, the active edge map-based registration method[45] has been proposed for multicontrast carotid MR images, which uses lumen and wall boundaries detected in 1 contrast weighting to optimally shift other contrast weightings (Fig. 4).

Plaque Component Segmentation

After the lumen/outer-wall segmentation and multicontrast images registration, trained experts have

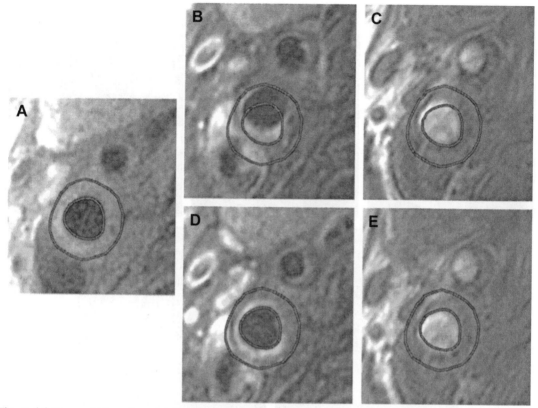

Fig. 4. (A) Segmented contours at black-blood T1-weighted image. (B) Black-blood T2-weighted image with contours from (A). (C) Bright-blood time-of-flight weighted image with contours from (A). (D) T2-weighted image with registered contours. (E) Time-of-flight weighted image with registered contours. (*From* Kerwin WS, Yuan C. Active edge maps for medical image registration. Med Imaging 2001 Image Process 2001;4320:516–26; with permission.)

been able to identify different plaque components based on different intensities in multiple MR weightings.[12] Numerous efforts have been made to automate this evaluation.[46–48] Based on the observed, implicit use of local wall morphology (eg, thickness) that trained manual reviewers use to identify components, the most successful algorithms have also added morphologic features and improve the segmentation performance.[48,49] The morphology-enhanced probabilistic plaque segmentation (MEPPS) algorithm is one of these methods (Fig. 5).[48] In addition to the 2-D sequences used in the original MEPPS development, Liu and colleagues[50] further used the MEPPS algorithm on 3-D carotid MR images, showing similar results (Fig. 6) compared with 2-D MEPPS algorithm.

Validation, Reproducibility, and Clinical Studies of Plaque Compositional Features

Quantification of plaque components has been validated primarily for manual analysis by expert image reviewers. For the identification of lipid-

rich/necrotic core and intraplaque hemorrhage, the results from multicontrast MR imaging agree with the histologic findings, with $\kappa = 0.69$, overall sensitivity of 85%, and specificity of 92%.[19] Compared with histologic results, MR imaging is able to distinguish juxtaluminal hemorrhage from intraplaque hemorrhage with an accuracy of 96%; sensitivity and specificity for identifying the appearance are 96% and 82%, respectively.[21] In another histology validated study,[12] the sensitivities and specificities of carotid MR imaging were 95% and 76% for lipid-rich/necrotic core, 84% and 91% for calcification, 87% and 84% for hemorrhage, and 79% and 77% for loose matrix, respectively. For characterization of the fibrous cap, the agreement of multicontrast MR imaging and histology can achieve $\kappa = 0.83$ and the Spearman correlation coefficient $= 0.88$,[17] whereas sensitivity and specificity are 0.81 and 0.90 for the unstable fibrous cap detection, respectively.[18]

Quantitatively, MR imaging measurements compare closely with histology when quantifying the area of lipid-rich/necrotic core (23.7% vs

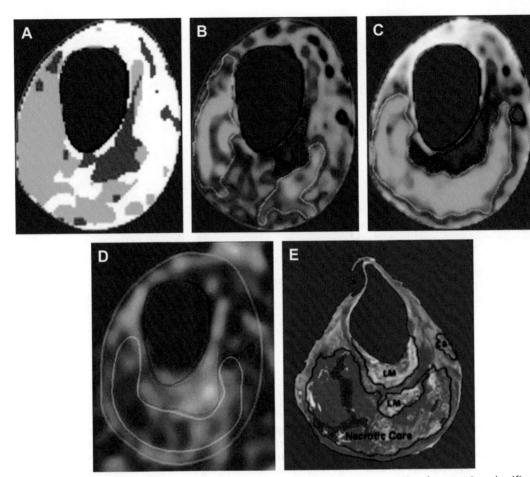

Fig. 5. Comparison of obtained plaque components: (*A*) automatic segmentation by gaussian classifier; (*B*) probability map and region contours based on intensity only—green is necrotic core, red is calcification, blue is loose matrix, and gray is fibrous tissue; (*C*) segmentation results based on the intensity and morphologic information; (*D*) manual segmentation results shown in T2-weighted image; and (*E*) the corresponding histology specimen. (*From* Liu F, Xu D, Ferguson MS, et al. Automated in vivo segmentation of carotid plaque MRI with Morphology-Enhanced probability maps. Magn Reson Med 2006;55(3):659–68; with permission.)

20.3%), loose matrix (5.1% vs 6.3%), fibrous tissue (66.3% vs 64%), and calcification (9.4% vs 5%).[12] Moderate to strong correlations between MR imaging and histology area measurements are found for lipid-rich/necrotic core ($r = 0.75$; $P<.001$), calcification ($r = 0.74$; $P<.001$), loose matrix ($r = 0.70$; $P<.001$), and hemorrhage ($r = 0.66$; $P<.001$).[12] In another study with histologic validation,[20] the mean percentage area of lipid-rich/necrotic core measured by MR imaging is also comparable with histology (30.1% vs 32.7%) and is highly correlated across locations ($r = 0.87$; $P<.001$). For intact fibrous cap quantification, MR images show a moderate to good correlation in length ($r = 0.73$; $P<.001$) and area ($r = 0.80$; $P<.001$) compared with histology. The intrareader and inter-reader reproducibilities of area measurements was good to excellent for lipid-rich/necrotic core (ICC = 0.89 and 0.92

respectively), calcification (ICC = 0.9 and 0.95 respectively), hemorrhage (ICC = 0.74 and 0.73 respectively), loose matrix (ICC = 0.79 and 0.79 respectively).[12] In a study with 4 scans, the measurement error of the volume is 11.1% for lipid-rich/necrotic core, and 18.6% for calcification.[14]

Automated component segmentation algorithms have also been validated and compare favorably to manual review. The MEPPS algorithm segmentation and the histologic drawing are highly associated.[51] Kerwin and colleagues[52] tested the MEPPS on 1.5T and 3.0T MR images; the correlation coefficients of average area were 0.91 (lipid-rich core), 0.93 (intraplaque hemorrhage), 0.95 (calcification), and 0.93 (fibrous tissue).

The plaque compositional features from MR imaging are widely used in clinical studies. Saam and colleagues[13] found that the symptomatic plaques had a higher incidence of fibrous cap rupture

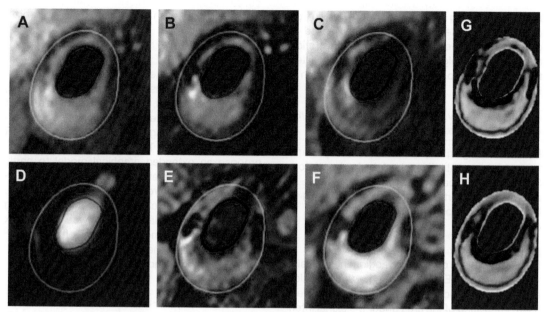

Fig. 6. (*A*) T1, (*B*) T2, (*C*) CET1, (*D*) TOF, (*E*) MP-RAGE, (*F*) MERGE, (*G*) segmentation using 2-D MEPPS, and (*H*) segmentation using 3-D MEPPS. (*G, H*) White color is fibrous, purple color is loose matrix, blue color is calcification, and yellow color is necrotic core. CET1, contrast-enhanced T1; TOF, time-of-flight; MP-RAGE, magnetization prepared rapid gradient echo; MERGE, motion sensitized driven equilibrium rapid gradient echo. (*From* Liu W, Balu N, Sun J, et al. Segmentation of carotid plaque using multicontrast 3D gradient echo, MRI. J Magn Reson Imaging 2012;35(4):812–9; with permission.)

(P = .007) and juxtaluminal hemorrhage or thrombus (P = .039) compared with asymptomatic plaques. By comparing patients with and without the subsequent symptoms, Takaya and colleagues[9] found that presence of a thin or ruptured fibrous cap has a hazard ratio of 17.0 ($P \leq .001$); intraplaque hemorrhage has a hazard ratio of 5.2 (P = .005). Yuan and colleagues[53] found that the ruptured fibrous cap is highly associated with a recent history of transient ischemic attack or stroke. In longitudinal studies, Zhao and colleagues[40] found a decreased lipid content can be observed by MR imaging in patients receiving intensive lipid-lowering therapy. In another 2-year study of rosuvastatin therapy using the MEPPS algorithm,[16] the mean area proportion of the vessel wall composed of lipid-rich/necrotic core decreased by 41.4% (P = .005).

What the Physician Needs to Know
- Effective differentiation of plaque components requires a combination of information from multiple contrast weightings.
- Several tools are available to facilitate plaque component segmentation.
- Image alignment is a necessary step for automated component segmentation.
- Plaque component measurements are reproducible and accurate.

PLAQUE ACTIVITY

A third aspect of atherosclerotic plaque vulnerability is inflammation, which is often associated with angiogenesis and referred to as *plaque activity*.[54,55] The accumulations of macrophages have been demonstrated to be associated with plaque instability.[22] Plaque vascularity is also a key feature of symptomatic carotid atherosclerosis.[23]

DCE–MR imaging provides an opportunity to quantify plaque inflammation and angiogenesis by using gadolinium contrast agents together with pharmacokinetic modeling.[24,56] DCE–MR imaging of the vessel wall is difficult to analyze because the vessel wall is a moving and small imaging target.

Imaging Protocols

For plaque activity assessment, the protocol should include: DCE imaging, 2-D acquisition, fat saturation, in-plane resolution less than 1 mm, slice thickness 3 mm or less, imaging rate 15 seconds per frame or less, and total imaging time at least 2 minutes.

Dynamic Contrast-Enhanced Image Registration and Filter

To overcome the analysis difficulties caused by patient motion and low signal-to-noise ratio in

DCE–MR imaging of carotid artery, Kerwin and colleagues[57] presented a Kalman filter–based algorithm called the Kalman filtering, registration, and smoothing algorithm, which not only filters the noise but also registers the image motion at the same time.

Parameters Derived from Vessel Wall Dynamic Contrast-Enhanced–MR Imaging

DCE–MR imaging results are ultimately transformed into quantitative physiologic descriptors. Several derived parameters have been used. All are related to perfusion characteristics, such as blood supply, permeability, and volume of distribution.

Integrated area under the curve

In quantification of plaque angiogenesis using vessel wall DCE–MR imaging, the simplest approach, a model-free parameter, has been used, consisting of the area under the signal intensity versus time curve (AUC) with different duration time (T).[58] The AUC can be calculated by the numeric integration:

$$AUC(T) = \int_0^T \left(SI(t) - SI_{precontrast} \right) dt$$

where $SI(t)$ is the signal curve at time t, $SI_{precontrast}$ is the average precontrast intensity. T can be 1, 2, 7, and 12 minutes after contrast agent injection to account for wash-in, wash-out, or both. As the integration time increases, this converges to a value proportional to the volume of distribution of the contrast agent.

Patlak model

Although the model-free parameter has the advantage of being simple and highly reproducible, it still suffers from no physiologic meaning. Thus, pharmacokinetic modeling has been proposed. Kerwin and colleagues[56] used the Patlak model[59] for DCE–MR imaging analysis, and validated with histology. The Patlak model assumes (1) the effect of contrast agent from the plaque back to the plasma is neglected and (2) the signal intensity reflects the contrast agent concentration. Then the tissue concentration $C_t(t)$ can be represented as

$$C_t(t) = v_p C_p(t) + K^{trans} \int C_p(u) du$$

where v_p represents the fractional plasma volume, K^{trans} is the transfer constant reflecting the permeability of neovessels, $C_p(t)$ and $C_t(t)$ are the contrast agent concentration curves in the plasma and tissue, which can be measured from the signal intensity curves of the plaque and blood.[60] Then,

the v_p and K^{trans} can be estimated for each pixel by linear fitting.

Extended graphical model

In the theory of the contrast agent dynamics, neglecting the contrast reflux from tissue to plasma, like the Patlak model, introduces bias in parameter estimation.[61] Considering the reflux effect, however, requires much longer total scan time in DCE–MR imaging acquisition. Thus, Chen and colleagues[25] propose an extended graphical model to partly model the contrast reflux effect to increase the accuracy without severely prolonging the scan time. The extended graphical model is found by exploring the mathematical relationship between the Patlak model[59] and the modified Kety/Tofts model,[60] which fully models the contrast reflux.

The equation of modified Kety/Tofts model is

$$C_t(t) = v_p C_p(t) + K^{trans} \int_0^t C_p(\tau) e^{\frac{K^{trans}}{v_e}(t-\tau)} d\tau$$

where v_e represents fractional extravascular extracellular space volume, and all other terms are as defined in the Patlak model. The Patlak model can be viewed as a 1-term expansion of the integral in this equation. To partly model the reflux, Chen and colleagues[25] proposed the extended graphical model, which uses a 2-term expansion of the integral:

$$C_t(t) = v_p C_p(t) + K^{trans} \int_0^t C_p(\tau) d\tau$$
$$- \frac{K^{trans^2}}{v_e} \int_0^t \int_0^{\tau_1} C_p(\tau_2) d\tau_2 d\tau_1$$

Reference region method in pharmacokinetic modeling

All these approaches assume knowledge of the blood plasma concentration or typically an intensity-based approximation. An imaging technique that preserves the blood signal cannot, however, evaluate the vessel wall with early lesions, due to the signal contamination from the adjacent blood. Thus, black-blood DCE–MR imaging techniques have been proposed[58,62–64] for thin vessel wall perfusion imaging. To deal with the missing blood concentration, some researchers has fallen back on using model-free parameters, as described previously. Chen and colleagues[64] proposed using the reference region method[65] in the pharmacokinetic modeling of black-blood vessel wall DCE–MR imaging. The reference region approach uses the knowledge that a suitable reference tissue, such as muscle, undergoes enhancement according to the same blood input function as the plaque. The estimated blood curve can then be deconvolved from the reference region enhancement pattern.

Validation, Reproducibility, and Clinical Studies of Plaque Activity

In a study based on animal atherosclerosis model,[58] the AUC (2 min) and AUC (7 min) were found correlated with neovessel count in histology, with $r = 0.89$ ($P = .016$) and $r = 0.91$ ($P = .011$), respectively. In another animal model investigation,[62] the interscan, interobserver, and intraobserver reproducibilities of AUC 1, 2, and 7 minutes were found good to excellent, with the interscan ICC larger than 0.76, intraobserver ICC larger than 0.99, and the interobserver ICC larger than 0.98 for all the parameters, respectively. In clinical studies, Vucic and colleagues[63] used the AUC parameter in a longitudinal study for therapeutic response investigation.

For model-based approaches, Kerwin and colleagues[56] validated v_p with the microvessels quantified on histology of human carotid plaque, and a significant correlation was found ($r = 0.8$; $P<.001$). In another study with a larger population, Kerwin and colleagues[24] found that K^{trans} and v_p are correlated with histologic features of inflammation and angiogenesis: K^{trans} and macrophage ($r = 0.75$; $P<.001$); K^{trans} and neovasculature ($r = 0.71$; $P<.001$); v_p and macrophages ($r = 0.54$; $P = .004$); and v_p and neovasculature ($r = 0.68$; $P<.001$). A further study also found that K^{trans} is significantly correlated with neovasculature ($r = 0.41$; $P = .04$) and macrophages ($r = 0.49$; $P = .01$) in histologic specimens.[66] Also, K^{trans} is found correlated with C-reactive protein levels ($r = 0.57$; $P = .01$) and elevated in active smokers compared with nonsmokers ($P = .02$). Gaens and colleagues[6] found a significant positive correlation between K^{trans} derived from Patlak model and the endothelial microvessel content on histology ($r = 0.72$; $P = .005$).

Kerwin and colleagues[66] have reported a high inter-reader reproducibility of K^{trans} with ICC of 0.95. The interscan reproducibility of v_p and K^{trans} calculated from Patlak model was also reported in a single-center study.[6] The CV for K^{trans} is 16% and for v_p is 26%. Chen and colleagues[67] have investigated the interscan reproducibility of Patlak model generated pharmacokinetic parameters in a multicenter setting. Moderate reproducibility was found for K^{trans} (ICC = 0.65 and CV = 25%), but a low reproducibility of v_p was found (ICC = 0.28 and CV = 62%). The reproducibility of v_p can be improved in larger lesions (ICC = 0.73 and CV = 28%), indicating current DCE–MR imaging and analysis techniques are more stable for large plaques.

The extended graphical model had lower noise sensitivity than the modified Kety/Tofts model. And compared with Patlak model, the extended graphical model bias is 74.4% to 99.8% less for K^{trans} estimation.[25] Gaens and colleagues[6] showed similar results, that the extended graphical model has lower relative fit uncertainty than the modified Kety/Tofts model. They also found a significant correlation between K^{trans} derived from the extended graphical model and the endothelial microvessel content in histology ($r = 0.69$; $P = .009$).[6] Moreover, the interscan reproducibility of the extended graphical model was also reported[6]: ICC = 0.73 and CV = 13% for K^{trans} estimation, which are better than for the modified Kety/Tofts model.

Chen and colleagues[64] demonstrated that the K^{trans} calculated the reference region method–based Patlak model has a significant correlation with macrophage content ($r = 0.70$; $P = .01$) in early atherosclerotic plaques. More importantly, the reference region method has the ability to monitor the early-stage plaque natural progression in vivo; K^{trans} showed a significant correlation with macrophage content ($r = 0.70$; $P = .01$).

The Patlak model is the most commonly used model in clinical studies of vessel wall DCE–MR imaging. Dong and colleagues[68] found a significant reduction in mean K^{trans} derived by Patlak model in 28 patients after 1 year of intensive lipid therapy. Sun and colleagues[69] found the presence of intraplaque hemorrhage was associated with a significantly higher K^{trans} value, demonstrating the independent physiologic link between the adventitial vasa vasorum and intraplaque hemorrhage. Truijman and colleagues[55] found that the macrophage activity measured by fludeoxyglucose F 18–PET (FDG-PET) and perfusion measured by DCE–MR imaging have a weak but significant positive correlation. Calcagno and colleagues[70] found a significant, weak inverse relationship between FDG-PET and DCE–MR imaging inflammation evaluation metrics. Wang and colleagues[71] found a moderate correlation only in symptomatic plaques but not in asymptomatic plaques, and the correlation between FDG-PET and DCE–MR imaging metrics varied with clinical conditions, indicating the complex interaction between macrophages and neovessels. Those studies show that the Patlak model can be used in therapeutic response investigation, plaque risk assessment, and atherosclerosis pathophysiologic research.

What the Physician Needs to Know
- DCE–MR imaging can be used to assess plaque inflammation and perfusion.
- Several choices of DCE–MR imaging approaches and corresponding quantitative analyses are available.
- Model-based methods provide physiologically meaningful descriptions of perfusion.

PLAQUE BIOMECHANICS

Previous discussions introduced plaque features that relate to vulnerability. In vivo, arteries always have blood flow inside, and the flow has some interactions with plaque. Thus, plaque vulnerability may depend not only on the inner features but also on the outer biomechanical forces.[72] Numerous studies have shown that there is a relation between biomechanical forces and pathogenesis of atherosclerotic plaque.[26,27,73]

There are 2 primary mechanical forces that have been studied for high-risk plaque identification: fluid WSS and tensile stress.[72] Several studies have shown that more plaque occurs in regions of low WSS compared with regions of high WSS.[26,74,75] WSS may be linked to vulnerable plaque features.[74] In regions where plaque rupture occurs, the tensile stresses are thought to be higher.[27] Thus, the increased tensile stress may be a key factor causing plaque rupture.[76]

Imaging Protocols

For plaque biomechanics assessment, the protocol should include: T1-weighted MR imaging (discussed previously) for vessel boundary evaluation and phase-contrast MR imaging for blood velocity measurements.

Wall Shear Stress

WSS is a major force imparted onto the boundary when fluids flow along a solid boundary, as a result of a loss of velocity.[77] Thus, the key to calculating WSS is to know the flow velocity at the boundary, that is, hemodynamic conditions. From carotid MR imaging, there are 2 ways to measure flow velocity: computational fluid dynamics (CFD) by modeling the artery geometry and flow boundary conditions[28–30] and direct velocity imaging by phase-contrast (PC) MR imaging.[31–33]

Computational fluid dynamics method

To obtain the hemodynamic data of carotid artery, there are processes that need to be carried out: (1) generating the geometry model from MR imaging data, (2) giving the velocity boundary condition, and (3) calculating the flow by CFD.

To generate the geometry model, the lumen surface is constructed from a series of 2-D carotid MR images or 3-D carotid images. The methods described previously can be used for lumen segmentation. After the segmentation, a 3-D lumen surface can be generated from 2-D contours or directly result from 3-D segmentation. Then, smoothing should be applied to the 3-D lumen surface for better CFD analysis,[78] especially for the segmentation from 2-D images **Figs. 7** and **8** illustrate an example of generated mesh.

For velocity boundary conditions, the flow velocity distribution of the inflow and outflow planes of the modeled artery in a cardiac cycle are needed. The boundary condition can be assumed but with inaccuracy and the lack of individual difference. The velocity conditions can also be acquired from the cine PC MR imaging, which can measure the 2-D flow velocity of a plane over time. To assure the measurement accuracy, the imaging plane of inflow boundary should be as far as possible from the bifurcation apex and remains within the region of interest.[28] The 2 outflow

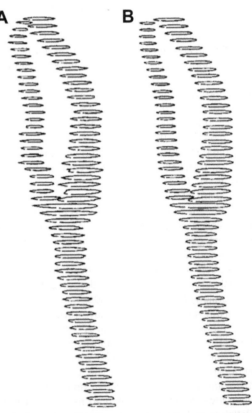

Fig. 7. (A) Original contours and (B) contours after smoothing. (From Long Q, Xu XY, Ariff B, et al. Reconstruction of blood flow patterns in a human carotid bifurcation: a combined CFD and MRI study. J Magn Reson Imaging 2000;11(3):299–311; with permission.)

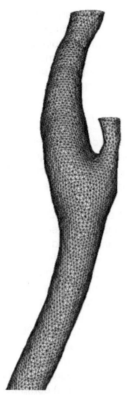

Fig. 8. An example of generated mesh. (*From* Steinman DA, Thomas JB, Ladak HM, et al. Reconstruction of carotid bifurcation hemodynamics and wall thickness using computational fluid dynamics and MRI. Magn Reson Med 2002;47(1):149–59; with permission.)

boundaries should be located at the internal carotid arteries and external carotid arteries superior to the bifurcation apex and in the relatively straight sections.[28] After imaging, the smoothing should be applied to exclude the influence of noise.

The CFD model can be simulated under the fluid flow equations with commercial software: CFX 4.2 (ANSYS, Canonsburg, PA), Automatic Dynamic Incremental Nonlinear Analysis (ADINA, Watertown, Massachusetts), Comsol Multiphysics (Stockholm, Sweden), or in-house finite element CFD code. The blood is assumed to be a newtonian fluid, the flow is considered laminar, and the vessel walls are assumed rigid. With the artery geometry and boundary condition, the hemodynamic conditions of the whole artery can be calculated by CFD. Then the WSS of the whole lumen boundary can be generated. **Fig. 9** illustrates an example of WSS results at the peak systole calculated by CFD.

Flow velocity imaging method
In addition to the CFD model, the WSS can be obtained directly from 3-D cine PC MR imaging. This

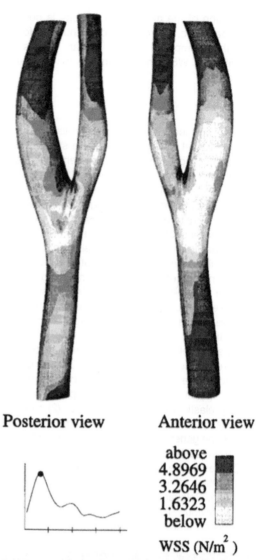

Posterior view   Anterior view

above
4.8969
3.2646
1.6323
below

WSS (N/m^2)

Fig. 9. WSS magnitude at peak systole. (*From* Long Q, Xu XY, Ariff B, et al. Reconstruction of blood flow patterns in a human carotid bifurcation: a combined CFD and MRI study. J Magn Reson Imaging 2000;11(3):299–311; with permission.)

method has the advantage of avoiding the inaccuracy of CFD model caused by the unrealistic assumption of newtonian fluid, laminar flow, and rigid lumen. But it has relatively low spatial resolution. The WSS calculation requires the flow velocity very near the boundary, which cannot be directly measured by the PC MR imaging method due to its low spatial resolution. Thus, Oyre and colleagues[31] proposed a fitting-based interpolation method to obtain a high spatial resolution flow velocity distribution from PC MR imaging. In this study, the velocity of the blood at the lumen boundary is assumed zero and the distribution of the axial blood velocity is considered parabolic. Oyre and colleagues[31] found that the computed result reveals errors of ±3.25% in WSS measurement in computer simulation.

Tensile Stress Model

The flowing blood inside the artery also pressurizes the vessel wall, causing tensile stress within the plaque. High tensile stress at certain location is found related to plaque rupture.[34] To quantify the tensile stress of plaque, finite element analysis can be used. Cheng and colleagues[34] divided the complex structure of a 2-D vessel wall slice into many smaller sections and estimated the distribution of tensile stress using finite element analysis. **Fig. 10** illustrates an example of the generated finite element meshes, where the meshing density is higher near the lumen to generate high accuracy in finite element analysis. Different components inside the plaque are assigned different mechanical properties.

In the finite element analysis to calculate the tensile stress inside plaque, there are 3 assumptions used to decide the component mechanical parameters[34]: (1) all components are approximated by linearly elastic material parameters, (2) the mechanical parameters do not change with time, and (3) the general structures of plaque and artery tissue are assumed to have identical mechanical properties in the circumferential and axial directions, which differ from properties in the radial direction. Relevant parameters can be estimated from previous literature[79–82] or limited based on previous knowledge during the analysis. These finite element models can be solved by mechanical analysis software, such as the ABAQUS (Simulia, Dassault Systèmes, Providence, RI) or ANSYS (Swanson Analysis Systems). Then the tensile stress map of the 2-D plaque slice can be calculated, as shown in **Fig. 11**.

Clinical Studies of Biomechanical Features

Biomechanical forces have been demonstrated to play an important role in plaque rupture by histology.[72,76] There are strong correlations between thickness and the reciprocal of maximum shear stress ($r = 0.90$; $P<.0005$) and the reciprocal of mean shear stress ($r = 0.82$; $P<.001$).[83] Moreover, a significant negative Pearson correlation between wall thickness increase and maximum shear stress was found ($r = -0.525$; $P<.0001$).[84] Cheng and colleagues[26] find that lesion size and vulnerability are highly determined by the pattern of fluid shear stress. Lower shear stress lesions are larger (1.38 ± 0.68 vs 0.22 ± 0.04); contain fewer smooth muscle cells ($1.9 \pm 1.6\%$ vs $26.3 \pm 9.7\%$), less collagen ($15.3 \pm 1.0\%$ vs $22.2 \pm 1.0\%$), and more lipids ($15.8 \pm 0.9\%$ vs $10.2 \pm 0.5\%$); and show more outward vascular remodeling ($214 \pm 19\%$ vs $117 \pm 9\%$) compared with oscillatory shear stress lesion.[26] Those results suggest the low WSS is associated with plaque development.

On the other hand, the maximum circumferential tensile stress in ruptured plaque is significantly higher than stress in stable plaque (4091 ± 1199 vs 1444 ± 485 mm Hg; $P<.0001$).[34] Richardson and colleagues[27] found that the position of maximum circumferential tensile stress is near

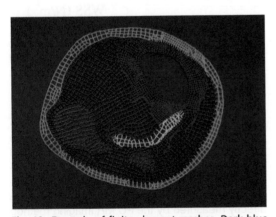

Fig. 10. Example of finite element meshes. Dark blue is calcium, red is fibrous plaque, yellow is lipid pool, and light blue is artery. (*From* Cheng GC, Loree HM, Kamm RD, et al. Distribution of circumferential stress in ruptured and stable atherosclerotic lesions. A structural analysis with histopathological correlation. Circulation 1993;87(4):1179–87; with permission.)

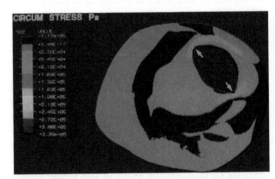

Fig. 11. An example of the tensile stress. The regions identified by the arrows have the highest circumferential (CIRCUM) stress (more than 200,000 Pascal [Pa]), which may be points vulnerable to rupture. (*Data from* Cheng GC, Loree HM, Kamm RD, et al. Distribution of circumferential stress in ruptured and stable atherosclerotic lesions. A structural analysis with histopathological correlation. Circulation 1993;87(4):1179–87.)

the lateral edge of the plaque cap in the plaque with a lipid pool, which is the most common location of rupture happens. Thus, high tensile stress is related to plaque rupture.

What the Physician Needs to Know
- Two biomechanical stresses play a role in atherosclerosis: WSS and plaque tensile stress.
- Estimating these stresses requires finite element modeling based on vessel structure.

REFERENCES

1. Kerwin WS. Carotid artery disease and stroke: assessing risk with vessel wall MRI. ISRN Cardiol 2012;2012:180710.
2. Dong L, Underhill HR, Yu W, et al. Geometric and compositional appearance of atheroma in an angiographically normal carotid artery in patients with atherosclerosis. AJNR Am J Neuroradiol 2010; 31(2):311–6.
3. Wasserman BA, Wityk RJ, Trout HH. Low-grade carotid stenosis: looking beyond the lumen with MRI. Stroke 2005;36(11):2504–13.
4. Saam T, Underhill HR, Chu B, et al. Prevalence of American Heart Association type vi carotid atherosclerotic lesions identified by magnetic resonance imaging for different levels of stenosis as measured by duplex ultrasound. J Am Coll Cardiol 2008; 51(10):1014–21.
5. Jander S, Sitzer M, Schumann R, et al. Inflammation in high-grade carotid stenosis a possible role for macrophages and t cells in plaque destabilization. Stroke 1998;29(8):1625–30.
6. Gaens ME, Backes WH, Rozel S, et al. Dynamic contrast-enhanced MR imaging of carotid atherosclerotic plaque: model selection, reproducibility, and validation. Radiology 2013;266(1):271–9.
7. Underhill HR, Kerwin WS, Hatsukami TS, et al. Automated measurement of mean wall thickness in the common carotid artery by MRI: a comparison to intima-media thickness by B-mode ultrasound. J Magn Reson Imaging 2006;24(2):379–87.
8. Li F, Yarnykh VL, Hatsukami TS, et al. Scan-rescan reproducibility of carotid atherosclerotic plaque morphology and tissue composition measurements using multicontrast MRI at 3T. J Magn Reson Imaging 2010;31(1):168–76.
9. Takaya N, Yuan C, Chu B, et al. Association between carotid plaque characteristics and subsequent ischemic cerebrovascular events: a prospective assessment with MRI - Initial results. Stroke 2006; 37(3):818–23.
10. Luo Y, Polissar N, Han C, et al. Accuracy and uniqueness of three in vivo measurements of atherosclerotic carotid plaque morphology with black blood MRI. Magn Reson Med 2003;50(1):75–82.
11. Yuan C, Beach KW, Smith LH, et al. Measurement of atherosclerotic carotid plaque size in vivo using high resolution magnetic resonance imaging. Circulation 1998;98(24):2666–71.
12. Saam T, Ferguson MS, Yarnykh VL, et al. Quantitative evaluation of carotid plaque composition by in vivo MRI. Arterioscler Thromb Vasc Biol 2005; 25(1):234–9.
13. Saam T, Cai J, Ma L, et al. Comparison of symptomatic and asymptomatic atherosclerotic carotid plaque features with in vivo MR imaging. Radiology 2006;240(2):464–72.
14. Saam T, Kerwin WS, Chu B, et al. Sample size calculation for clinical trials using magnetic resonance imaging for the quantitative assessment of carotid atherosclerosis. J Cardiovasc Magn Reson 2005; 7(5):799–808.
15. Phan AP, Chu B, Polissar N, et al. Association of high-density lipoprotein levels and carotid atherosclerotic plaque characteristics by magnetic resonance imaging. Int J Cardiovasc Imaging 2007; 23(3):337–42.
16. Underhill HR, Yuan C, Zhao XQ, et al. Hatsukami, Effect of rosuvastatin therapy on carotid plaque morphology and composition in moderately hypercholesterolemic patients: a high-resolution magnetic resonance imaging trial. Am Heart J 2008;155(3): 584.e1–8.
17. Hatsukami TS, Ross R, Polissar NL, et al. Visualization of fibrous cap thickness and rupture in human atherosclerotic carotid plaque in vivo with high-resolution magnetic resonance imaging. Circulation 2000;102(9):959–64.
18. Mitsumori LM, Hatsukami TS, Ferguson MS, et al. In vivo accuracy of multisequence MR imaging for identifying unstable fibrous caps in advanced human carotid plaques. J Magn Reson Imaging 2003;17(4):410–20.
19. Yuan C, Mitsumori LM, Ferguson MS, et al. In vivo accuracy of multispectral magnetic resonance imaging for identifying lipid-rich necrotic cores and intraplaque hemorrhage in advanced human carotid plaques. Circulation 2001;104(17):2051–6.
20. Cai J, Hatsukami TS, Ferguson MS, et al. In vivo quantitative measurement of intact fibrous cap and lipid-rich necrotic core size in atherosclerotic carotid plaque: comparison of high-resolution, contrast-enhanced magnetic resonance imaging and histology. Circulation 2005;112(22):3437–44.
21. Kampschulte A, Ferguson MS, Kerwin WS, et al. Differentiation of intraplaque versus juxtaluminal hemorrhage/thrombus in advanced human carotid atherosclerotic lesions by in vivo magnetic resonance imaging. Circulation 2004;110(20): 3239–44.

22. Husain T, Abbott CR, Scott DJA, et al. Macrophage accumulation within the cap of carotid atherosclerotic plaques is associated with the onset of cerebral ischemic events. J Vasc Surg 1999;30(2):269–76.

23. Mofidi R, Crotty TB, McCarthy P, et al. Association between plaque instability, angiogenesis and symptomatic carotid occlusive disease. Br J Surg 2001; 88(7):945–50.

24. Kerwin WS, Brien KDO, Ferguson MS, et al. Inflammation in Carotid atherosclerotic plaque: a dynamic contrast-enhanced mr imaging study. Radiology 2006;241(2):459–68.

25. Chen H, Li F, Zhao X, et al. Extended graphical model for analysis of dynamic contrast-enhanced MRI. Magn Reson Med 2011;66(3):868–78.

26. Cheng C, Tempel D, van Haperen R, et al. Atherosclerotic lesion size and vulnerability are determined by patterns of fluid shear stress. Circulation 2006; 113(23):2744–53.

27. Richardson PD, Davies MJ, Born GVR. Influence of plaque configuration and stress distribution on fissuring of coronary atherosclerotic plaques. Lancet 1987;334(8669):941–4.

28. Long Q, Xu XY, Ariff B, et al. Reconstruction of blood flow patterns in a human carotid bifurcation: a combined CFD and MRI study. J Magn Reson Imaging 2000;11(3):299–311.

29. KAAazempur-Mofrad MR, Isasi AG, Younis HF, et al. Characterization of the atherosclerotic carotid bifurcation using MRI, finite element modeling, and histology. Ann Biomed Eng 2004;32(7):932–46.

30. Steinman DA, Thomas JB, Ladak HM, et al. Reconstruction of carotid bifurcation hemodynamics and wall thickness using computational fluid dynamics and MRI. Magn Reson Med 2002;47(1):149–59.

31. Oyre S, Ringgaard S, Kozerke S, et al. Quantitation of circumferential subpixel vessel wall position and wall shear stress by multiple sectored three-dimensional paraboloid modeling of velocity encoded cine MR. Magn Reson Med 1998;40(5): 645–55.

32. Stalder AF, Russe MF, Frydrychowicz A, et al. Quantitative 2D and 3D phase contrast MRI: optimized analysis of blood flow and vessel wall parameters. Magn Reson Med 2008;60(5):1218–31.

33. Efstathopoulos EP, Patatoukas G, Pantos I, et al. Measurement of systolic and diastolic arterial wall shear stress in the ascending aorta. Phys Med 2008;24(4):196–203.

34. Cheng GC, Loree HM, Kamm RD, et al. Distribution of circumferential stress in ruptured and stable atherosclerotic lesions. A structural analysis with histopathological correlation. Circulation 1993;87(4): 1179–87.

35. Kerwin W, Xu D, Liu F, et al. Magnetic resonance imaging of carotid atherosclerosis: plaque analysis. Top Magn Reson Imaging 2007;18(5):371–8.

36. Underhill H, Kerwin W. Markov shape models: object boundary identification in serial magnetic resonance images, in proceedings 14th scientific meeting, International Society for Magnetic Resonance in Medicinevol. Seattle, WA, May 6–12, 2006.

37. Ukwatta E, Yuan J, Rajchl M, et al. 3-D carotid multi-region MRI segmentation by globally optimal evolution of coupled surfaces. IEEE Trans Med Imaging 2013;32(4):770–85.

38. Han C, Yuan C. Plaque morphological quantitation. In: Suri J, Laximarayan S, editors. Angiography and plaque imaging. Boca Raton (FL): 2003; p. 365–96.

39. Varghese A, Crowe LA, Mohiaddin RH, et al. Interstudy reproducibility of three-dimensional volume-selective fast spin echo magnetic resonance for quantifying carotid artery wall volume. J Magn Reson Imaging 2005;21(2):187–91.

40. Zhao XQ, Yuan C, Hatsukami TS, et al. Effects of prolonged intensive lipid-lowering therapy on the characteristics of carotid atherosclerotic plaques in vivo by MRI: a case-control study. Arterioscler Thromb Vasc Biol 2001;21(10):1623–9.

41. Takaya N, Yuan C, Chu B, et al. Presence of intraplaque hemorrhage stimulates progression of carotid atherosclerotic plaques: a high-resolution magnetic resonance imaging study. Circulation 2005; 111(21):2768–75.

42. Virmani R, Ladich ER, Burke AP, et al. Histopathology of carotid atherosclerotic disease. Neurosurgery 2006;59(5):S3–219.

43. Redgrave JNE, Lovett JK, Gallagher PJ, et al. Histological assessment of 526 symptomatic carotid plaques in relation to the nature and timing of ischemic symptoms: the Oxford plaque study. Circulation 2006;113(19):2320–8.

44. Cappendijk VC, Cleutjens KB, Kessels AGH, et al. Assessment of Human atherosclerotic carotid plaque components with multisequence mr imaging: initial experience. Radiology 2005; 234(2):487–92.

45. Kerwin WS, Yuan C. Active edge maps for medical image registration. Med Imaging 2001 Image Process 2001;4320:516–26.

46. Boekhorst BT, van 't Klooster R, Bovens SM, et al. Evaluation of multicontrast MRI including fat suppression and inversion recovery spin echo for identification of intra-plaque hemorrhage and lipid core in human carotid plaque using the mahalanobis distance measure. Magn Reson Med 2012;67(6): 1764–75.

47. Adame IM, Van Der Geest RJ, Wasserman BA, et al. Automatic segmentation and plaque characterization in atherosclerotic carotid artery MR images. MAGMA 2004;16(5):227–34.

48. Liu F, Xu D, Ferguson MS, et al. Automated in vivo segmentation of carotid plaque MRI with

Morphology-Enhanced probability maps. Magn Reson Med 2006;55(3):659–68.

49. Van Engelen A, Niessen WJ, Klein S, et al. Atherosclerotic plaque component segmentation in combined carotid MRI and CTA data incorporating class label uncertainty. PLoS One 2014;9(4):1–14.

50. Liu W, Balu N, Sun J, et al. Segmentation of carotid plaque using multicontrast 3D gradient echo, MRI. J Magn Reson Imaging 2012;35(4):812–9.

51. Liu F, Xu D, Chu B, et al. Reproducibility assessment of morphology-enhanced probabilistic plaque segmentation (MEPPS) on two baseline magnetic resonance scans. Proc. 14th Sci. Meet. Int. Soc. Magn. Reson. Med. 2006. p. 1277.

52. Kerwin WS, Liu F, Yamykh V, et al. Signal features of the atherosclerotic plaque at 3.0 Tesla versus 1.5 Tesla: impact on automatic classification. J Magn Reson 2008;28(4):987–95.

53. Yuan C, Zhang SX, Polissar NL, et al. Identification of fibrous cap rupture with magnetic resonance imaging is highly associated with recent transient ischemic attack or stroke. Circulation 2002;105(2):181–5.

54. Libby P, Ridker PM, Maseri A. Inflammation and atherosclerosis. Circulation 2002;105(9):1135–43.

55. Truijman MT, Kwee RM, Van Hoof RHM, et al. Combined 18F-FDG PET-CT and DCE-MRI to assess inflammation and microvascularization in atherosclerotic plaques. Stroke 2013;44(12):3568–70.

56. Kerwin W, Hooker A, Spilker M, et al. Quantitative magnetic resonance imaging analysis of neovasculature volume in carotid atherosclerotic plaque. Circulation 2003;107(6):851–6.

57. Kerwin WS, Cai J, Yuan C. Noise and motion correction in dynamic contrast-enhanced MRI for analysis of atherosclerotic lesions. Magn Reson Med 2002; 47(6):1211–7.

58. Calcagno C, Cornily J-C, Hyafil F, et al. Detection of neovessels in atherosclerotic plaques of rabbits using dynamic contrast enhanced MRI and 18F-FDG PET. Arterioscler Thromb Vasc Biol 2008;28(7): 1311–7.

59. Patlak CS, Blasberg RG, Fenstermacher JD. Graphical evaluation of blood-to-brain transfer constants from multiple-time uptake data. J Cereb Blood Flow Metab 1983;3(1):1–7.

60. Tofts PS. Modeling tracer kinetics in dynamic Gd-DTPA MR imaging. J Magn Reson Imaging 1997;7(1):91–101.

61. Li KL, Jackson A. New hybrid technique for accurate and reproducible quantitation of dynamic contrast-enhanced MRI data. Magn Reson Med 2003;50(6): 1286–95.

62. Calcagno C, Vucic E, Mani V, et al. Reproducibility of black blood dynamic contrast-enhanced magnetic resonance imaging in aortic plaques of atherosclerotic rabbits. J Magn Reson Imaging 2010;32(1): 191–8.

63. Vucic E, Calcagno C, Dickson SD, et al. Regression of inflammation in atherosclerosis by the LXR agonist R211945: a noninvasive assessment and comparison with atorvastatin. JACC Cardiovasc Imaging 2012;5(8):819–28.

64. Chen H, Ricks J, Rosenfeld M, et al. Progression of experimental lesions of atherosclerosis: assessment by kinetic modeling of black-blood dynamic contrast-enhanced MRI. Magn Reson Med 2013; 69(6):1712–20.

65. Wu YG. Noninvasive quantification of local cerebral metabolic rate of glucose for clinical application using positron emission tomography and 18F-fluoro-2-deoxy-D-glucose. J Cereb Blood Flow Metab 2008;28(2):242–50.

66. Kerwin WS, Oikawa M, Yuan C, et al. MR imaging of adventitial vasa vasorum in carotid atherosclerosis. Magn Reson Med 2008;59(3):507–14.

67. Chen H, Sun J, Kerwin WS, et al. Scan-rescan reproducibility of quantitative assessment of inflammatory carotid atherosclerotic plaque using dynamic contrast-enhanced 3T CMR in a multicenter study. J Cardiovasc Magn Reson 2014; 16(1):51.

68. Dong L, Kerwin WS, Chen H, et al. Carotid artery atherosclerosis: effect of intensive lipid therapy on the vasa vasorum — evaluation by using dynamic contrast-enhanced MR imaging. Radiology 2011; 260(1):224–31.

69. Sun J, Song Y, Chen H, et al. Adventitial perfusion and intraplaque hemorrhage: a dynamic contrast-enhanced MRI study in the carotid artery. Stroke 2013;44(4):1031–6.

70. Calcagno C, Ramachandran S, Izquierdo-Garcia D, et al. The complementary roles of dynamic contrast-enhanced MRI and 18F-fluoro-deoxyglucose PET/CT for imaging of carotid atherosclerosis. Eur J Nucl Med Mol Imaging 2013;40(12):1884–93.

71. Wang J, Liu H, Sun J, et al. Varying correlation between 18F-fluorodeoxyglucose positron emission tomography and dynamic contrast-enhanced MRI in carotid atherosclerosis: implications for plaque inflammation. Stroke 2014;45(6):1842–5.

72. Kerwin WS, Canton G. Advanced techniques for MRI of atherosclerotic plaque. Top Magn Reson Imaging 2009;20(4):217–25.

73. Canton G, Chiu B, Chen H, et al. A framework for the co-registration of hemodynamic forces and atherosclerotic plaque components. Physiol Meas 2013; 34(9):977.

74. Malek AM, Alper SL, Izumo S. Hemodynamic shear stress and its role in atherosclerosis. JAMA 1999; 282(21):2035–42.

75. Caro CG. Discovery of the role of wall shear in atherosclerosis. Arterioscler Thromb Vasc Biol 2009;29(2):158–61.

76. Arroyo LH, Lee RT. Mechanisms of plaque rupture: mechanical and biologic interactions. Cardiovasc Res 1999;41(2):369–75.

77. Qian Y, Takao H, Umezu M, et al. Risk analysis of unruptured aneurysms using computational fluid dynamics technology: preliminary results. AJNR Am J Neuroradiol 2011;32(10):1948–55.

78. Long Q, Xu XY, Collins MW, et al. Magnetic resonance image processing and structured grid generation of a human abdominal bifurcation. Comput Methods Programs Biomed 1998;56(3):249–59.

79. Lee RT, Grodzinsky AJ, Frank EH, et al. Structure-dependent dynamic mechanical behavior of fibrous caps from human atherosclerotic plaques. Circulation 1991;83(5):1764–70.

80. Lee RT, Richardson SG, Loree HM, et al. Prediction of mechanical properties of human atherosclerotic tissue by high-frequency intravascular ultrasound imaging. An in vitro study. Arterioscler Thromb 1992;12(1):1–5.

81. Born GV, Richardson PD. Mechanical properties of human atherosclerotic lesions. New York: Springer New York; 1990. p. 413–23.

82. Patel DJ, Janicki JS, Carew TE. Static anisotropic elastic properties of the aorta in living dogs. Circ Res 1969;25(6):765–79.

83. Ku DN, Giddens DP, Zarins CK, et al. Pulsatile flow and atherosclerosis in the human carotid bifurcation. Positive correlation between plaque location and low oscillating shear stress. Arteriosclerosis 1985;5(3):293–302.

84. Tang D, Yang C, Mondal S, et al. A negative correlation between human carotid atherosclerotic plaque progression and plaque wall stress: in vivo mri-based 2D/3D FSI models. J Biomech 2008;41(4):727–36.

Incorporating Carotid Plaque Imaging into Routine Clinical Carotid Magnetic Resonance Angiography

Alan R. Moody, FRCR, FRCP*, Navneet Singh, MD

KEYWORDS

- Imaging • Carotid plaque • Intraplaque hemorrhage • Magnetic resonance angiography
- MR imaging

KEY POINTS

- The incorporation of a simple, short, and easy-to-acquire sequence to visualize the vessel wall and detect intraplaque hemorrhage (IPH) is achievable now.
- Assessment of carotid disease should include baseline imaging to show stenosis, such as time of flight or contrast-enhanced magnetic resonance angiography, and commonly includes simple brain imaging to assess prior neuroischemic disease.
- Total imaging time is therefore likely to be in the order of 15 to 20 minutes.
- The addition of an IPH-detecting vessel wall sequence only adds a further 5 to 6 minutes to a baseline examination, which overall translates into 30 to 40 minutes of scanner table time.

INTRODUCTION

Over the last 20 years magnetic resonance(MR) imaging has become established as one of the mainstays of noninvasive imaging of carotid artery disease. Almost all investigations of the carotid artery are for the detection of the effects of atherosclerotic plaque at or around the carotid artery bifurcation. Investigation of the carotid artery may be triggered in the search for potentially symptomatic lesions as part of primary prevention, or in response to a neuroischemic event to secondarily prevent further brain ischemia.

Routine clinical carotid artery imaging comprises techniques that attempt to quantify vessel stenosis, which can be used to decide whether the patient is eligible for a nonmedical intervention.

Interventions to reduce future cerebroischemic events have been shown to be warranted when the carotid vessel reaches a certain significant stenosis.[1] However, although patients with significant stenosis are at higher risk of events, patients without such degrees of vessel narrowing may also be prone to transient ischemic attack or stroke, which suggests that the culprit vascular lesion is defined not only by stenosis but by other, currently hidden, features that make the vessel wall disease more prone to cause thromboembolic events.

In the same time period in which MR angiography (MRA) of the carotid artery has gained clinical acceptance as an accurate and clinically useful technique for detecting and measuring carotid artery stenosis, there has also been an active

Disclosure: The investigators have nothing to disclose.
Department of Medical Imaging, University of Toronto, Toronto, Ontario, Canada
* Corresponding author.
E-mail address: alan.moody@sunnybrook.ca

1052-5149/16/$ – see front matter Crown Copyright © 2016 Published by Elsevier Inc. All rights reserved.

research agenda to use MR imaging to provide more information regarding vessel wall disease in an attempt to add to the MRA data already available.[2] This work has added greatly to the understanding of the natural history of vessel wall disease in vivo. By identifying vessel wall components of atherosclerotic disease, an understanding of what is now known to be the complex pathobiology of atherosclerosis has informed the development of imaging biomarkers. One characteristic of high-risk plaque that has such an imaging surrogate is intraplaque hemorrhage (IPH).[3] This article discusses the opportunity for introducing vessel wall imaging into clinical practice using a single sequence to detect IPH. Reluctance to do so earlier, despite the development of vessel wall MR imaging techniques, has likely stemmed from the perceived notion that implementation is a complex process requiring specialized equipment and sequences, and needing the addition of long imaging protocols with off-line postprocessing for interpretation. In addition, evidence that the information provided by such imaging is useful clinically has previously been sparse. This article therefore addresses some of these issues and positions the current and future role of clinical vessel wall MR imaging to detect IPH, and discusses the use of time-efficient imaging protocols to provide additional, clinically relevant information on current MR imaging platforms.

PATHOLOGY

Atherosclerosis is initiated by several factors that disturb endothelial function, including aging, hyperglycemia, hypercholesterolemia, hypertension, and smoking.[4] Endothelial dysfunction manifests as loss of normal antiinflammatory, antithrombotic, and vasoreactive functions. Normal cholesterol handling at the interface between the vessel wall and lumen is disturbed such that there is a net ingress of cholesterol into the intima and increased cholesterol residency. Over time, cholesterol coalesces into lipid pools. The intraplaque environment results in lipid oxidation with the production of oxygen free radicals.

In response to these changes, circulating white cells are attracted within the plaque through endothelial activation and expression of surface receptors. Circulating monocytes enter the plaque and transform into tissue macrophages. Phagocytosis of plaque lipids by macrophages results in foam cell formation commonly leading to macrophage apoptosis rather than removal of lipid from the vessel wall. A reparative response to disease within the plaque results in stimulation of smooth muscle cell proliferation and the development of intima-medial thickening in an attempt to stabilize the inflammatory process.

An indirect effect of plaque surface thickening is loss of the usual oxygen diffusion from the lumen into the vessel wall once the thickening increases to more than 200 μm. In response to this, secondary to release of factors such as HIF-1 (hypoxic inducible factor), and the presence of intraplaque macrophages, there is a release of VEGF (vascular endothelial growth factor), which stimulates neovessel growth within the plaque predominantly from the normal vasa vasorum within the adventitia. However, the new vessel growth results in leaky, friable vessels, vulnerable to red cell deposition and frank hemorrhage within the vessel wall. The trigger for plaque hemorrhage is not clearly understood but plaque morphology, hemodynamics, or changes in systemic blood pressure, particularly the pulse pressure,[5] may result in repeated microhemorrhages within the plaque (**Fig. 1**).

The delivery of red blood cells within the plaque has several deleterious effects. First, if the volume of blood deposited in the atherosclerotic plaque is large it can result in a significant change in volume of vessel wall disease and potential encroachment on the lumen. This process has been seen as one of the causes of rapid changes in stenosis; rapid reduction can also occur with blood resorption. Likely, and more common, are repeated small hemorrhages, not causing a significant change in plaque volume. These hemorrhages result in repeated delivery of red cells deep within the vessel wall lesion, which has 2 significant and related effects. Red blood cell membranes have one of the highest cholesterol contents of any cell in the human body, and this is further increased in states of hypercholesterolemia. Each red cell delivered into the plaque therefore adds to the lipid core. Following red cell lysis, the other major component directly introduced within the plaque is hemoglobin. As this undergoes degradation, free heme is released. Heme is highly inflammatory and through the Fenton reaction drives the repetitive production of oxygen free radicals, which continue to feed the hostile plaque environment.

The combination of cholesterol and heme delivered with every red cell therefore provides an inflammatory combination driving the atherosclerotic process. In response there is further monocyte/macrophage migration into the plaque, which results in further inflammatory cytokines, angiogenesis, lipid oxidation, and cell death causing enlargement of the plaque's necrotic core, neovascularization, and subsequent hemorrhage. This vicious cycle likely accounts for the acceleration in atherosclerotic disease from a

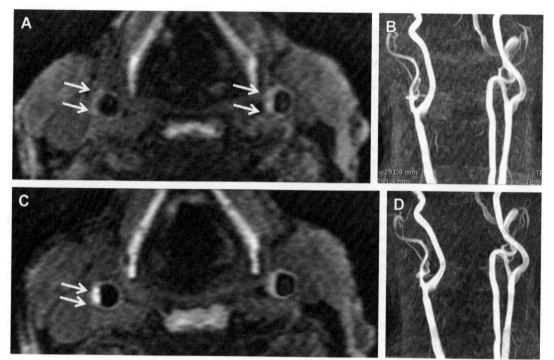

Fig. 1. (*A*) Vessel wall imaging shows bilateral vessel wall thickening (*arrows*). (*B*) Time of flight (TOF) MRA shows no significant luminal narrowing. (*C*) One year later, intense high signal is seen in the right common carotid vessel wall thickening in keeping with the occurrence of IPH in the interim period (*arrows*). (*D*) TOF MRA 1 year later is unchanged.

slow, predictable progression to more rapid, unpredictable plaque progression and disruption. The presence of plaque hemorrhage therefore denotes a more advanced atherosclerotic state (American Heart Association [AHA] type VI) in keeping with increased plaque vulnerability and plaque progression[6].

Targeting of many of these plaque characteristics with imaging can provide significant information about the state of vessel wall disease, but, at the present time, the clinical need is evidence that, in addition to their theoretic credentials, one or more of these imaging markers can provide useful information to further guide patient management. One of these markers, IPH, has come under particular scrutiny because of its many pathobiological and imaging features[7] that make it attractive as a biomarker of plaque vulnerability. The World Health Organization has broadly defined a biomarker as "any substance, structure, or process that can be measured in the body, or its products, that influence or predict the incidence of outcome or disease."[8] IPH could represent such a substance/process provided that it predicts outcomes related to carotid disease. Accepting this, there are still several barriers to adoption that must be overcome in order for this to be introduced into routine clinical imaging of carotid disease.

INTRODUCTION TO CLINICAL PRACTICE

Introduction of IPH MR imaging to clinical carotid artery imaging has few real barriers to adoption. The sequences required to apply this technique are readily available on all scanner platforms; they are rapidly acquired; IPH detection is accurate and interpretation is simple, presently comprising dichotomization into presence or absence of IPH. Furthermore, MR imaging at present is the only readily available imaging technique for the detection of plaque hemorrhage, and MR imaging is already a technique used for investigating carotid artery disease, thus making the addition of this 1 sequence to the standard carotid artery imaging protocol simple, with little time-cost impact.

CLINICAL APPLICATIONS

Addition of IPH imaging to routine carotid artery MR imaging assessment has the potential to affect patient management in several clinical settings: whether the patient is asymptomatic but at high risk of vascular disease; symptomatic and being assessed for risk of future event; or in the work-up before carotid artery intervention. Newer applications may include identifying high-risk disease requiring modified, intensive, or costly therapy; identification of patients requiring increased monitoring; entry criteria for therapeutic trials; and phenotyping of high-risk patients who may require more comprehensive vascular investigation and potentially therapy modification.

PRIMARY PREVENTION

In the absence of organized vascular screening programs, asymptomatic carotid arteries are most commonly imaged because of high-risk atherosclerotic vascular disease in another vascular bed, such as the coronary or peripheral vascular circulation.[9] Alternatively, asymptomatic vessels are commonly imaged in conjunction with a symptomatic contralateral carotid artery. Despite the silent nature of these carotid vessels, study of asymptomatic cohorts has repeatedly shown an increased risk of future clinical events, irrespective of the degree of stenosis, in those patients with MR-demonstrated IPH rather than in those without[10,11] (Fig. 2). Importantly, the very low rate of events in the IPH-negative groups is probably an even more compelling reason to investigate patients using IPH MR imaging. The absence of IPH seems to confer a level of low risk that might be useful in managing patients, even those with significant carotid artery stenosis,

potentially allowing the withholding of invasive interventions[12,13] Carotid vessels with no stenosis are also found to contain IPH, suggesting that, despite representing advanced vessel wall disease, IPH can occur even when vessel wall thickening is minimal (Fig. 3A). Large cohort trials currently underway may provide information on the relevance of finding this high-risk biomarker in otherwise normal people, potentially confirming whether this can act as an early marker of future events even in the absence of other more established risk markers.

Asymptomatic patients found to have IPH may be candidates for more intensive management despite the lack of recognized risk factors such as luminal stenosis. Patients screened for carotid disease because of vascular disease elsewhere are known to have asymptomatic normal or nonstenotic carotid disease identified with IPH MR imaging.[14] Knowing that IPH is a stimulus for plaque progression[15] and potentially carotid stenosis progression[16] these patients could be identified for more follow-up in order to better detect the occurrence of significant stenosis (which may then be eligible for surgical intervention). Before the need for surgical intervention, the risk/benefit ratio of more intensive medical therapy can be weighed, in the knowledge that these patients are at higher risk of disease progression (Fig. 3B).

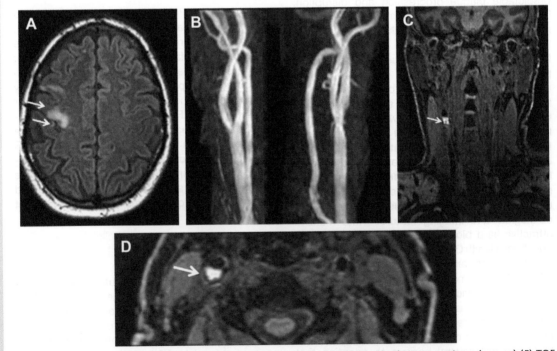

Fig. 2. (A) An area of mature infarction is seen within the right middle cerebral artery territory (arrows) (B) TOF MRA shows no significant stenosis. (C, D) Vessel wall imaging in the coronal and reconstructed axial plane show intense high signal intensity within the vessel wall in keeping with IPH (arrows).

The concept of identifying high-risk patients by identifying high-risk lesions could be further expanded. From the prospective study of clinical outcomes of patients with histologically proven IPH in their carotid endarterectomy specimens[17] and the retrospective review of comorbid cardiovascular conditions in patients with and without carotid IPH,[18] it seems that the status of the carotid artery, and in particular the presence or absence of IPH, provides a useful biomarker of the patients' vascular phenotypes. IPH in the carotid bed therefore seems to associate with symptomatic vascular disease peripherally and in the coronary circulation, and is also able to predict risk of future cardiovascular events. It could be argued that medical therapy for 1 vascular bed (ie, carotid) has an equally beneficial effect in all vascular beds and therefore no further investigation is required elsewhere. However, a case could be made for the investigation and exclusion of other high risk, silent lesions (eg, in the proximal coronary arteries) once carotid IPH has been detected.

Knowing that IPH represents a marker of increased risk of atherosclerotic progression and clinical outcomes, the technique could be used to improve the selection of patients for proof-of-principle trials of new interventions. Using MR imaging–detected IPH as a predictive classifier to select those patients at greater risk of events, smaller recruitment numbers will be required, allowing the demonstration of effect more efficiently.

SECONDARY PREVENTION

Patients with symptoms referable to the carotid artery circulation should always undergo carotid artery investigation. First, defining the cause of a cerebral event affects future therapy or intervention and accurate diagnosis of carotid artery disease as the source of thromboemboli excludes other sources such as the heart. However, the current diagnostic criteria for diagnosing significant carotid artery disease rely on the identification of a 50% stenosis or more.[19] Less than this and the carotid artery is considered asymptomatic. Degrees of stenosis less than 50% can cause cerebral thromboemboli; however, the incidence of events decreases with the level of stenosis. However, the cumulative number of cerebral events in the nonstenotic group is significant. MR IPH has been shown to be present even in low-grade (<50%) carotid artery stenosis and associated with symptoms. Although prospective outcome trials of this biomarker in this nonstenotic group are yet to be performed, identification of IPH with MR imaging in these patients may be useful

in identifying symptom-causing carotid artery disease. However, because there is not a direct cause-and-effect relationship between IPH and cerebral symptoms, further study of the significance of IPH detection in these patients with cerebrovascular symptoms is required.

However, patients are often investigated for the causes of stroke and none, using current criteria, are found; the diagnosis remains as cryptogenic stroke. Although a direct causal relationship between IPH and stroke cannot be made, one of the first descriptions of MR imaging–detected IPH[20] was in patients with acute stroke, which noted that 5 of 11 patients with MR imaging high signal that indicated IPH had carotid stenosis less than 50%. Using MR imaging to detect IPH may identify culprit lesions associated with stroke, which otherwise would be classified as cryptogenic. More recently[21] similar results were shown in patients with stroke that had been proved on diffusion-weighted imaging without significant (>50%) stenosis who showed IPH ipsilateral to the index cerebral infarct in 6 of 27 patients (22.2%), but none on the contralateral side. Like in many areas of carotid artery investigation, imaging for IPH has the potential to add to the knowledge already provided by the current imaging techniques.

Because of the increasing interest in IPH there are now sufficient studies that allow meta-analysis of multiple trials concerning the relationship of IPH and cerebroischemic symptoms. Studies by Hosseini and colleagues[22] (odds ratio, 12.2), Saam and colleagues[23] (hazard ratio [HR], 5.69) and Gupta and colleagues[24] (HR, 4.59) all showed an increased association of symptoms with IPH.

A recent article by Treiman and colleagues[13] (2015) projected the probability of stroke occurrence assuming an annual rate of symptomatic stroke of 2.2% and 4.0% of silent cerebral infarction in the setting of a 5.2 HR for stroke in the presence of IPH. Projections to 4 years showed that the probability of symptomatic stroke with IPH was 18% and symptomatic/asymptomatic stroke combined was 43%. This finding compares with projections of 3% and 8% respectively for IPH-negative patients (Fig. 4).

PROGRESSION OF VESSEL WALL DISEASE

From the pathobiology of IPH it can be seen that the proinflammatory nature of free hemoglobin within the plaque is a stimulus for plaque growth, through a mixture of attempted repair and healing, lipid accumulation, and repeated plaque hemorrhage. Plaque growth initially may be through

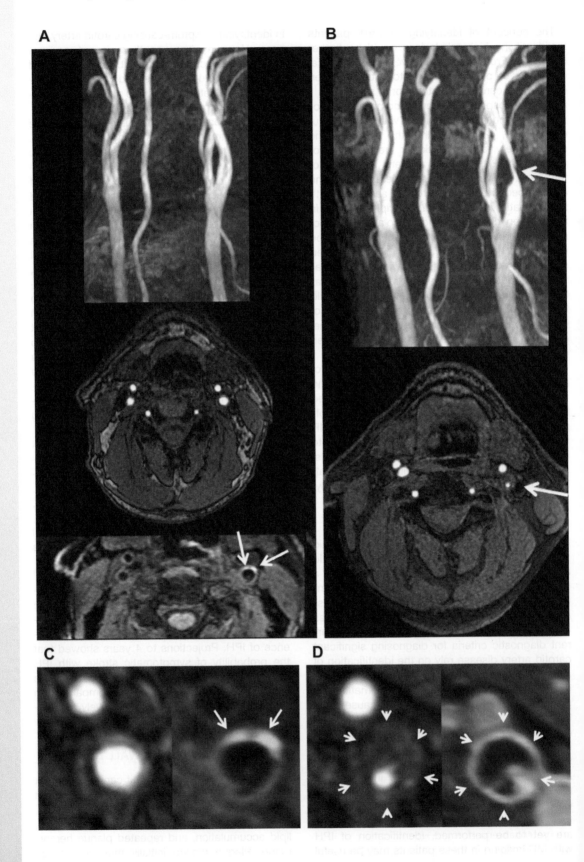

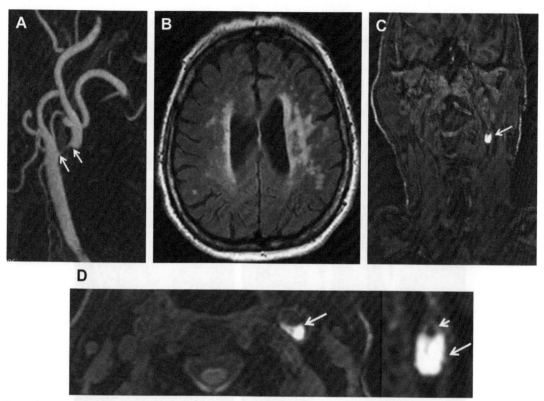

Fig. 4. (*A*) TOF MRA shows a stenosis at the origin of the left internal carotid artery (*arrows*). (*B*) Fluid-attenuated inversion recovery brain imaging shows widespread deep white matter hyperintensities, greater on the left. (*C*) Coronal and axial vessel wall images show intense high signal intensity at the site of the stenosis (*arrows*). (*D*) Close-up view of the stenosis shows the vessel wall hemorrhage (*arrow*) and the extremely small residual lumen (*arrowhead*).

positive remodeling with no encroachment on the lumen, but eventually this is expressed as an increasing degree of luminal stenosis. During the positive remodeling phase, measurement of stenosis is therefore a poor means of detecting vessel wall disease. Detection of vessel wall disease when there is no lumen stenosis, by the addition of vessel wall imaging, is therefore particularly important.

IPH has been shown in several studies to predict progression of vessel wall disease. More recently this has been shown to be translated into progression of clinical stenosis as well[16] (see **Fig. 3**). The importance of IPH therefore seems amplified, because not only may it result in plaque

destabilization, potential plaque rupture, and end organ ischemia but it can produce a more gradual and persistent effect by driving plaque progression. The driving of plaque progression eventually reaches a stage at which clinical events become manifest. The persistent presence of IPH can therefore be thought of as acting as a slow, continual stimulus for plaque growth, likely leading to further bleeding within the plaque and then punctuated with more sporadic and unpredictable plaque rupture. The sporadic, unpredictable plaque rupture is likely to depend on local features of the plaque, including geometry, hemodynamics, plaque composition, circulating factors, and vascular function. The presence of IPH during

Fig. 3. (*A*) Baseline imaging shows no stenosis and only minimal vessel wall thickening in the left internal carotid artery. However, high signal in keeping with IPH is already present (*arrows*). (*B*) At 2-year follow-up the site of IPH has undergone significant narrowing to approximately 50%, well seen on the axial source data and coronal maximal intensity projection (MIP) (*arrows*). (*C*) Baseline TOF (*left*) and vessel wall (*right*) images show normal-caliber lumen and IPH high signal anteriorly (*arrows*). (*D*) At 2-year follow-up the lumen on TOF is reduced and associated with significant vessel wall thickening (*left*) (*arrowheads*). Postcontrast images (*right*) show intense enhancement of the adventitial surface (*arrowheads*), likely caused by increased neovessels, and low-signal-intensity material replacing the lumen, in keeping with extensive lipid deposition.

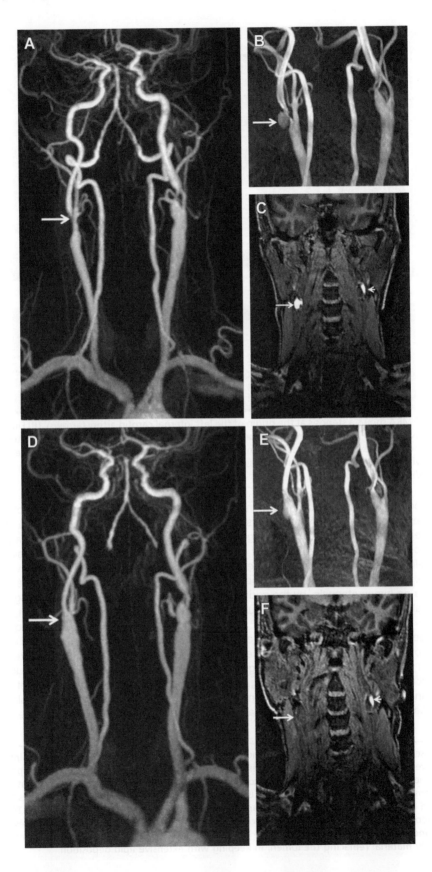

the nonstenotic phase may therefore provide a useful marker of those lesions that are more prone to increases in plaque volume and thus eventual increased risk of future events. This marker provides a theoretic opportunity to target patients for more intensive follow-up and medical therapy in an attempt to halt or potentially reverse the vessel wall disease. However, these trials have not yet been undertaken using the presence of IPH as the entry criterion for treatment.

PREINTERVENTION IMAGING

The relationship of IPH, as shown by MR imaging, to periprocedural outcomes for carotid interventions has been studied. Overall, as might be expected, the presence of IPH confers an increased risk for patients undergoing carotid intervention because the presence of plaque hemorrhage indicates a more advanced and complex morphology, such that any manipulation of the carotid artery may result in thromboembolic disease (Fig. 5). Even before surgery there is evidence that the resting rate of high-intensity signals (HITS) on transcranial Doppler is increased from carotid arteries containing IPH.[25] During endarterectomy surgery, manipulation of carotid arteries containing IPH also results in more perioperative HITS.[26]

Carotid stenting might seem an attractive alternative to avoid the IPH risks associated with carotid endarterectomy. However, the presence of IPH also increases the risks associated with carotid artery stenting, resulting in more periprocedural cerebroischemic events compared with endarterectomy.[27] Because the presence IPH seems to confer increased risk during carotid interventions, preprocedural imaging may be of use in interventional planning and provide insight into potential risks on a lesion-by-lesion basis.

TECHNIQUES

Most of the techniques for imaging plaque hemorrhage rely on the T1 shortening effects induced by methemoglobin. While in the circulation, both oxyhemoglobin and deoxyhemoglobin contain heme iron in the reduced (ferrous) state. Once hemoglobin extravasates and becomes extravascular within the plaque the normal mechanisms for maintaining the ferrous state are lost, allowing oxidation to the ferric state ($Fe+++$) producing methemoglobin. Methemoglobin is a paramagnetic species with 5 unpaired electrons, which, when in close proximity to water molecules, causes rapid T1 relaxation and high signal on a T1-weighted sequence. This effect is seen whether the red cell has lysed or not owing to the ability of water to enter the red cell despite an intact membrane.

Understanding the evolution of the MR imaging signal caused by red cell extravasation and oxidative denaturation of hemoglobin suggests that when high signal is seen within an atheromatous plaque the minimum time the hemoglobin has been present within the plaque before high signal develops is 3 to 4 days. In the acute setting of a patient presenting with stroke, the generation of the high signal is presumably temporally removed from the original plaque hemorrhage, which happened at least some days earlier. This process supports the notion that hemorrhage, detected as high signal on T1-weighted MR imaging, is not directly causative of the event leading to stroke presentation, but likely generates the intraplaque environment that sets in play a cascade of events that result in thromboembolism and the subsequent acute neurologic event. The timing of such events at present remains theoretic.

Similarly, high signal within plaque has been observed to persist for months if not years after first being detected.[28] This observation suggests that either there is a unique environment with the plaque allowing methemoglobin to persist without undergoing further oxidation and removal, or there is a process of repeated microbleeds that maintains the methemoglobin levels within the plaque.

In order to incorporate vessel wall imaging and IPH detection into routine clinical imaging protocols, the technique should require little in the way of additional software, hardware, or protracted imaging time. Most trials cited earlier have used either T1-weighted two-dimensional fast spin echo or three-dimensional (3D)magnetization prepared gradient echo sequences, the

Fig. 5. (A) Contrast-enhanced MRA shows a stenosis at the origin of the right internal carotid artery (arrow). (B) TOF MRA confirms the stenosis and a large area of adjacent high signal representing IPH (arrow). (C) Vessel wall imaging clearly defines the right carotid IPH (arrow) and a smaller region within the proximal left internal carotid artery (arrowhead). IPH on the presurgical imaging is associated with increased risk of intraoperative embolization. (D) At 1-year follow-up following endarterectomy the right carotid stenosis has resolved on the contrast-enhanced MRA (arrow). (E) TOF MRA confirms repair of the stenosis and removal of the region of high-signal IPH on the right (arrow) but a residual stenosis on the left side. (F) Vessel wall imaging shows no high signal on the right (arrow) and only shows the residual left-sided carotid IPH (arrowhead).

latter having previously been shown to have improved detection of IPH for similar or shorter imaging times, of around 5 to 6 minutes[29] (see **Fig. 8**A). The detection of IPH is accentuated by suppressing the normal high signal from surrounding fat and nulling the signal from blood by adjusting the inversion time (**Fig. 6**). Addition of one such IPH sequence to routine carotid artery imaging, which is usually in the order of 30 to 40 minutes,

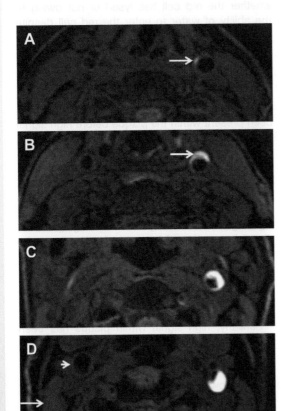

Fig. 6. Areas of high signal intensity secondary to IPH are clearly seen against the T1-weighted low-signal background. Background fat signal is suppressed and the lumen is of low signal intensity by using an appropriate inversion time to null the T1 of blood. (A) Despite the lack of stenosis and little vessel wall thickening, a small area of high signal in keeping with IPH (AHA type VI disease) is already present in this asymptomatic diabetic patient (*arrow*). (B) Extensive vessel wall high signal is present but the vessel lumen remains maintained because of positive remodeling (*arrow*). (C, D) Extensive high signal intensity with secondary moderate (C) and severe (D) luminal stenosis. The normal vessel wall signal intensity and thickness are well seen on the contralateral side (D, *arrowhead*). The vessel wall intensity is seen to return similar signal as the adjacent sternocleidomastoid (SCM) muscle, which is used as an internal control to identify high signal intensity (defined as 1.5–2.0 times that of the SCM) (*arrow*).

therefore potentially has little time impact. The 3D MPRAGE (Magnetisation Prepared Rapid Acquisition Gradient Echo) sequence has a further advantage in that it can be acquired in the coronal plane and therefore has greater coverage of the carotid vessels from the aortic arch to the circle of Willis. This greater coverage may be advantageous when complicated atheromatous disease is located away from the carotid artery bifurcation.[30]

Carotid vessel wall imaging has now gravitated largely to 3-T MR imaging scanners exploiting the increased signal/noise ratio, and improved time of flight (TOF) effects used with accompanying MRA sequences. However, because IPH detection is fundamentally a contrast rather than spatial resolution technique, lower field strength scanners can still be used to detect the presence of IPH, although usually at lower image spatial resolution. Although dedicated surface coils can be used if just the carotid artery bifurcation is targeted, the use of neurovascular array coils gives greater coverage and homogeneity of signal. Using nonspecialized sequences and hardware allows the techniques to be easily applied on all vendor platforms, making widespread application more feasible.

Interpretation of IPH images has largely been a matter of dichotomizing images into presence or absence of IPH. Carotid artery imaging trials incorporating IPH imaging have largely identified patients as IPH positive or negative by detecting IPH anywhere within the index carotid artery. Very high signal intensity within the hemorrhage or large volume usually makes identification simple. However, when plaque hemorrhage volume is small or the intensity is reduced, this can be more problematic. The use of an internal standard, commonly the sternocleidomastoid muscle adjacent to the carotid vessel, provides a means by which abnormal vessel wall signal, usually taken as 1.5 to 2 times the muscle signal, can be used to provide more quantitative assessment (see **Fig. 6**D). Incorporation of such measures into more automated detection of IPH will not only help in the more uniform detection of vessel wall IPH (potentially across sites) but will provide quantitative IPH volume measurements, which may be useful as part of carotid artery assessment, although this has yet to be proved.

Few causes for IPH false-positive results have been reported. Susceptibility artifact from heavy calcification can give a bright, blooming artifact that is difficult to differentiate from small areas of hemorrhage.[29] Hemorrhage adjacent to the vessel in an adjacent structure or postoperatively may cause some confusion. Similarly, any flow artifact

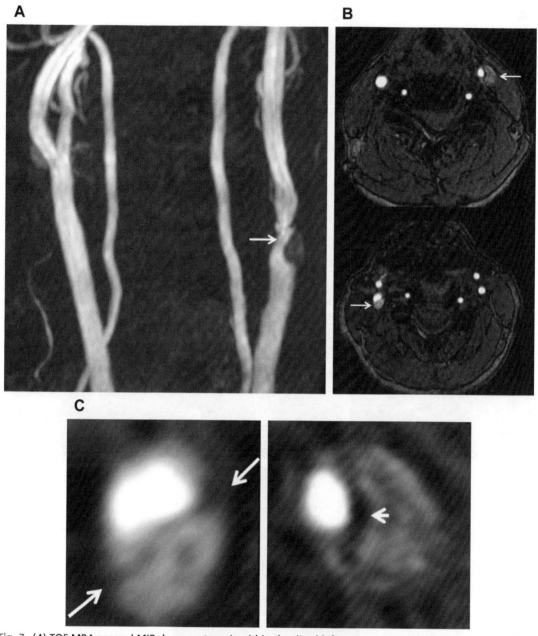

Fig. 7. (*A*) TOF MRA coronal MIP shows a stenosis within the distal left common carotid artery (*arrow*), but little narrowing on the right side. (*B*) Axial source images from the TOF acquisition show extensive positive remodeling in the left common carotid artery (*top*) and right internal carotid artery (*bottom*). Both regions show an increase in signal intensity in keeping with IPH (*arrows*). (*C*) Close-up views of the vessel wall disease. Left common carotid artery disease (*right*) shows the lumen partially separated from the vessel wall disease (IPH) by a band of low signal, which may represent thickening of the fibrous cap or early calcification (*arrowhead*). The right internal carotid disease (*left*) shows a thin line covering the vessel wall high signal, which may be a thin fibrous cap (*arrows*).

that interferes with the normally suppressed luminal signal can give misleading results. False-negative results may relate to hemorrhage of different ages, either during the hyperacute stage while hemoglobin is still in the oxyhemoglobin or deoxyhemoglobin form, or once methemoglobin has further matured into hemosiderin and hemichromes. High-signal intraluminal flow artifact may obscure adjacent IPH, as may insufficient fat suppression adjacent to the adventitial surface.

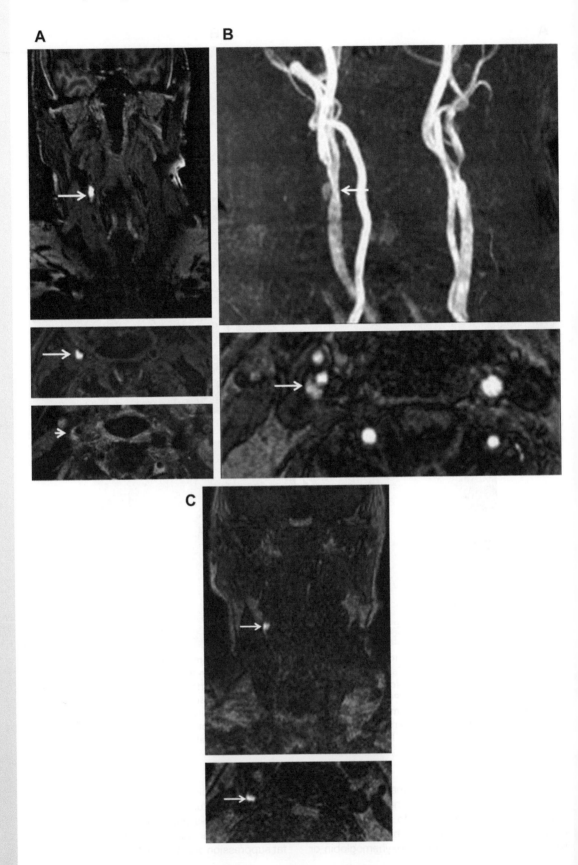

Most prospective and retrospective trials investigating the impact of MR imaging–detected IPH on patient outcomes and plaque progression have used fast spin echo or MPRAGE sequences. Simple applications of old techniques have exploited properties similar to the magnetization prepared gradient echo sequences. TOF MRA uses gradient echo sequences and as such is also able to detect the T1 shortening species within methemoglobin. Careful inspection of TOF images therefore can depict high-intensity signal within the vessel wall[29,31] (Fig. 7). Drawbacks of this technique include differentiating juxtaluminal IPH signal from lumen TOF signal; detection of small quantities of IPH; and obscuration of IPH by perivascular fat, which is not actively suppressed. A similar approach, again using gradient echo sequences, has used the mask images from contrast-enhanced MRA[31] (Fig. 8C), and these too are capable of detecting methemoglobin high signal, and the rapid acquisition with short repetition time leads to increased background and fat suppression. TOF MRA and the use of mask images have the advantage of being acquired as part of routine carotid artery imaging and so the acquisition of IPH data has no added time penalty.

However, there has been significant interest in developing new sequences dedicated to the detection of IPH and other plaque characteristics. Techniques have exploited the benefits of 3D imaging (eg, isotropic voxels, increased signal/noise ratio, improved postprocessing) and more reliable positioning for comparative or follow-up studies. These benefits have been achieved in conjunction with reasonable imaging times and extracting additional plaque characteristics.

Three-dimensional Sequence for Hemorrhage Assessment Using Inversion Recovery and Multiple Echoes

The 3D sequence for hemorrhage assessment using inversion recovery and multiple echoes (SHINE) uses the combination of a 3D gradient recalled echo sequence with inversion recovery preparation and multiple echo times provides a time-efficient acquisition not only for the detection

of IPH but with the potential to age the hemorrhage from its T2* properties.[32]

Multicontrast Atherosclerosis Characterization

Multicontrast atherosclerosis characterization (MATCH) uses a fast low-angle shot technique with a nonselective inversion pulse, and 3 inversion times following the initial 180° pulse result in images selective for IPH, intermediate gray blood signal to improve detection of calcification, and T2 prepared vessel wall images, all combined with flow and fat suppression. Despite the prolonged total inversion time to complete the acquisition the total scan time for high in-plane resolution and carotid bifurcation coverage is only in the order of 5 minutes.[33]

Simultaneous Noncontrast Angiography and Intraplaque Hemorrhage

Simultaneous noncontrast angiography and intraplaque hemorrhage (SNAP) uses an inversion recovery technique that differentiates between flowing blood and IPH by using a phase-sensitive technique during the inversion recovery, making it possible to separate the high signal of IPH from flowing blood such that both elements can be extracted from the same image acquisition. This technique reduces the overall imaging time to provide a time-efficient acquisition.[34]

SUMMARY

The incorporation of simple, short, and easy-to-acquire sequences to visualize the vessel wall and detect IPH is achievable now. Assessment of carotid disease is likely to include baseline imaging to show stenosis, such as TOF or contrast-enhanced MRA, and some simple brain imaging to assess prior neuroischemic disease. Total imaging time is therefore likely in the order of 15 to 20 minutes. The addition of an IPH-detecting vessel wall sequence will only add a further 5 to 6 minutes to this examination, which overall translates into 30 to 40 minutes of scanner table time. The time impact is therefore small and the

Fig. 8. (A) Dedicated vessel wall imaging reveals intense high signal within the proximal right internal carotid artery on the coronal (upper, arrow) and reformatted axial (middle, arrow) images. The fast spin echo T1-weighted image at the same level is also included for reference (lower), showing increased but less intense signal at the same site (arrowhead). (B) Coronal MIP TOF MRA shows minor narrowing within the proximal right internal carotid artery (arrow). There is also an area of high signal intensity adjacent to the lumen seen on the axial source image (lower) in keeping with vessel wall IPH (arrow). (C) Precontrast mask images from a contrast-enhanced MRA acquisition show an area of high signal (IPH) within the right side of the neck (arrow) on the coronal source image (upper) and reformatted axial image (lower, arrow). Background tissues are brighter because fat is not specifically suppressed in this sequence.

A

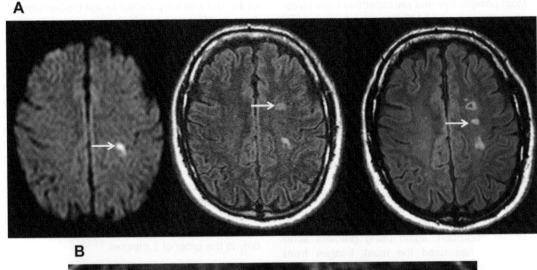

B

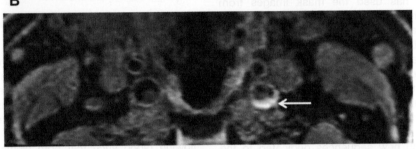

Fig. 9. (*A*) Baseline brain imaging reveals an area of restricted diffusion within the left middle cerebral artery territory (*left, arrow*) in keeping with acute cerebral ischemic injury, as well as a mature area of ischemic damage more anteriorly (*middle, arrow*). Four years later a further area of ischemic damage (*right, arrow*) in the same territory has appeared. The findings therefore suggest 3 discrete ischemic episodes resulting in the final appearances. (*B*) Vessel wall imaging at the final time point reveals high signal intensity within the left internal carotid artery in keeping with IPH (*arrow*), which may in part account for the repetitive left-sided events (although vessel wall imaging from earlier time points was not available).

additional new information provided is potentially clinically useful in the setting of carotid artery disease investigation (**Fig. 9**). Recent studies have shown that MR imaging investigation of carotid disease including a sequence for IPH detection is theoretically a cost-effective means of improving patient outcome.[35]

REFERENCES

1. Barnett HJ, Taylor DW, Eliasziw M, et al. Benefit of carotid endarterectomy in patients with symptomatic moderate or severe stenosis. N Engl J Med 1998; 339:1415–25.
2. Toussaint JF, LaMuraglia GM, Southern JF, et al. Magnetic resonance images lipid, fibrous, calcified, hemorrhagic, and thrombotic components of human atherosclerosis in vivo. Circulation 1996;94: 932–8.
3. Virmani R, Kolodgie FD, Burke AP, et al. Atherosclerotic plaque progression and vulnerability to rupture: angiogenesis as a source of intraplaque hemorrhage. Arterioscler Thromb Vasc Biol 2005;25: 2054–61.
4. Michel JB, Virmani R, Arbustini E, et al. Intraplaque haemorrhages as the trigger of plaque vulnerability. Eur Heart J 2011;32:1977–85, 1985a, 1985b, 1985c.
5. Selwaness M, van den Bouwhuijsen QJ, Verwoert GC, et al. Blood pressure parameters and carotid intraplaque hemorrhage as measured by magnetic resonance imaging: the Rotterdam Study. Hypertension 2013;61:76–81.
6. Stary HC, Chandler AB, Dinsmore RE, et al. A definition of advanced types of atherosclerotic lesions and a histological classification of atherosclerosis: a report from the Committee on Vascular Lesions of the Council on Arteriosclerosis, American Heart Association. Circulation 1995;92:1355–74.
7. Leung G, Moody AR. MR imaging depicts oxidative stress induced by methemoglobin. Radiology 2010; 257:470–6.

8. WHO International Programme on Chemical Safety. Biomarkers in risk assessment: Validity and validation. 2001. Available at: http://www.inchem.org/documents/ehc/ehc/ehc222.htm.Accessed June 15, 2015.

9. Brott TG, Halperin JL, Abbara S, et al. 2011 ASA/ACCF/AHA/AANN/AANS/ACR/ASNR/CNS/SAIP/SCAI/SIR/SNIS/SVM/SVS guideline on the management of patients with extracranial carotid and vertebral artery disease: executive summary. A report of the American College of Cardiology Foundation/American Heart Association Task Force on Practice Guidelines, and the American Stroke Association, American Association of Neuroscience Nurses, American Association of Neurological Surgeons, American College of Radiology, American Society of Neuroradiology, Congress of Neurological Surgeons, Society of Atherosclerosis Imaging and Prevention, Society for Cardiovascular Angiography and Interventions, Society of Interventional Radiology, Society of NeuroInterventional Surgery, Society for Vascular Medicine, and Society for Vascular Surgery. Circulation 2011;124:489–532.

10. Singh N, Moody AR, Gladstone DJ, et al. Moderate carotid artery stenosis: MR imaging-depicted intraplaque hemorrhage predicts risk of cerebrovascular ischemic events in asymptomatic men. Radiology 2009;252:502–8.

11. Altaf N, MacSweeney ST, Gladman J, et al. Carotid intraplaque hemorrhage predicts recurrent symptoms in patients with high-grade carotid stenosis. Stroke 2007;38:1633–5.

12. Gupta A, Marshall RS. Moving beyond luminal stenosis: imaging strategies for stroke prevention in asymptomatic carotid stenosis. Cerebrovasc Dis 2015;39:253–61.

13. Treiman GS, McNally JS, Kim SE, et al. Correlation of carotid intraplaque hemorrhage and stroke using 1.5 T and 3 T MRI. Magn Reson Insights 2015;8:1–8.

14. Cheung HM, Moody AR, Singh N, et al. Late stage complicated atheroma in low-grade stenotic carotid disease: MR imaging depiction–prevalence and risk factors. Radiology 2011;260:841–7.

15. Takaya N, Yuan C, Chu B, et al. Presence of intraplaque hemorrhage stimulates progression of carotid atherosclerotic plaques: a high-resolution magnetic resonance imaging study. Circulation 2005;111:2768–75.

16. Singh N, Moody A. Persistent intraplaque hemorrhage is associated with the progression of preexisting low and moderate grade carotid stenosis: results of a 10-year 3D carotid MRI clinical experience. In: Malhotra A, Liu BP, editors. ASNR 53rd Annual Meeting. Chicago (IL), April 25–30, 2015.

17. Hellings WE, Peeters W, Moll FL, et al. Composition of carotid atherosclerotic plaque is associated with cardiovascular outcome: a prognostic study. Circulation 2010;121:1941–50.

18. Singh N, Moody AR, Rochon-Terry G, et al. Identifying a high risk cardiovascular phenotype by carotid MRI-depicted intraplaque hemorrhage. Int J Cardiovasc Imaging 2013;29:1477–83.

19. Adams HP Jr, Bendixen BH, Kappelle LJ, et al. Classification of subtype of acute ischemic stroke. Definitions for use in a multicenter clinical trial. TOAST. Trial of Org 10172 in Acute Stroke Treatment. Stroke 1993;24:35–41.

20. Moody AR, Allder S, Lennox G, et al. Direct magnetic resonance imaging of carotid artery thrombus in acute stroke. Lancet 1999;353:122–3.

21. Gupta A, Gialdini G, Lerario MP, et al. Magnetic resonance angiography detection of abnormal carotid artery plaque in patients with cryptogenic stroke. J Am Heart Assoc 2015;4(6):e002012.

22. Hosseini AA, Kandiyil N, Macsweeney ST, et al. Carotid plaque hemorrhage on magnetic resonance imaging strongly predicts recurrent ischemia and stroke. Ann Neurol 2013;73:774–84.

23. Saam T, Hetterich H, Hoffmann V, et al. Meta-analysis and systematic review of the predictive value of carotid plaque hemorrhage on cerebrovascular events by magnetic resonance imaging. J Am Coll Cardiol 2013;62:1081–91.

24. Gupta A, Baradaran H, Schweitzer AD, et al. Carotid plaque MRI and stroke risk: a systematic review and meta-analysis. Stroke 2013;44:3071–7.

25. Altaf N, Goode SD, Beech A, et al. Plaque hemorrhage is a marker of thromboembolic activity in patients with symptomatic carotid disease. Radiology 2011;258:538–45.

26. Altaf N, Beech A, Goode SD, et al. Carotid intraplaque hemorrhage detected by magnetic resonance imaging predicts embolization during carotid endarterectomy. J Vasc Surg 2007;46:31–6.

27. Yoshimura S, Yamada K, Kawasaki M, et al. High-intensity signal on time-of-flight magnetic resonance angiography indicates carotid plaques at high risk for cerebral embolism during stenting. Stroke 2011;42:3132–7.

28. Simpson RJ, Akwei S, Hosseini AA, et al. MR imaging-detected carotid plaque hemorrhage is stable for 2 years and a marker for stenosis progression. AJNR Am J Neuroradiol 2015;36:1171–5.

29. Ota H, Yarnykh VL, Ferguson MS, et al. Carotid intraplaque hemorrhage imaging at 3.0-T MR imaging: comparison of the diagnostic performance of three T1-weighted sequences. Radiology 2010;254:551–63.

30. Moody AR, Murphy RE, Morgan PS, et al. Characterization of complicated carotid plaque with magnetic resonance direct thrombus imaging in patients with cerebral ischemia. Circulation 2003;107:3047–52.

31. Qiao Y, Etesami M, Malhotra S, et al. Identification of intraplaque hemorrhage on MR angiography images: a comparison of contrast-enhanced mask

and time-of-flight techniques. AJNR Am J Neuroradiol 2011;32:454–9.

32. Zhu DC, Vu AT, Ota H, et al. An optimized 3D spoiled gradient recalled echo pulse sequence for hemorrhage assessment using inversion recovery and multiple echoes (3D SHINE) for carotid plaque imaging. Magn Reson Med 2010;64:1341–51.

33. Fan Z, Yu W, Xie Y, et al. Multi-contrast atherosclerosis characterization (MATCH) of carotid plaque with a single 5-min scan: technical development and clinical feasibility. J Cardiovasc Magn Reson 2014;16:53.

34. Wang J, Bornert P, Zhao H, et al. Simultaneous non-contrast angiography and intraplaque hemorrhage (SNAP) imaging for carotid atherosclerotic disease evaluation. Magn Reson Med 2013;69:337–45.

35. Gupta A, Mushlin AI, Kamel H, et al. Cost-effectiveness of carotid plaque MR imaging as a stroke risk stratification tool in asymptomatic carotid artery stenosis. Radiology 2015;274(2):142843.

FDG PET/CT Imaging of Carotid Atherosclerosis

Abdelrahman Ali, MD[a], Ahmed Tawakol, MD[a,b],*

KEYWORDS

- FDG-PET • Arterial inflammation • Atherosclerosis • Stroke • CVD

KEY POINTS

- PET with ^{18}F fluorodeoxyglucose. (^{18}F FDG)-PET/computed tomography (CT) is a noninvasive imaging modality that can quantify carotid inflammation.
- Carotid ^{18}F FDG uptake correlates with inflammation, predicts plaque progression and subsequent cerebrovascular events.
- [18]F FDG-PET/CT can be used to evaluate the impact of therapies on arterial inflammation.
- Future studies should determine if carotid ^{18}F FDG-PET/CT imaging can be used to risk stratify individuals with stenotic carotid disease to decide whether to pursue optimized medical therapy or revascularization.

INTRODUCTION

Atherosclerosis, a complex inflammatory process, is an integral component of myocardial infarction and stroke and thus is implicated as the most common cause of death in developed countries.[1,2] The presence of atherosclerotic plaques can be detected using several well-established techniques such as ultrasonography, myocardial perfusion imaging, coronary angiography, multidetector computed tomography (CT), and MR imaging. These modalities assess the luminal encroachment of the plaques or the structural features and do not directly report on the biological processes present within the atheroma. Because atherosclerotic disease is driven by a dynamic biological process (with inflammation as a key component) imaging plaque biology in concert with plaque structure may provide important insights. PET scanning using [18]F Fluorodeoxyglucose. (^{18}F FDG-PET) is a molecular imaging modality that is commonly combined with CT scanning to characterize oncological processes. [18]F FDG-PET imaging has been well-demonstrated to greatly improve the characterization of tumors and has transformed the imaging approach in cancer.[3,4] This review examines the role of ^{18}F FDG-PET/CT imaging in the characterization of atherosclerotic plaque biology.

PATHOGENESIS OF ATHEROSCLEROSIS

Atherosclerosis, although previously considered an indolent lipid storage disorder, is now well-recognized to be an active inflammatory condition.[1] Inflammation seems to play a role in all phases of plaque development, from initiation, to plaque progression, and eventually to plaque rupture.[5,6] One of the initial steps in atherosclerotic plaque development is endothelial dysfunction. Several cardiovascular risk factors are associated with heightened expression of selective adhesion molecules (vascular cell adhesion molecule-1) on the endothelial cell surface, which prompts leukocytes to bind to the arterial wall. Once monocytes attach to the wall, they migrate to the intima

Disclosure: The authors have nothing to disclose.
[a] Cardiac MR PET CT Program, Massachusetts General Hospital, Harvard Medical School, Boston, MA, USA;
[b] Division of Cardiology, Massachusetts General Hospital, Harvard Medical School, Boston, MA, USA
* Corresponding author. Cardiac MR PET CT Program, Massachusetts General Hospital, 165 Cambridge Street, Suite 400, Boston, MA 02114-2750.
E-mail address: atawakol@partners.org

Neuroimag Clin N Am 26 (2016) 45–54
http://dx.doi.org/10.1016/j.nic.2015.09.004
1052-5149/16/$ – see front matter © 2016 Elsevier Inc. All rights reserved.

through diapedesis, which is stimulated by chemoattractant molecules such as monocyte chemoattractant protein-1.[6,7] Once monocytes invade the arterial intima, they differentiate into proinflammatory macrophages (**Fig. 1A, E**).[8] There, they release inflammatory mediators, which attract additional inflammatory cells to the developing plaque, causing a vicious cycle of inflammation.

Plaque inflammation stimulates progression and growth of the atheroma and prompts the development of several features that renders the plaque more prone to rupture. First, macrophages contribute importantly to the development and enlargement of the lipid-rich necrotic core. Macrophages engulf accumulated oxidized low-density lipoprotein (LDL) molecules and turn into foam cells.[9,10] Eventually, foam cells undergo apoptosis and apoptotic bodies accumulate within the core of atheromatous plaque, leading to expansion of the lipid core. Additionally, macrophages release proteolytic enzymes such as matrix metalloproteinases, which thin and weaken the fibrous cap, rendering it more susceptible to rupture.[11,12] The proteolytic milieu also participates in the positive remodeling of the atheroma,[12] another feature of

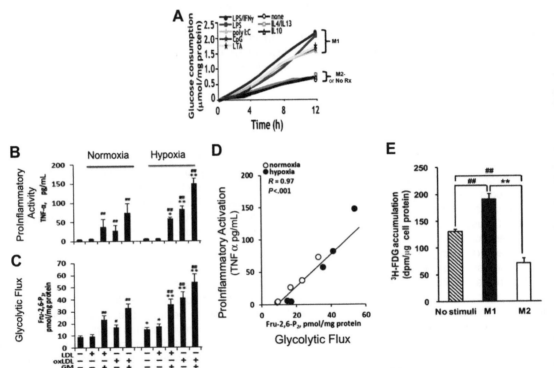

Fig. 1. (A) Macrophage glycolysis increased after M1 activation. Macrophage glycolysis increases substantially after proinflammatory (M1) but not antiinflammatory (M2) stimulation. (B–D) Inflammation and metabolism in an atherosclerotic environment. Macrophage proinflammatory stimulation (B), as tumor necrosis factor (TNF)-α production, and macrophage glycolysis (C), a fructose 2,6p2 production were assessed in response to constituent found in an atherosclerotic environment, including oxidized low-density lipoprotein (LDL), granulocyte macrophage colony stimulating factor, and hypoxia **P<.01 vs the same condition under normoxia. ##P<.01 vs the same O₂ in the absence of LDL or oxLDL. Across a range of stimuli, glycolytic flux keeps pace with proinflammatory activation (D). (E) 18F Fluorodeoxyglucose. (18F FDG) uptake is linked with proinflammatory activation. 3H-FDG accumulates 2.6 times more in proinflammatory macrophages subtype (M1) compared with M2 macrophages (antiinflammatory subtype) **P<.01, comparison between M1 and M2. ##P<.01, compared with no stimuli by Tukey test. IFN, interferon; IL, interleukin; LPS, lipopolysaccharide; LPA, Lipoteichoic acid. (Adapted from [A] Rodríguez-Prados JC, Través PG, Cuenca J, et al. Substrate fate in activated macrophages: a comparison between innate, classic, and alternative activation. J Immunol 2010;185(1):609, with permission. Copyright 2010. The American Association of Immunologists, Inc. and [B–D] Tawakol A, Singh P, Mojena M, et al. HIF-1α and PFKFB3 mediate a tight relationship between proinflammatory activation and anaerobic metabolism in atherosclerotic macrophages. Arterioscler Thromb Vasc Biol 2015;35(6):1463–71, with permission; and From [E] Satomi T, Ogawa M, Mori I, et al. Comparison of contrast agents for atherosclerosis imaging using cultured macrophages: FDG versus ultrasmall superparamagnetic iron oxide. J Nucl Med 2013;54(6):999–1001, with permission.)

rupture-prone plaques.[13] As the inflammatory condition continues over decades, plaques progression continues, and often results in clinical manifestations owing to luminal narrowing (either from gradual encroachment or from or sudden plaque rupture).[5]

18F FLUORODEOXYGLUCOSE UPTAKE AS A MARKER OF TISSUE INFLAMMATION

18F FDG, an analog of glucose, enters the cells via glucose transporter protein (GLUT) and is subsequently phosphorylated to become 18F FDG-6-phosphate by hexokinase, a glycolytic enzyme. However, in contrast to glucose-6-phosphate, 18F FDG-6-phosphate cannot be further metabolized through the glycolytic pathway; thus, it becomes trapped inside the cell and accumulates at a rate that is proportionate to the cell's glycolytic rate.[14] This link to glycolysis facilitates the identification of inflamed tissues. Inflammatory cells (such as macrophages) have a relatively high rate of glycolysis at rest, relative to other tissues, and increase their glycolytic rate further upon proinflammatory stimulation.[15] Additionally, recent studies also show a tight relationship between 18F FDG uptake and macrophage (MØ) activation in an atheromatous environment. Uptake of radiolabeled 2-deoxyglucose by human MØ in vitro is increased by cytokine activation and by oxidized LDL. Moreover, across oxygen tensions and varied stimuli, MØ activation and glycolytic flux are tightly and linearly related, resulting in calibration of glycolysis to keep pace with proinflammatory activation (tumor necrosis factor production) via a mechanism that depends on the ubiquitous PFK-2 isoenzyme and hypoxia inducible factor-1α[16] (Fig. 1B–D).

In concert with the strong associations between glycolysis and MØ activation, several studies have demonstrated that arterial 18F FDG uptake correlates with MØ density within the artery wall. Preclinical studies reported high correlations between 18F FDG uptake and the density of MØ in atherosclerotic lesions and that anti-inflammatory therapies can reduce the arterial 18F FDG-PET signal.[17–19] Moreover, several groups have shown in human studies that 18F FDG uptake in the carotid artery, which can be quantified noninvasively using PET, provides and index of atherosclerotic inflammation. Rudd and colleagues[20] demonstrated that 18F FDG uptake in carotid plaques was higher in symptomatic carotid lesions compared with the contralateral healthy asymptomatic lesions, which was confirmed later by autoradiography of carotid plaques after carotid endarterectomy. Several groups demonstrated

that 18F FDG uptake within carotid plaque correlates with the amount of macrophages in the inflamed plaque, by staining with anti-CD68 antibodies[15,21,22] (Fig. 2A–G). Further, the inflammatory signal is reproducible, as was shown in a study in which patients with known atherosclerotic disease underwent PET/CT imaging twice (2 weeks apart).[23]

The measure of arterial inflammation correlates with risk factor prevalence and seems to predict subsequent structural changes within the artery wall. Arterial inflammation as assessed by 18F FDG-PET/CT correlates with the Framingham Risk Score as well as with inflammatory biomarkers. In a study of 137 patients who underwent PET/CT imaging, arterial 18F FDG uptake predicted the subsequent rate of arterial calcification within the underlying segment.[24] Moreover, arterial 18F FDG uptake has been repeatedly shown to provide an independent measure of risk for subsequent cardiovascular disease (CVD) events. Rominger and colleagues[25] observed, in a retrospective study of 932 patients who underwent 18F FDG-PET/CT imaging for cancer, that the 18F FDG uptake (as a target-to-background ratio) predicted the risk of subsequent vascular events. In another retrospective study, Figueroa and colleagues[26] in a study of 513 subjects who were followed for a median 4.2 years showed that arterial 18F FDG uptake significantly and independently improved the prediction of cardiovascular events apart from Framingham Risk Score, resulting in a net reclassification improvement of approximately 27.5% (Fig. 3). Furthermore, Marnane and colleagues[27] showed in a prospective study of individuals with recent cerebrovascular accidents that carotid 18F FDG uptake was associated with the risk of subsequent cerebrovascular accident (Fig. 4). Accordingly, a growing body of retrospective as well as prospective studies shows that arterial 18F FDG uptake independently predicts atherothrombotic events.

EVALUATION OF THE PATHOPHYSIOLOGY OF ATHEROSCLEROTIC DISEASES

Several chronic conditions are associated with both increased immune system activity and a heightened risk of atherosclerosis. PET/CT imaging is increasingly being used to examine the interplay between those inflammatory conditions and atherosclerosis. One such chronic inflammatory disorder, rheumatoid arthritis (RA), is associated with a substantially increased risk of CVD. A recent study using PET/CT imaging in individuals with RA reported that individuals with RA have substantially heightened arterial inflammation relative to

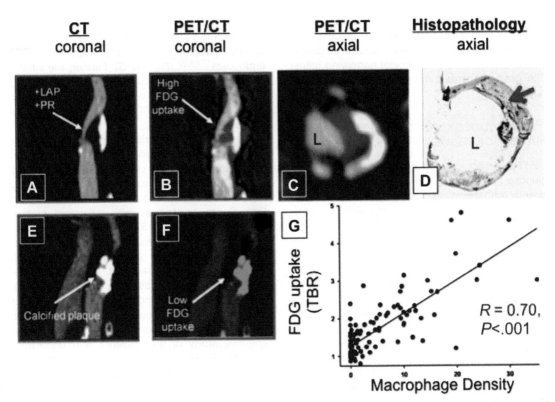

Fig. 2. (*A–G*) Arterial ^{18}F Fluorodeoxyglucose. (^{18}F FDG) uptake relates to plaque inflammation. (*A, E*) Computed tomography (CT) and (*B, C, F*) PET/CT images are shown for 2 individuals with severe carotid stenosis. The images from the upper panel were taken from an individual who proved to have substantial inflammation within his carotid plaque (the *red arrow* highlights the macrophage staining on histology). That same individual had intense ^{18}F FDG uptake related to the same plaque (*red* activity on images *B* and *C*). In contrast, the images from an individual who had little inflammation on histology had little ^{18}F FDG uptake on his PET (*F*). (*G*) Across the study population, there is a significant correlation between carotid target-to-background ratio (TBR) and the percentage of CD68 staining of the excised plaques. LAP, low-attenuation plaque; PR, positive remodeling.

carefully matched controls, and that inflammation in the artery wall correlates with the degree of inflammatory activity in the joints.[28] Further, another study in patients with RA showed that 8 weeks of treatment with an antibody targeting tumor necrosis factor-α (used for the purpose of reducing joint inflammation), resulted in a reduction in atherosclerotic inflammation.[29] These observations suggest a potential communication between the synovial and atherosclerotic inflammatory milieus, and supports the hypothesis that treating synovial inflammation may also benefit atherosclerosis.

Infection with the human immunodeficiency virus (HIV) is also associated with a heightened risk of atherosclerosis. Although the exact mechanisms underlying this risk have not been well-established, chronic up-regulation of immune system activity is believed to represent an important potential mechanism. To further evaluate the relationship between inflammation and HIV, Subramanian and colleagues[30] performed ^{18}F FDG-

PET/CT imaging in 81 subjects, including 27 with HIV infection and 54 matched controls. They found that individuals with HIV infection have increased arterial inflammation compared with noninfected individuals who were matched according to age, gender, and Framingham Risk Score. Furthermore, the arterial ^{18}F FDG signal was found to correlate with CD163 (a soluble marker of monocyte activation), suggesting that upregulation of the monocyte cellular niche may represent an important pathobiological mechanism of atherosclerosis in HIV. In a separate study, the same group evaluated whether arterial inflammation was associated with structural lesions within the coronary tree of individuals with HIV. They observed that individuals with increased arterial inflammation (greater than median values for aortic ^{18}F FDG uptake) had a 4-fold higher risk of having high-risk coronary plaques on CT (coronary atherosclerotic plaques with positive remodeling or low attenuation).[31] Together, the findings link

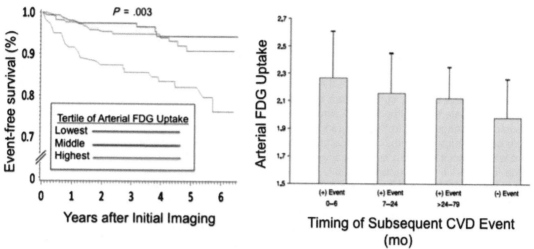

Fig. 3. Arterial ¹⁸F Fluorodeoxyglucose. (¹⁸F FDG) provides data on risk and timing of future cardiovascular disease (CVD) events. Kaplan–Meier survival analysis graph (*left*) illustrates that subjects in the highest target-to-background ratio (TBR) tertile had a higher risk for CVD compared with participants in the lowest TBR tertile. The magnitude of arterial inflammation (TBR) is inversely proportional to the timing of cardiovascular events. (*Adapted from* Figueroa AL, Abdelbaky A, Truong QA. Measurement of arterial activity on routine FDG PET/CT images improves prediction of risk of future CV events. JACC Cardiovasc Imaging 2013;6(12):1256; with permission.)

monocyte activation, to arterial inflammation, to the presence of high-risk coronary structural features, thus providing some mechanistic clues linking HIV to atherothrombosis.

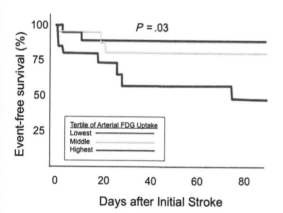

Fig. 4. ¹⁸F Fluorodeoxyglucose. (¹⁸F FDG)-PET imaging of carotid inflammation predicts stroke recurrence. When patients were grouped into tertiles according to the carotid ¹⁸F FDG uptake, the actuarial stroke recurrence rates were 19.8% (95% CI, 6.7–50.4) in the lowest tertile, 13% (95% CI, 3.4–42.7) in the middle tertile, and 58.5% (95% CI, 33.4–85.1) in the highest tertile (log-rank; $P = .03$). (*From* Marnane M, Merwick A, Sheehan OC, et al. Carotid plaque inflammation on 18F-fluorodeoxyglucose positron emission tomography predicts early stroke recurrence. Ann Neurol 2012;71(5):713; with permission.)

The evaluation of arterial inflammation has provided insights into the pathobiology of milder inflammatory conditions as well. For example, asthma, which is associated with a very long duration of mild chronic inflammation, associates with atherosclerotic inflammation even after correcting for cardiovascular risk factors.[32] Moreover, the degree of arterial inflammation correlates with the severity of the pulmonary condition. Along similar lines, another study observed a relationship between periodontal and carotid inflammation.[33] In a later study, the same group used PET/CT imaging to study the impact of statin therapy on periodontal inflammation, and observed a substantial reduction in periodontal inflammation, which correlated significantly with changes in arterial inflammation.[34]

PET/COMPUTED TOMOGRAPHIC IMAGING TO ASSESS IMPACT OF THERAPY ON ARTERIAL INFLAMMATION

The efficacy of different medications on arterial inflammation (assessed using ¹⁸F FDG-PET/CT imaging) has been evaluated in several clinical trials. A question of substantial interest is whether findings on ¹⁸F FDG-PET/CT imaging provide insight into the clinical efficacy of the compounds. Although additional studies are continuing to provide more data to answer that question, currently there are 4 classes of drugs for which both PET/CT imaging data and clinical endpoint data are available (statins, thiazolidinediones, cholesteryl ester transfer protein modulator, and lipoprotein-associated phospholipase A2 inhibitors). Thus far, the ^{18}F FDG-PET/CT data seem to align with the clinical endpoint trial data.

In one of the first studies to evaluate the impact of therapy on the arterial signal, Tahara and colleagues evaluated the impact of simvastatin versus diet management. In this non-randomized single-center study, 3 months of simvastatin treatment was associated with a substantial reduction in the arterial ^{18}F FDG uptake relative to diet only.[35] More recently, in a double-blinded, multicenter ^{18}F FDG-PET/CT imaging trial comparing high-dose with low-dose atorvastatin, high-dose atorvastatin rapidly reduce arterial inflammation (as early as 4 weeks after randomization) (Fig. 5A, B).[36] Such studies are in concert with the findings of clinical endpoint studies,[37] which have reproducibly proven a clinical benefit for statins. Interestingly, the ^{18}F FDG-PET/CT studies did not observe a relationship between changes in LDL concentrations and reductions in arterial inflammation. However, it is also noteworthy that studies of nonpharmacologic LDL lowering (with LDL apheresis) did report a relationship between changes in LDL and changes in inflammation.[38]

Similarly, the effect of thiazolidinediones on arterial inflammation was evaluated. In a study of 56 subjects (with a history of diabetes or impaired glucose intolerance and carotid atherosclerosis) who were randomized to pioglitazone versus glimepiride (a sulfonylurea) for 4 months. Despite achieving a similar blood glucose concentration, pioglitazone reduced arterial wall ^{18}F FDG uptake whereas glimepiride did not.[39] In concert with those findings, prior clinical trials have shown that thiazolidinediones reduce clinical CVD events relative to sulfonylureas.[40,41]

[18]F FDG-PET/CT has been actively used for the evaluation of novel therapies targeting atherosclerosis. Dalcetrapib, a cholesteryl ester protein modulator, was evaluated in the dal-PLAQUE (Safety and Efficacy of Dalcetrapib on Atherosclerotic Disease Using Novel Noninvasive Multimodality Imaging) trial, was a multicenter PET/CT imaging study in which 130 subjects were randomized either to dalcetrapib or placebo. In that study, dalcetrapib was not associated with any change in the prespecified PET/CT imaging endpoints.[42] Subsequently, the dal-OUTCOMES study, which randomized nearly 16,000 individuals to dalcetrapib versus placebo, concluded that dalcetrapib failed to decrease the risk of recurrent cardiovascular events in patients with history of recent coronary syndrome.[43]

More recently, ^{18}F FDG-PET/CT was used to evaluate the impact of lipoprotein-associated

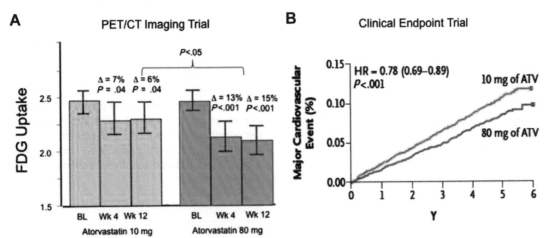

Fig. 5. Measurement of changes in arterial inflammation: assessing the impact of treatment. (*A*) In a multicenter PET/computed tomography (CT) imaging trial, statin therapy decreased arterial inflammation (target-to-background ratio [TBR]) as early as 4 weeks after randomization to atorvastatin (ATV). By 12 weeks, there was a significant decrease in TBR from baseline in subjects treated with 80 mg compared with subjects who received atorvastatin 10 mg. (*B*) The findings of the PET/CT imaging trial are consistent with the observation from large randomized clinical endpoint trials showing that high-dose statins are more effective fro reducing cardiovascular disease (CVD) events when compared with low-dose statins. FDG, ^{18}F fluorodeoxyglucose; HR, hazard ratio. (*Adapted from* [*A*] Tawakol A, Fayad ZA, Mogg R. Intensification of statin therapy results in a rapid reduction in atherosclerotic inflammation: results of a multicenter fluorodeoxyglucose-positron emission tomography/computed tomography feasibility study. J Am Coll Cardiol 2013;62(10):913, with permission; and *From* [*B*] LaRosa JC, Grundy SM, Waters DD, et al. Intensive lipid lowering with atorvastatin in patients with stable coronary disease. N Engl J Med 2005;352(14):1431; with permission.)

phospholipase A2 inhibition on arterial inflammation. In that study 83 patients who were randomly given either rilapladib or placebo for 3 months. Although active treatment resulted in an 80% reduction in phospholipase A2 activity, there was no change in arterial inflammation.[44] In concert with those findings, 2 large clinical endpoint trials (of 15,828 and 13,026 subjects) subsequently reported that lipoprotein-associated phospholipase A2 inhibition had no beneficial impact on CVD events.[45,46]

CLINICAL IMAGING OF INFLAMMATION USING ¹⁸F FLUORODEOXYGLUCOSE PET

Although ¹⁸F FDG-PET/CT is not routinely used clinically to image atherosclerotic inflammation, it is being used to evaluate the inflammation of other body tissues. Evaluation of cardiac sarcoidosis using ¹⁸F FDG-PET/CT is currently a routine procedure. Patients with cardiac sarcoidosis are at higher risk of death or fatal arrhythmias such as ventricular tachycardia. Blankstein and colleagues[47] investigated the capability of ¹⁸F FDG-PET/CT to identify the subset of individuals with sarcoidosis who are at greatest risk for adverse events. They observed that the presence of focal ¹⁸F FDG uptake identifies patients who are at greater risk of adverse events.[47] That group also demonstrated that a reduction in the intensity of myocardial ¹⁸F FDG uptake (through antiinflammatory therapies) is associated with improvements in left ventricular ejection fraction, supporting the idea of using serial PET/CT scanning to guide titration of immunosuppressive therapy.[48]

Infective endocarditis (IE) is another serious medical condition associated with significant morbidity and mortality. Although the revised Duke criteria are used most commonly to diagnose IE, there is little doubt that more accurate methods to identify IE are needed. To that end, several studies have investigated the role that ¹⁸F FDG-PET/CT imaging might play in improving the accuracy of diagnosing IE. Although ¹⁸F FDG-PET/CT does not seem to improve the evaluation of IE in native valves,[49] several studies have shown that PET/CT imaging may facilitate diagnosis of IE in prosthetic valves.[50,51] Beyond prosthetic valves, ¹⁸F FDG-PET/CT is being used increasingly to evaluate for active infection of an implanted device or prosthesis.[52] In those cases, ¹⁸F FDG uptake may not be limited to macrophages, because it is well-known that neutrophils also avidly accumulate ¹⁸F FDG, using mechanisms that are similar to those seen in macrophages. Hence ¹⁸F FDG uptake may be enhanced within tissues that are rich in either proinflammatory macrophages or neutrophils.[53]

FUTURE DIRECTIONS

The potential clinical application of PET/CT imaging for assessment of atherosclerotic disease may be facilitated by 1 or more of several scientific advances. One area of rapid advances is the development of additional PET tracers beyond ¹⁸F FDG. To that end, tracers such as ¹⁸F-fluorodeoxymanose (FDM), FMISO, and ¹⁸F-sodium fluoride (¹⁸F-NaF) might provide unique data. In a recent clinical trial, Joshi and colleagues[54] showed that ¹⁸F-NaF localized to culprit lesions within coronary arteries. It is possible that NaF imaging could be similarly useful for identifying symptomatic carotid lesions. A more recently developed tracer, 2-deoxy-2-[18F] fluoro-D-mannose (¹⁸FDM), binds to the mannose receptor. Because the mannose receptor is classically used to identify M2-polarized macrophages, FDM (unlike ¹⁸F FDG) might be useful for identifying antiinflammatory macrophage subsets.[55]

Beyond novel tracers, important gains are being made in camera technology. New time-of-flight technology and new, more sensitive detector systems are improving the ability to quantify the PET signal. Moreover, new PET/MR systems, which combine the exquisite quantitative capabilities of PET with the excellent tissue characterization of MR imaging, may be particularly well-suited for carotid plaque characterization. Prospective studies will be needed to assess whether the combination of PET and MR data will indeed improve the ability to characterize risk associated with carotid atheromatous lesions. For example, in moderate carotid stenosis, there is relative equipoise in choosing between invasive revascularization versus optimal medical therapy. A question of substantial importance is whether ¹⁸F FDG-PET/CT imaging (either alone or in combination with MR imaging data) could assist in choosing between medical therapy versus revascularization in carotid stenotic disease. Future studies are needed to evaluate the impact of PET/MR or PET/CT imaging for occlusive carotid disease.

SUMMARY

For over a decade, ¹⁸F FDG-PET/CT imaging has provided an enhanced ability to study atherosclerotic inflammation and its contribution to atherothrombotic syndromes. ¹⁸F FDG-PET/CT has been well-validated, has been shown to be reproducible, and shown to predict atherosclerotic disease progression and the risk of atherothrombotic complications, including stroke. Additional studies are urgently needed to assess whether ¹⁸F FDG-PET/CT imaging may play an effective role in the clinical management of carotid atherosclerotic diseases.

REFERENCES

1. Libby P. Inflammation in atherosclerosis. Nature 2002;420:868–74.
2. Rosamond W, Flegal K, Friday G, et al. Heart disease and stroke statistics—2007 update: a report from the American Heart Association statistics committee and stroke statistics subcommittee. Circulation 2007;115:e69–171.
3. Lardinois D, Weder W, Hany TF, et al. Staging of non-small-cell lung cancer with integrated positron-emission tomography and computed tomography. N Engl J Med 2003;348:2500–7.
4. Antoch G, Vogt FM, Freudenberg LS, et al. Whole-body dual-modality PET/CT and whole-body MRI for tumor staging in oncology. JAMA 2003;290: 3199–206.
5. Ross R. Atherosclerosis is an inflammatory disease. Am Heart J 1999;138:S419–20.
6. Faxon DP, Fuster V, Libby P, et al. Atherosclerotic vascular disease conference: writing group III: pathophysiology. Circulation 2004;109:2617–25.
7. Libby P, Ridker PM, Maseri A. Inflammation and atherosclerosis. Circulation 2002;105:1135–43.
8. Johnson JL, Newby AC. Macrophage heterogeneity in atherosclerotic plaques. Curr Opin Lipidol 2009; 20:370–8.
9. Kruth HS. Sequestration of aggregated low-density lipoproteins by macrophages. Curr Opin Lipidol 2002;13:483–8.
10. Newby AC, George SJ, Ismail Y, et al. Vulnerable atherosclerotic plaque metalloproteinases and foam cell phenotypes. Thromb Haemost 2009;101: 1006–11.
11. Tarkin J, Joshi F, Rudd J. PET imaging of inflammation in atherosclerosis. Nat Rev Cardiol 2014;11(8): 443–57.
12. Galis ZS, Sukhova GK, Lark M, et al. Increased expression of matrix metalloproteinases and matrix degrading activity in vulnerable regions of human atherosclerotic plaques. J Clin Invest 1994;94: 2493–503.
13. Figueroa AL, Subramanian SS, Cury RC, et al. Distribution of inflammation within carotid atherosclerotic plaques with high-risk morphological features: a comparison between positron emission tomography activity, plaque morphology, and histopathology. Circ Cardiovasc Imaging 2012;5(1):69–77.
14. Rudd JH, Narula J, Strauss HW, et al. Imaging atherosclerotic plaque inflammation by fluorodeoxyglucose with positron emission tomography: ready for prime time? J Am Coll Cardiol 2010;55(23): 2527–35.
15. Font MA, Fernandez A, Carvajal A, et al. Imaging of early inflammation in low-to-moderate carotid stenosis by 18-FDG-PET. Front Biosci (Landmark Ed) 2009;14:3352–60.
16. Tawakol A, Singh P, Mojena M, et al. HIF-1α and PFKFB3 mediate a tight relationship between proinflammatory activation and anaerobic metabolism in atherosclerotic macrophages. Arterioscler Thromb Vasc Biol 2015;35(6):1463–71.
17. Ogawa M, Ishino S, Mukai T, et al. (18) F-FDG accumulation in atherosclerotic plaques: immunohistochemical and PET imaging study. J Nucl Med 2004;45:1245–50.
18. Tawakol A, Migrino RQ, Hoffmann U, et al. Noninvasive in vivo measurement of vascular inflammation with F-18 fluorodeoxyglucose positron emission tomography. J Nucl Cardiol 2005;12:294–301.
19. Ogawa M, Magata Y, Kato T, et al. Application of 18F-FDG PET for monitoring the therapeutic effect of antiinflammatory drugs on stabilization of vulnerable atherosclerotic plaques. J Nucl Med 2006;47: 1845–50.
20. Rudd JH, Warburton EA, Fryer TD, et al. Imaging atherosclerotic plaque inflammation with [18 F]-fluorodeoxyglucose positron emission tomography. Circulation 2002;105:2708–11.
21. Tawakol A, Migrino RQ, Bashian GG, et al. InVivo 18 F-fluorodeoxyglucose positron emission tomography imaging provides a noninvasive measure of carotid plaque inflammation in patients. J Am Coll Cardiol 2006;48:1818–24.
22. Taqueti VR, Di Carli MF, Jerosch-Herold M, et al. Increased microvascularization and vessel permeability associate with active inflammation in human atheromata. Circ Cardiovasc Imaging 2014;7(6): 920–9.
23. Rudd JH, Myers KS, Bansilal S, et al. (18)Fluorodeoxyglucose positron emission tomography imaging of atherosclerotic plaque inflammation is highly reproducible: implications for atherosclerosis therapy trials. J Am Coll Cardiol 2007;50:892–6.
24. Abdelbaky A, Corsini E, Figueroa AL, et al. Focal arterial inflammation precedes subsequent calcification in the same location: a longitudinal FDG-PET/CT study. Circ Cardiovasc Imaging 2013;6:747–54.
25. Rominger A, Saam T, Wolpers S, et al. 18F-FDG PET/CT identifies patients at risk for future vascular events in an otherwise asymptomatic cohort with neoplastic disease. J Nucl Med 2009;50:1611–20.
26. Figueroa AL, Abdelbaky A, Truong QA, et al. Measurement of arterial activity on routine FDG PET/CT images improves prediction of risk of future CV events. JACC Cardiovasc Imaging 2013;6:1250–9.
27. Marnane M, Merwick A, Sheehan OC, et al. Carotid plaque inflammation on 18F-fluorodeoxyglucose positron emission tomography predicts early stroke recurrence. Ann Neurol 2012;71:709–18.
28. Emami H, Vijayakumar J, Subramanian S, et al. Arterial inflammation in rheumatoid arthritis correlates with synovial activity. JACC Cardiovasc Imaging 2014;7:959–60.

29. Maki-Petaja KM, Elkhawad M, Cheriyan J, et al. Anti-tumor necrosis factor alpha therapy reduces aortic inflammation and stiffness in patients with rheumatoid arthritis. Circulation 2012;126:2473–80.

30. Subramanian S, Tawakol A, Burdo TH, et al. Arterial inflammation in patients with HIV. JAMA 2012;308: 379–86.

31. Tawakol A, Lo J, Zanni MV, et al. Increased arterial inflammation relates to high-risk coronary plaque morphology in HIV-infected patients. J Acquir Immune Defic Syndr 2014;66(2):164–71.

32. Vijayakumar J, Subramanian S, Singh P, et al. Arterial inflammation in bronchial asthma. J Nucl Cardiol 2013;20(3):385–95.

33. Fifer KM, Qadir S, Subramanian S, et al. Positron emission tomography measurement of periodontal 18F-fluorodeoxyglucose uptake is associated with histologically determined carotid plaque inflammation. J Am Coll Cardiol 2011;57:971–6.

34. Subramanian S, Emami H, Vucic E, et al. High-dose atorvastatin reduces periodontal inflammation: a novel pleiotropic effect of statins. J Am Coll Cardiol 2013;62:2382–91.

35. Tahara N, Kai H, Ishibashi M, et al. Simvastatin attenuates plaque inflammation: evaluation by fluorodeoxyglucose positron emission tomography. J Am Coll Cardiol 2006;48:1825–31.

36. Tawakol A, Fayad ZA, Mogg R, et al. Intensification of statin therapy results in a rapid reduction in atherosclerotic inflammation: results of a multicenter fluorodeoxyglucose-positron emission tomography/computed tomography feasibility study. J Am Coll Cardiol 2013;62:909–17.

37. LaRosa JC, Grundy SM, Waters DD, et al, Treating to New Targets (TNT) Investigators. Intensive lipid lowering with atorvastatin in patients with stable coronary disease. N Engl J Med 2005;352(14):1425–35.

38. van Wijk DF, Sjouke B, Figueroa A, et al. Nonpharmacological lipoprotein apheresis reduces arterial inflammation in familial hypercholesterolemia. J Am Coll Cardiol 2014;64(14):1418–26.

39. Mizoguchi M, Tahara N, Tahara A, et al. Pioglitazone attenuates atherosclerotic plaque inflammation in patients with impaired glucose tolerance or diabetes a prospective, randomized, comparator-controlled study using serial FDG PET/CT imaging study of carotid artery and ascending aorta. JACC Cardiovasc Imaging 2011;4:1110–8.

40. Erdmann E, Dormandy JA, Charbonnel B, et al. The effect of pioglitazone on recurrent myocardial infarction in 2445 patients with type 2 diabetes and previous myocardial infarction: results from the PROactive (PROactive 05) Study. J Am Coll Cardiol 2007;49:1772–80.

41. Dormandy JA, Charbonnel B, Eckland DJ, et al. Secondary prevention of macrovascular events in patients with type 2 diabetes in the PROactive Study (PROspective pioglitAzone Clinical Trial In macroVascular Events): a randomized controlled trial. Lancet 2005;366:1279–89.

42. Fayad ZA, Mani V, Woodward M, et al. Safety and efficacy of dalcetrapib on atherosclerotic disease using novel noninvasive multimodality imaging (dal-PLAQUE): a randomised clinical trial. Lancet 2011;378:1547–59.

43. Schwartz GG, Olsson AG, Abt M, et al. Effects of dalcetrapib in patients with a recent acute coronary syndrome. N Engl J Med 2012;367:2089–99.

44. Tawakol A, Singh P, Rudd JH, et al. Effect of treatment for 12 weeks with rilapladib, a lipoprotein-associated phospholipase A2 inhibitor, on arterial inflammation as assessed with 18F- fluorodeoxyglucose-positron emission tomography imaging. J Am Coll Cardiol 2014;63:86–8.

45. O'Donoghue ML, Braunwald E, White HD, et al, SOLID-TIMI 52 Investigators. Effect of darapladib on major coronary events after an acute coronary syndrome: the SOLID-TIMI 52 randomized clinical trial. JAMA 2014;312(10):1006–15.

46. STABILITY Investigators, White HD, Held C, et al. Darapladib for preventing ischemic events in stable coronary heart disease. N Engl J Med 2014;370(18): 1702–11.

47. Blankstein R, Osborne M, Naya M, et al. Cardiac positron emission tomography enhances prognostic assessments of patients with suspected cardiac sarcoidosis. J Am Coll Cardiol 2014;63:329–36.

48. Osborne MT, Hulten EA, Singh A, et al. Reduction in 18F fluorodeoxyglucose uptake on serial cardiac positron emission tomography is associated with improved left ventricular ejection fraction in patients with cardiac sarcoidosis. J Nucl Cardiol 2014;21(1):166–74.

49. Kouijzer IJ, Vos FJ, Janssen MJ, et al. The value of 18F-FDG PET/CT in diagnosing infectious endocarditis. Eur J Nucl Med Mol Imaging 2013;40(7): 1102–7.

50. Ricciardi A, Sordillo P, Ceccarelli L, et al. 18-Fluoro-2-deoxyglucose positron emission tomography-computed tomography: an additional tool in the diagnosis of prosthetic valve endocarditis. Int J Infect Dis 2014;28:219–24.

51. Saby L, Laas O, Habib G, et al. Positron emission tomography/computed tomography for diagnosis of prosthetic valve endocarditis: increased valvular 18F-fluorodeoxyglucose uptake as a novel major criterion. J Am Coll Cardiol 2013;61(23):2374–82.

52. Sarrazin JF, Philippon F, Tessier M, et al. Usefulness of fluorine-18 positron emission tomography/computed tomography for identification of cardiovascular implantable electronic device infections. J Am Coll Cardiol 2012;59(18):1616–25.

53. Hara T, Truelove J, Tawakol A, et al. 18F-fluorodeoxyglucose positron emission tomography/computed tomography enables the detection of recurrent

same-site deep vein thrombosis by illuminating recently formed, neutrophil-rich thrombus. Circulation 2014;130(13):1044–52.

54. Joshi NV, Vesey AT, Williams MC, et al. 18F-fluoride positron emission tomography for identification of ruptured and high-risk coronary atherosclerotic plaques: a prospective clinical trial. Lancet 2014; 383:705–13.

55. Tahara N, Mukherjee J, de Haas HJ, et al. 2-deoxy-2-[18F]fluoro-D-mannose positron emission tomography imaging in atherosclerosis. Nat Med 2014; 20:215–9.

Utility of Combining PET and MR Imaging of Carotid Plaque

Alex T. Vesey, MD[a], Marc R. Dweck, MD, PhD[a,b,c],
Zahi A. Fayad, PhD[b,c],*

KEYWORDS

- PET • MR imaging • Carotid plaque imaging

KEY POINTS

- By harnessing the versatility and soft tissue imaging capabilities of MR imaging alongside the unmatched sensitivity and biomolecular flexibility of PET, the potential to provide detailed multiparametric plaque characterization in the carotid arteries is clear.
- Both these modalities already have a proven track record in vascular imaging and the capability to cross validate one against the other is attractive, particularly in an era in which obtaining good tissue for image validation is becoming more difficult.
- The ability to acquire simultaneous, and dynamic multimodal data is perhaps PET/MR's greatest strength that will be of major interest to researchers investigating carotid and coronary atherosclerosis alike.

INTRODUCTION

Stroke remains a major global cause of morbidity and mortality,[1] while controversy and debate as to the best method for imaging and treating carotid atherosclerosis endures. Anatomic measures of carotid luminal stenoses remain the imaging gold standard and are widely used to risk stratify patients and guide invasive management. Carotid stenosis is conceptually straightforward and measured easily, cheaply, and reliably on a variety of platforms; yet, it is also profoundly limited as a biomarker, as we know that most patients even with a high-grade (70% to 99% by the criteria of the North American Symptomatic Carotid Endarterectomy Trial Collaborators[2]) symptomatic anatomic stenosis will *not* go on to have further events.[3] With this problem in mind, an expert group has described the search for reliable molecular imaging of the extracranial carotid arteries as "critical."[4] Unfortunately it has proven challenging to identify such a technique capable of improving the current paradigm.

Imaging the carotids is not just about identifying the high-risk plaque or patient but also concerns measuring and monitoring pathologic disease burden and activity. This can provide not only mechanistic insight but also a method for monitoring response to therapy and for testing the biological plausibility of novel treatments. In the

Disclosure: The authors have nothing to disclose.
[a] British Heart Foundation Centre for Cardiovascular Science, College of Medicine and Veterinary Medicine, University of Edinburgh, Room Suite 305, The Chancellor's Building, 49 Little France Crescent, Edinburgh EH16 4SB, UK; [b] Imaging Science Laboratories, Department of Radiology, Translational and Molecular Imaging Institute, Mount Sinai School of Medicine, 1 Gustave L. Levy Place, New York, NY 10029, USA; [c] Imaging Science Laboratories, Department of Medicine, Translational and Molecular Imaging Institute, Mount Sinai School of Medicine, 1 Gustave L. Levy Place, New York, NY 10029, USA
* Corresponding author. Translational and Molecular Imaging Institute, Icachn School of Medicine at Mount Sinai, 1 Gustave L. Levy Place, New York, NY 10029.
E-mail address: zahi.fayad@mssm.edu

1052-5149/16/$ – see front matter © 2016 Elsevier Inc. All rights reserved.

cardiovascular field, ultrasound, computed tomography (CT), MR imaging, and more recently PET have all demonstrated promise in these respects and in several instances been used successfully in interventional trials.[5,6] Each has their own individual strengths and limitations, leading to major interest in the use of hybrid imaging systems capable of harnessing the information provided by 2 or more approaches. In this regard, PET/CT has for many years led the field; however, more recently hybrid PET/MR systems have been brought to market with the intention of combining PET with the advantages that MR imaging holds over CT, principally the improved soft tissue contrast and the lack of radiation exposure.

The aim of this review was to summarize the current status of dedicated hybrid PET/MR imaging; to crystallize the rationale for and advantages of this technique with respect to carotid atherosclerosis; and to discuss current limitations, challenges, and future directions.

CURRENTLY AVAILABLE PLATFORMS, TECHNICAL CONSIDERATIONS, AND FEASIBILITY

Fully integrated hybrid PET/MR systems are a compromise, with the MR component of the scanner necessitating alteration of the PET component and vice versa. PET detectors were not originally conceived to function in strong magnetic fields and photomultiplier tubes cannot operate in such an environment. Initial approaches to hybrid PET/ MR imaging therefore simply consisted of attempting to fuse images acquired separately on different PET/CT and MR scanners. This technique can work well in nondeformable regions of anatomy, such as the skull, in which rigid registration can take place off-line; however, it is less straightforward in soft tissue structures, particularly ones that are mobile. To advance the field, different manufacturers have taken different approaches: the first systems maintained separation of the MR imaging and PET components (eg, Philips Ingenuity TF PET/MR [Phillips, The Netherlands]) but used a dedicated rail-based shuttle table to transfer the patient between scanners in an attempt to minimize movement and facilitate coregistration. The first ever installed worldwide was in 2009 at Mount Sinai Medical Center in New York. However, in practice this approach was suboptimal and lacked the advantages associated with a truly synchronous imaging system.

More recently, genuinely integrated hybrid scanners have come to market (Fig. 1). Incorporating significant alterations to both the MR and PET components of these systems has allowed both imaging modalities to be combined into a single gantry. The Siemens Biograph mMR device (Siemens, Erlangen Germany) uses an avalanche photodiode detector, whereas the more recently available GE system (General Electric, New York, USA) (Signa PET/MR) uses a silicon-based photomultiplier tube, both of which are capable of functioning within a magnetic field and therefore allow the simultaneous acquisition of PET and MR imaging data. The challenges of adequately shielding the PET components without negatively impacting on MR quality have been met principally thanks to developments in gradient design, making increasing bore sizes possible.[7]

Many studies have now been published in various domains showing that the use of these devices is feasible (for a recent review, refer to Tudisca and colleagues[8]), but it goes without saying that they are expensive, require a large interdisciplinary support staff, and represent a significant ongoing financial commitment.

RATIONALE FOR COMBINING PET WITH MR FOR CAROTID PLAQUE IMAGING

MR offers multiple key advantages to CT when imaging the carotid arteries, supporting PET/MR as the hybrid system of choice for molecular imaging of these regions. Although previously this was tempered by problems in acquiring and quantifying the PET data, recent technological advances have ensured that solutions to these issues have largely been found. The potential advantages of PET/MR imaging compared with PET/CT fall into several domains (Table 1).

Carotid Angiography

In terms of plaque visualization and segmentation, although CT is able to achieve submillimeter spatial resolution in combination with a very short acquisition time, soft tissue contrast is poor and 1-dimensional (ie, plaque segmentation is based purely on photon attenuation). CT carotid imaging is also hampered by blooming artifact from dense calcification. Both these factors make visualization of the luminal and adventitial borders for region of interest analysis difficult. By comparison, MR with black-blood imaging offers superior soft tissue detail that provides excellent contrast at the adventitial and luminal borders (see Fig. 1). Iodinated contrast enhancement does improve visualization on CT but may be contraindicated in renal failure or with previous contrast reactions and does nothing to abrogate blooming from calcium. Although MR angiography with gadolinium remains a concern in patients with advanced renal failure, alternative technique can be performed

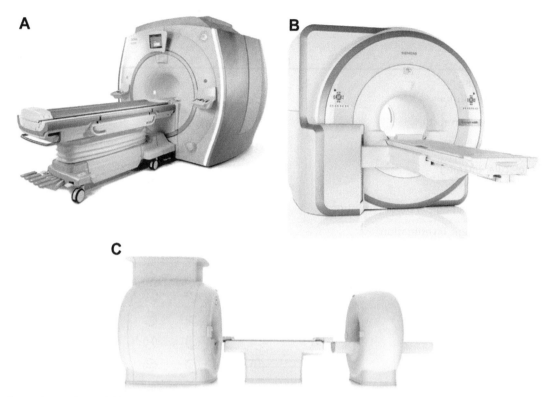

Fig. 1. Currently available systems. Three examples of available PET/MR systems. Only the Siemens and GE systems are truly hybrid permitting synchronous imaging. (*A*) GE Signa PET/MR. (*B*) Siemens Biograph mMR. (*C*) Philips Ingenuity TF PET/MR (this system only permits sequential imaging. The patient needs to be transferred between MR imaging and PET on a dedicated system that minimizes patient movement between scans).

safely in these patients either via the use of alternative contrast agents (iron oxide nanoparticles[9]) or using standard time of flight (TOF) MR sequences.

Limitations of Histologic Validation and Cross Validation with MR Imaging

A standard and productive model for cardiovascular PET research has been to scan patients just before carotid endarterectomy (CEA). The excised plaque can then be collected and used to validate the PET radiotracer in question using histologic[10–12] or even gene expression techniques.[13] This model is, however, becoming difficult to deliver as a result of the increasing impetus to intervene expeditiously on patients with symptomatic carotid stenosis[14–16] and a greater reluctance to intervene on asymptomatic lesions.[17] A further consideration is that the role of carotid artery stenting may increase,[16,18,19] reducing the role of endarterectomy and the opportunity to use this valuable approach. Histologic examination also has its limitations: patients undergoing endarterectomy are invariably at the severe end of the

disease spectrum, biasing such studies against the earlier phases of the condition. Moreover, the processing of the heterogeneous and calcified necrotic tissue that emerges from surgery is notoriously difficult, and further complicated by trauma to the specimen at the time of its excision. Finally, histologic sampling is necessarily limited to small regions of the plaque and thus prone to sampling bias. Critically, these regions do not include the outer tunica media and tunica adventitia of the carotid artery (because of the way the plaque is excised), tissues that are increasing recognized to play central roles in atherogenesis.[20]

Alternative methods of validating novel PET radiotracers and imaging techniques are therefore required. Because of the limitations previously discussed, CT is not able to adequately resolve carotid plaque for detailed compositional and phenotypic analysis. By contrast, MR provides much greater information with respect to plaque morphology, with the ability to identify multiple key plaque characteristics, including an intact or ruptured fibrous cap, a necrotic lipid-rich core, intraplaque hemorrhage, thrombus, intraplaque neovascularization, macrophage infiltration,

Table 1
Strengths and weaknesses of PET, computed tomography (CT), MR imaging, and combined modalities

	MR Imaging	CT	PET	PET/CT	PET/MR
Anatomic imaging					
Spatial resolution	☺	☺	☹	☺	☺
Soft tissue contrast	☺	☹	—	☹	☺
Versatility	☺	😐	☺	😐	☺
Molecular imaging					
Sensitivity	😐	☹	☺	☺	☺
Dynamic imaging/temporal resolution	☺	😐	😐	😐	☺
Pharmacologic investigation	😐	☹	☺	☺	☺
Feasibility					
Complexity	😐	☺	☹	☹	☹
Scanning time	☹	☺	😐	😐	☹
Ease of scheduling	😐	☺	☹	😐	☹
Cost	😐	☺	☹	☹	☹
Patient acceptability	😐	☺	😐	😐	?
Other					
Research potential	☺	😐	☺	☺	☺
Translatability	😐	☺	☹	☹	☹
Potential for PET data motion correction	☺	☹	☹	☹	☺
Quality of attenuation correction	😐	☺	—	☺	😐
Susceptibility to artifact/variability	☹	☺	😐	😐	☹

☺ = favorable, 😐 = neutral, ☹ = unfavorable.

biomechanical stress, and others (**Fig. 2**) (a recent review by Makris and colleagues is recommended[21]). Although obviously not as "definitive" as histology, MR is an excellent alternative and complementary technique with the key advantage that plaques can be assessed in situ at multiple stages in their development. MR also permits serial and 3-dimensional volumetric assessment of the carotid artery in its entirety, including the layers missed with histologic validation. On this basis, hybrid PET/MR offers the opportunity to cross validate a wide range of novel PET tracers, providing mechanistic information beyond simple anatomic coregistration (**Table 2**).

Indeed, the feasibility of this approach has already been demonstrated in several clinical studies using sequentially acquired [18F]-FDG PET/CT and MR,[22–31] studies that would have been greatly simplified by a hybrid system.

Moreover, 2 elegant preclinical studies have recently been published in this domain, the first cross-validating a fibrin-targeted probe (EP-2104R)[32] and the second comparing ultrasmall superparamagnetic iron oxide–enhanced MR with [18F]-FDG as alternative markers of plaque inflammation. The availability of such preclinical PET/MR systems, capable of scanning human specimens ex vivo and small animals in vivo, is likely to accelerate the development and clinical translation of this imaging technique.

Simultaneous Scanning and Motion Correction

CT and PET datasets are necessarily acquired sequentially and are frequently either degraded if not frankly spoiled by movement. The nature of this movement can either be *intrinsic* (ie, cardiac

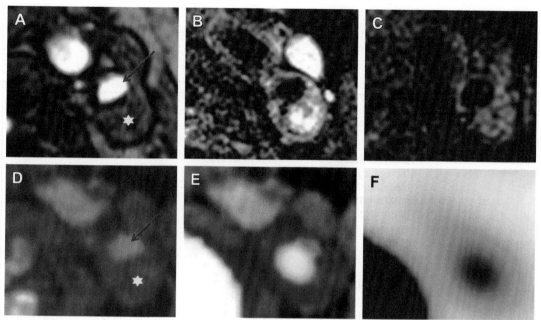

Fig. 2. Example of atheromatous carotid plaque on multicontrast MR (3T) and [18F]-fluoride PET/CT. Images are all from the same left proximal internal carotid artery (ICA) in a neurologically symptomatic patient. The red arrow denotes the lumen of the ICA and the yellow star denotes the hemorrhagic plaque. (*A*) Axial TOF MR angiogram. (*B*) T2-weighted image. (*C*) T1-weighted image. (*D*) CT carotid angiogram. (*E*) Fused PET/CT. (*F*) [18F]-fluoride PET. (*Data from* authors' institution.)

motion, respiratory motion, swallowing, hollow viscus peristalsis) or *extrinsic* (ie, an uncomfortable patient who squirms or shifts position). The ability to simultaneously acquire PET and MR data is a critical advantage that modern hybrid PET/MR systems hold. This opens up the possibility of accurate motion correction with huge potential benefits for imaging of the coronary arteries and the myocardium in addition to the carotids (**Fig. 3**).

With PET/CT, the only options for tackling motion relate either to measures aimed at controlling such movement (ie, asking patients to lie still, ensuring their comfort, or using neck collars and blocks to provide gentle restraint) or to postprocessing the PET data in an attempt to correct for it. Postprocessing may involve either registration (manual or automated, rigid or nonrigid) that is limited by poor PET spatial resolution (~4.5–5 mm) and a lack of fiducial landmarks or, in the case of cardiac and respiratory motion, retrospective gating. Retrospective gating is accomplished by acquiring PET data in list mode (analogous to using a video camera instead of a photographic camera) and simultaneously acquiring electrocardiogram and respiratory cycle data. This permits retrospective exclusion of PET data acquired during portions of the cardiac and/or respiratory cycle where the region of interest is unacceptably mobile. Unfortunately, discarding most PET events with retrospective gating has a major

negative impact on the signal-to-noise ratio (SNR) that can presently only be abrogated by increasing radiotracer dose or patient bed-times. Additionally, this retrospective approach does not typically attempt to correct for the effects of patient motion when constructing the attenuation correction maps, leading to the potential for systematic biases in PET quantification.

Hybrid PET/MR can permit improved retrospective gating either by directly measuring organ location (eg, by using a diaphragmatic navigator) or far more elegantly, by obtaining continuous and synchronous MR and PET data. Indeed, the latter approach offers the theoretic and enticing possibility of correcting for both intrinsic and extrinsic movement without having to discard any emission data. Not only would this significantly enhance image quality by minimizing motion blur and improving SNR, it would also have major cost implications, as scanning times could be reduced allowing more patients to be scanned in a given scanning session or production run on the cyclotron. Ultimately, such economic factors could prove crucial in translating cardiovascular PET imaging into the clinical environment.

Robust motion correction using PET/MR might also make accurate dynamic PET imaging of moving tissues a possibility. The general principle of MR-based motion correction involves recording

Table 2
Examples of molecular and structural PET and MR imaging targets in carotid atherosclerosis: complementarity and potential for cross validation

Process	Target	PET Radiotracer	MR Technique (Molecular or Structural)
Inflammation/cell recruitment	VCAM-1	—	VCAM-1-BP + USPIO[53] VCAM-1-BP + Gd[54]
	ICAM-1	—	ICAM-1 ligand + MPIO[55]
	Glycolysis	[18F]-FDG[10,56]	—
	TSPO receptor	[11C]-PK11195[11]	—
	Macrophage scavenger receptor	[124I]-CD86-Fc[57]	SR-A1 ligand + USPIO[58]
	Somatostatin Receptor 2	[68Ga]-DOTATATE[59]	—
	Phagocytosis	—	Unconjugated USPIO[60]
		—	Emulsified perfluorocarbons[39]
Matrix and proteinases	MMP	Various[61]	P947 + Gd[62]
	Elastin	—	BMS753951 + Gd[63]
Lipid-rich core	Lipid pool	—	LDL particles + Gd[64]
	Hypoxic cells	[18F]-FMISO[65] [18F]-FDG[66]	—
Cell death	Phosphatidylserine	—	Phosphatidylserine targeting peptide + Gd[67]
	Caspase 3 activity	[18F]-CP18[68]	
Angiogenesis	$\alpha_v\beta_3$-integrins	[18F]-galacto-RGD[69]	RGD-peptide mimetic + Gd[70]
	Neovessels	—	DCE-MR imaging
Intraplaque hemorrhage	Methemoglobin	—	Multicontrast MR imaging[71,72]
Calcification process	Active micro-calcification	[18F]-Fluoride[12]	—
Thrombosis	Fibrin	[64Cu]-EP-2104R[32] [64Cu]-FPB7[74]	EP-2104R + Gd[32,73] —

Abbreviations: BP, binding protein; DCE, delayed contrast enhancement; FMISO, fluoromisonidazole; Gd, gadolinium; ICAM, intercellular adhesion molecule; LDL, low-density lipoprotein; MMP, matrix metalloproteinase; TSPO, translocator protein; USPIO, ultrasmall superparamagnetic iron oxide; VCAM, vascular cell adhesion molecule.

the displacements of the relevant anatomy in space and time (ie, in 4 dimensions) using MR and then using these data to either retrospectively "deconvolve" the reconstructed and time-binned PET data, or better still, to achieve this prospectively by including the 4-dimensional MR data in the reconstruction algorithm. In principle, the same methods also may be used to reduce the impact of movement on attenuation correction, thus further improving data quality. It is beyond the scope of this review to discuss these methods in detail but the reader is referred to excellent articles by Catana[33] and Petibon and colleagues.[34,35] Although the biggest impact of these advances may well apply to PET imaging of the heart, such motion correction also will be of direct relevance to carotid imaging. Indeed, little can presently be done to control for small extrinsic movements or the effects of swallowing and jaw movement, which can have a major impact on PET quantification in small-volume carotid plaques.

Radiation Exposure, Serial Imaging, and Multiprocess Imaging

One of the major attractions of PET is that it is able to resolve specific biological pathways and physiologic activity in vivo with exquisite sensitivity and without disturbing the subjects' biology. This had led to a new model for phase 2 clinical trials in which novel pharmacologic agents are tested for biological efficacy in vivo using serial PET examinations, before proceeding to large and expensive phase 3 trials. Indeed, we successfully used this approach in the recent dal-PLAQUE study[5] and are currently conducting several other similar studies in our institutions.[36,37] One of the major concerns relating to this approach is the large cumulative dose of radiation that may accrue with multiple PET/CT examinations. The ability to remove CT from the equation will go a long way to allaying anxiety on this front, and in opening up the possibility of examining disease activity at 3

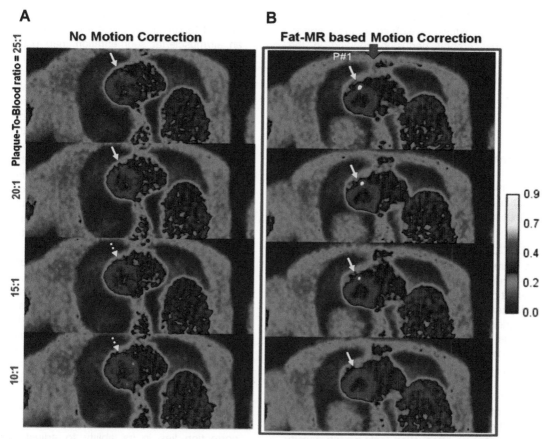

Fig. 3. The potential for motion correction using PET/MR. Each image is the same [18F]-FDG PET slice (with simulated "hot plaque") reconstructed with and without motion correction using a method based on fat segmentation. A variety of target-to-blood activity ratios are demonstrated. Motion correction can be clearly seen to significantly improve the ability to resolve the increased intraplaque uptake (*yellow arrows*). (*Data from* Petibon Y, Fakhri El G, Nezafat R, et al. Towards coronary plaque imaging using simultaneous PET-MR: a simulation study. Phys Med Biol 2014;59(5):1203–22; with permission.)

or 4 different time points, or investigating several disease processes simultaneously.

Potential for Multiprocess Imaging and PET Sensitivity and Specificity

As well as permitting cross validation, PET/MR offers the opportunity to combine the functional information of PET with emerging molecular MR techniques, rendering true multimodality, multiprocess imaging possible. This would allow for studies, incorporating a wide array of both PET and MR techniques, capable of investigating multiple pathologic processes simultaneously. A complete discussion of emerging molecular MR techniques is beyond the scope of this review, but includes the design of specific molecular MR tracers incorporating either paramagnetic (gadolinium) or superparamagnetic (coated iron oxide nanoparticles) reporters (see **Table 2**), dual-tuned coils to enable simultaneous [1H] and [19F]

imaging of perfluorocarbon tracers,[38,39] MR spectroscopy,[40] and hyperpolarized MR[41] (indeed, the concept of "HyperPET" has already entered the lexicon[42]). The opportunity also exists to design imaging nanoparticles with reporters for both PET and MR. Although promising, several of these MR techniques are currently limited either by the nonlinearity of reporter accumulation and signal change or by low sensitivity. Indeed, PET is generally quoted to be 3 to 4 orders of magnitude more sensitive than MR, which of course is a key attraction of PET.

Versatility and Concurrent Imaging of Other Relevant Organ Systems

MR imaging is currently the gold standard technique for imaging the brain, and many of the radiotracers of interest in the carotid also will be of interest in the brain (eg, [18F]-FDG). The ability to do a full simultaneous vasculo-cerebral PET/MR assessment using multiple complementary sequences (eg, diffusion-weighted imaging abnormalities or cerebral perfusion imaging in the context of a carotid stenosis) and PET acquisitions will therefore be of major interest to stroke and vasculopathy researchers, especially as it will not involve additional radiation exposure.

CURRENT LIMITATIONS OF HYBRID PET/MR

As well as the usual contraindications to MR imaging, such as the presence of pacemakers and certain metallic implants, there are several areas of actual and potential limitation to hybrid PET/MR that merit consideration.

Attenuation Correction

The paired photons generated by positron/electron annihilation are variably attenuated by different body tissues and by scanner components (table, head/neck stabilizers). To gain an accurate estimation of tracer distribution, photon attenuation must be adjusted for. CT is suited to this, as it itself directly measures attenuation (ie, electron density). Moreover, it is easy to convert 80 to 140 keV x-ray photon attenuation values into linear attenuation coefficients (LAC) at the 511-keV annihilation photon level. These can then be used to adjust the PET data. By contrast, MR does not directly measure attenuation (only proton density and T1/T2/T2* tissue properties) and, as such, finding new ways of achieving accurate attenuation correction represents perhaps the greatest current challenge in hybrid PET/MR.

Several approaches to this problem have been investigated. A detailed description is not within the purview of this article, but excellent reviews of the challenges and potential solutions by Boellaard and Quick,[43] Quick,[44] and Boss and colleagues[45] are available. Several issues are, however, worthy of consideration:

- Attenuation by scanner components is accounted for by either integrating fixed and rigid components with known attenuation properties (ie, the patient table and spinal coils or head coils) into the reconstruction algorithm or, for mobile components (chest coils, breast coils), using versions specifically designed to be minimally attenuating.
- Body tissue is highly heterogeneous and mobile, making it difficult to generate a valid MR-based attenuation map. One approach is to use atlases of attenuation data[43,46] derived from archived CT data (for example) but these require off-line registration and do not work if subject anatomy is abnormal (eg, in the

context of implants, previous surgery). The favored technique at present is to generate an air/muscle/fat segmentation map based on 3-dimensional Dixon-VIBE (volume interpolated breath hold examination) sequences and to assign a tissue relevant LAC (derived from CT) to the MR voxels (Fig. 4). This Dixon technique is limited as it cannot segment bone separately and as such there is evidence that uptake in bone and surrounding tissue may be systematically underestimated.[47] New ultrashort echo time (UTE) or zero-echo time (ZTE) sequences capable of rendering bone and generating "pseudo-CT" attenuation maps are promising but are limited by small fields-of-view (FOV) and long acquisition times, and remain in development.[48,49]

- The limited FOV associated with MR can also be problematic for attenuation correction, as tissue lying outside the FOV will not be accounted for in the attenuation map. This is particularly the case for bony tissue in the arms and more generally in obese subjects (see Fig. 4), although these effects can be abrogated somewhat using an MR sequence called HUGE (homogenization using gradient enhancement).[50]
- The one key area in which MR holds a potential advantage over CT for attenuation correction lies in its ability to adjust for motion. CT attenuation maps are not necessarily ideal, as there is an unavoidable spatial and temporal mismatch between CT and PET. As discussed, MR has the potential to provide a 4-dimensional attenuation correction map, adjusting for the effects of motion and improving the accuracy of PET quantification.

In terms of carotid imaging, the most significant concern that will need to be addressed is that the Dixon-based segmentation attenuation maps, as implemented on current systems, assign bone or calcification an inappropriately low LAC (that of soft tissue). As a consequence, PET/MR may systematically underestimate radiotracer uptake in heavily calcified vessels. Although the UTE sequences described previously may go some way to addressing this problem, further work is required to assess the true impact of this effect.

Cost and Logistics

A significant obstacle to the widespread uptake of PET/MR will be the associated costs and logistical challenges. As well as the formidable investment in hardware and maintenance overheads, personnel costs are high given the requirement for a

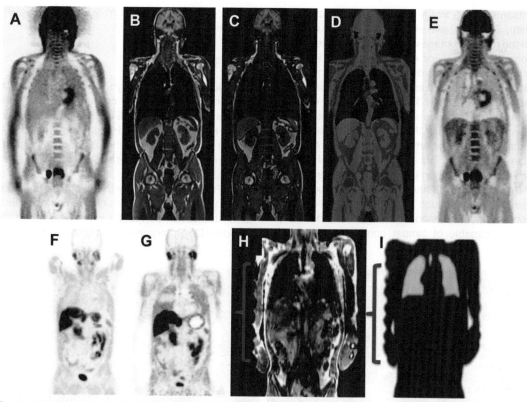

Fig. 4. Attenuation correction and PET/MR. The upper panel shows the method for obtaining an attenuation map using MR imaging. (*A*) The uncorrected PET. (*B, C*) The Dixon sequence images used to generate the soft tissue segmentation map (*D*). Different tissue groups are then assigned attenuation coefficients (although bone is assigned a soft tissue value by this method). A corrected PET image can then be generated (*E*). The lower panel shows 2 sources of artifact in PET/MR imaging. On the left, (*F*) and (*G*) are of the same patient imaged by [18F]-FDG PET/CT and PET/MR, respectively. The PET/MR attenuation correction results in an overestimation of lung activity. (*H*) and (*I*) show a Dixon sequence and the resulting MR-based attenuation correction map, respectively. The truncation artifact on MR (*red bracket*) is translated to the attenuation correction map. (*From* Boellaard R, Quick HH. Current image acquisition options in PET/MR. Semin Nucl Med 2015;45(3):192–200; with permission.)

close-knit multidisciplinary team of nuclear medicine physicians, physicists, image analysis specialists, radiologists, oncologists, vascular surgeons, radiographers, radio-chemists, neurologists, cardiologists, and others. Maintaining grant funding in the medium to long-term to sustain such ventures will be challenging and likely to require close cooperation with industry. These costs must of course be balanced against the rich vein of research work that will be facilitated and it should also be recalled that significant advances in MR technology, unlike CT, rarely require replacement of the magnet or major components, but rather rely on relatively inexpensive developments in software sequences and body coils.

In terms of logistics, PET/CT is already highly challenging as a result of the mandatory pharmacologic and radiation regulations, as well as the issues surrounding scheduling of the scans in synchronization with the activity of the cyclotron.

Adding the complexity of MR and magnetic field safety will certainly not diminish this burden.

Standardization and Artifact Susceptibility

The ability of MR to induce and measure a wide variety of different effects on a multitude of tissues (merely by altering MR sequences and coils) confers on it great versatility. This is at once a singular strength and a significant weakness. Variation between scanning protocols, sequences, contrast agents, magnets, coils, manufacturers, and coverage mean that it is difficult to standardize scanning between centers, rendering robust comparisons difficult. Moving forward it will be essential to achieve consensus on the optimal methods for assessing anatomy, function, and molecular information so that multicenter imaging studies will be feasible.

The intrinsic properties of MR also render it highly susceptible to sources of potential artifact (ie, implants, flow, image geometry, and chemical shift). This can have an adverse impact not only on the resultant images but also on the attenuation correction maps. For example, metallic implants will create signal voids on standard sequences, rendering the correct assignation of LAC very difficult if not impossible. This is of particular concern in the carotid arteries with the likely future expansion of endovascular therapy and the insertion of metallic stents. The artifact associated with these stents will directly impact on the tissue of interest and will be an important issue to resolve both in the carotid and coronary vasculature. Importantly, new sequences, such as MAVRIC (multi-acquisition variable-resonance image combination), appear capable of almost completely reversing

metal-related artifact and may ultimately provide a solution.[45]

PUBLISHED RESEARCH

One recent study using hybrid PET/MR of the carotid arteries by Ripa and colleagues[51] compared the results of [18F]-FDG PET/MR and PET/CT analysis of the carotid arteries in 6 patients with chronic human immunodeficiency virus infection, a group at high risk of atherosclerosis. Subjects were fasted as standard and given a 400-MBq does of [18F]-FDG. PET/MR scanning (Siemens Biograph mMR) was performed 2 hours after isotope injection. Attenuation correction was achieved by the standard Dixon segmentation technique described

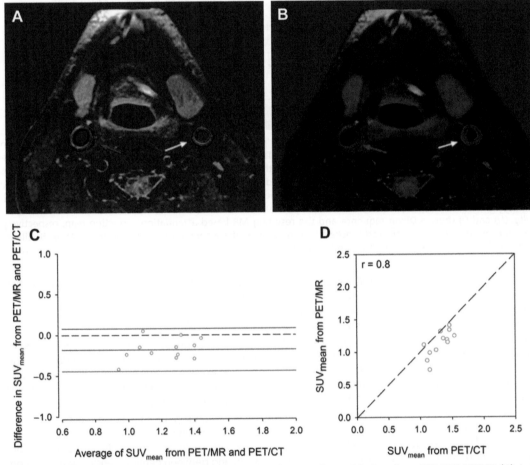

Fig. 5. Example of dedicated carotid 18F-FDG PET/MR and comparison with data from 18F-FDG PET/CT. (A) Axial section through the neck using a black-blood, T1-weighted, turbo spin-echo sequence with fat suppression. The regions of interest drawn by the authors are also on the image. (B) Fused PET and MR image data (MR attenuation map generated using the standard Dixon water-fat sequence described in the text). (C, D) Bland-Altman and scatter plots, respectively, for mean SUV as assessed by PET/MR versus PET/CT. As expected, there is a small but systematic underestimation of uptake with PET/MR compared with PET/CT. Red arrows point to the carotid arteries. (From Ripa RS, Knudsen A, Hag AMF, et al. Feasibility of simultaneous PET/MR of the carotid artery: first clinical experience and comparison to PET/CT. Am J Nucl Med Mol Imaging 2013;3(4):361–71; with permission.)

previously. TOF angiography and axial stacks incorporating standard 2-dimensional black-blood and fat-suppressed T1-weighted and T2-weighted high-resolution sequences were obtained. Following the PET/MR, PET/CT imaging was performed, alongside contrast angiography. Image analysis was performed on both the PET/MR and PET/CT data sets and comparisons made between tracer activity in the carotids measured using the standardized uptake value (SUV_{mean} and SUV_{max}). The key findings were that 18F-FDG uptake (whole-vessel SUV_{mean}) as assayed by the 2 hybrid systems was very similar with correlation coefficients of $r = 0.8$ and Bland-Altman analysis showing a mean bias of -0.2 with 95% limits of agreement of -0.4 to 0.1 (Fig. 5). This slight systematic underestimation by PET/MR is not unexpected given the underestimation of bone density by the MR Dixon-based method for attenuation correction and is consistent with the data in nonatherosclerotic tissue. This study therefore demonstrated the feasibility of PET/MR in the carotids and looks set to herald a new era of studies investigating the utility of this novel imaging approach. These include the PESA study,[52] a prospective observational cohort study of 4000 employees at the Santander Bank Headquarters in Madrid, Spain. Subjects aged between 40 and 54 will be recruited and undergo extensive baseline phenotyping including standard clinical assessment, a variety of blood analyses, and imaging analysis. A subset of 1300 patients with documented carotid plaque on duplex examination will undergo advanced imaging with [18F]-FDG PET/MR. Follow-up will be for 6 years and will help establish whether PET/MR has a role in predicting future adverse cardiovascular events.

SUMMARY

This review has focused on the potential advantages and limitations of hybrid PET/MR in assessing carotid atherosclerotic disease. By harnessing the versatility and soft tissue imaging capabilities of MR imaging alongside the unmatched sensitivity and biomolecular flexibility of PET, the potential to provide detailed multiparametric plaque characterization in the carotid arteries is clear. Both these modalities already have a proven track record in vascular imaging and the capability to cross validate one against the other is attractive, particularly in an era in which obtaining good tissue for image validation is becoming more difficult. The ability to acquire simultaneous and dynamic multimodal data is perhaps PET/MR's greatest strength that will be of major interest to researchers investigating

carotid and coronary atherosclerosis alike. In particular, this capability is likely to permit more accurate delineation of regions of interest in the carotids, reduce partial volume effects, and improve our ability to correct for motion without excluding PET counts. The latter has the potential to substantially improve signal to noise and will be useful in improving the efficiency and reducing the costs and radiation exposure associated with vascular PET.

Despite the promise of this exciting and highly complex new technology, the field remains in its infancy and several challenges must be met so as to convince physicians of PET/MR's clinical and translational utility. For now, caution must be exercised in interpreting quantitative PET data based on MR attenuation maps, given that they do not take into consideration bony attenuation and are based on fairly crude and occasionally truncated segmentation maps. The bar to demonstrating cost-effectiveness is also high. The requirement for a large interdisciplinary team, a radiochemistry suite, a major capital investment, and significant overhead costs will mean that currently only a limited number of centers will be able to deliver this platform. Finally, it is worth remembering that despite the encouraging results in cardiovascular PET/CT over the past 13 years, the technique is not routinely used in the clinic. That being said, the advantages of PET/MR are clear, and if the relevant barriers can be overcome, then this imaging modality has the potential to greatly improve our understanding of carotid atherosclerosis and improve patient risk stratification.

REFERENCES

1. Feigin VL, Forouzanfar MH, Krishnamurthi R, et al. Global and regional burden of stroke during 1990-2010: findings from the Global Burden of Disease Study 2010. Lancet 2014;383(9913):245–54.
2. North American Symptomatic Carotid Endarterectomy Trial Collaborators. Beneficial effect of carotid endarterectomy in symptomatic patients with high-grade carotid stenosis. N Engl J Med 1991;325(7): 445–53.
3. Rerkasem K, Rothwell PM. Carotid endarterectomy for symptomatic carotid stenosis. Cochrane Database Syst Rev 2011;(4):CD001081.
4. Buxton DB, Antman M, Danthi N, et al. Report of the National Heart, Lung, and Blood Institute Working Group on the Translation of Cardiovascular Molecular Imaging. Circulation 2011;123(19):2157–63.
5. Fayad ZA, Mani V, Woodward M, et al. Safety and efficacy of dalcetrapib on atherosclerotic disease using novel non-invasive multimodality imaging

(dal-PLAQUE): a randomised clinical trial. Lancet 2011;378(9802):1547–59.

6. Tang TY, Howarth SPS, Miller SR, et al. The ATHEROMA (atorvastatin therapy: effects on reduction of macrophage activity) study. J Am Coll Cardiol 2009;53(22):2039–50.

7. Catana C, Guimaraes AR, Rosen BR. PET and MR imaging: the odd couple or a match made in heaven? J Nucl Med 2013;54(5):815–24.

8. Tudisca C, Nasoodi A, Fraioli F. PET-MRI: nuclear medicine communications. Nucl Med Commun 2015;36(7):666–78.

9. Neuwelt EA, Hamilton BE, Varallyay CG, et al. Ultra-small superparamagnetic iron oxides (USPIOs): a future alternative magnetic resonance (MR) contrast agent for patients at risk for nephrogenic systemic fibrosis (NSF)? Kidney Int 2008;75(5):465–74.

10. Tawakol A, Migrino RQ, Bashian GG, et al. In vivo 18F-fluorodeoxyglucose positron emission tomography imaging provides a noninvasive measure of carotid plaque inflammation in patients. J Am Coll Cardiol 2006;48(9):1818–24.

11. Gaemperli O, Shalhoub J, Owen DRJ, et al. Imaging intraplaque inflammation in carotid atherosclerosis with 11C-PK11195 positron emission tomography/computed tomography. Eur Heart J 2012;33(15):1902–10.

12. Joshi NV, Vesey AT, Williams MC, et al. 18F-fluoride positron emission tomography for identification of ruptured and high-risk coronary atherosclerotic plaques: a prospective clinical trial. Lancet 2014;383(9918):705–13.

13. Pedersen SF, Graebe M, Fisker Hag AM, et al. Gene expression and 18FDG uptake in atherosclerotic carotid plaques. Nucl Med Commun 2010;31(5):423–9.

14. Naylor AR. Occam's razor: intervene early to prevent more strokes! J Vasc Surg 2008;48(4):1053–9.

15. National Collaborating Centre for Chronic Conditions (UK). Stroke: national clinical guideline for diagnosis and initial management of acute stroke and transient ischaemic attack (TIA). London: Royal College of Physicians (UK); 2008.

16. Brott TG, Halperin JL, Abbara S, et al. 2011 ASA/ACCF/AHA/AANN/AANS/ACR/ASNR/CNS/SAIP/SCAI/SIR/SNIS/SVM/SVS guideline on the management of patients with extracranial carotid and vertebral artery disease. J Neurointerv Surg 2011;57(8):e16–94.

17. Abbott AL. Medical (nonsurgical) intervention alone is now best for prevention of stroke associated with asymptomatic severe carotid stenosis: results of a systematic review and analysis. Stroke 2009;40(10):e573–83.

18. Brott TG, editor. CREST-2: The carotid revascularization and medical management for asymptomatic carotid artery stenosis study. Available at: http://www.crest2trial.org/. Accessed April 23, 2015.

19. Bonati LH, Dobson J, Featherstone RL, et al. Long-term outcomes after stenting versus endarterectomy for treatment of symptomatic carotid stenosis: the International Carotid Stenting Study (ICSS) randomised trial. Lancet 2015;385(9967):529–38.

20. Libby P, Hansson GK. Inflammation and immunity in diseases of the arterial tree: players and layers. Circ Res 2015;116(2):307–11.

21. Makris GC, Teng Z, Patterson AJ, et al. Advances in MR imaging for the evaluation of carotid atherosclerosis. Br J Radiol 2015;88(1052):20140282.

22. Davies JR, Rudd JHF, Fryer TD, et al. Identification of culprit lesions after transient ischemic attack by combined 18F fluorodeoxyglucose positron-emission tomography and high-resolution magnetic resonance imaging. Stroke 2005;36(12):2642–7.

23. Tang TY, Moustafa RR, Howarth SP, et al. Combined PET-FDG and USPIO-enhanced MR imaging in patients with symptomatic moderate carotid artery stenosis. Eur J Vasc Endovasc Surg 2008;36(1):53–5.

24. Izquierdo-Garcia D, Davies JR, Graves MJ, et al. Comparison of methods for magnetic resonance-guided [18-F]fluorodeoxyglucose positron emission tomography in human carotid arteries: reproducibility, partial volume correction, and correlation between methods. Stroke 2008;40(1):86–93.

25. Silvera SS, Aidi HE, Rudd JHF, et al. Multimodality imaging of atherosclerotic plaque activity and composition using FDG-PET/CT and MRI in carotid and femoral arteries. Atherosclerosis 2009;207(1):139–43.

26. Kwee RM, Teule GJJ, van Oostenbrugge RJ, et al. Multimodality imaging of carotid artery plaques: 18F-fluoro-2-deoxyglucose positron emission tomography, computed tomography, and magnetic resonance imaging. Stroke 2009;40(12):3718–24.

27. Calcagno C, Ramachandran S, Izquierdo-Garcia D, et al. The complementary roles of dynamic contrast-enhanced MRI and 18F-fluorodeoxyglucose PET/CT for imaging of carotid atherosclerosis. Eur J Nucl Med Mol Imaging 2013;40(12):1884–93.

28. Mani V, Woodward M, Samber D, et al. Predictors of change in carotid atherosclerotic plaque inflammation and burden as measured by 18-FDG-PET and MRI, respectively, in the dal-PLAQUE study. Int J Cardiovasc Imaging 2014;30(3):571–82.

29. Truijman MTB, Kwee RM, van Hoof RHM, et al. Combined 18F-FDG PET-CT and DCE-MRI to assess inflammation and microvascularization in atherosclerotic plaques. Stroke 2013;44(12):3568–70.

30. Saito H, Kuroda S, Hirata K, et al. Validity of dual MRI and F-FDG PET imaging in predicting vulnerable and inflamed carotid plaque. Cerebrovasc Dis 2013;35(4):370–7.

31. Lei-xing X, Jing-jing G, Jing-xue N, et al. Combined application of 18F-fluorodeoxyglucose positron

emission tomography/computed tomography and magnetic resonance imaging in early diagnosis of vulnerable carotid atherosclerotic plaques. J Int Med Res 2014;42(1):213–23.

32. Uppal R, Catana C, Ay I, et al. Bimodal thrombus imaging: simultaneous PET/MR imaging with a fibrin-targeted dual PET/MR Probe—feasibility study in rat model. Radiology 2011;258(3):812–20.

33. Catana C. Motion correction options in PET/MRI. Semin Nucl Med 2015;45(3):212–23.

34. Petibon Y, Ouyang J, Zhu X, et al. Cardiac motion compensation and resolution modeling in simultaneous PET-MR: a cardiac lesion detection study. Phys Med Biol 2013;58(7):2085–102.

35. Petibon Y, Fakhri El G, Nezafat R, et al. Towards coronary plaque imaging using simultaneous PET-MR: a simulation study. Phys Med Biol 2014;59(5): 1203–22.

36. DIAMOND. Dual antiplatelet therapy to reduce myocardial injury. Available at: http://clinicaltrials. gov/ct2/show/NCT02110303. Accessed April 24, 2015.

37. SALTIRE II Study. Investigating the effect of drugs used to treat osteoporosis on the progression of calcific aortic stenosis. Available at: http://clinicaltrials.gov/ct2/show/NCT02132026. Accessed April 24, 2015.

38. Ruiz-Cabello J, Barnett BP, Bottomley PA, et al. Fluorine (19F) MRS and MRI in biomedicine. NMR Biomed 2010;24(2):114–29.

39. Temme S, Bönner F, Schrader J, et al. 19F magnetic resonance imaging of endogenous macrophages in inflammation. Wiley Interdiscip Rev Nanomed Nanobiotechnol 2012;4(3):329–43.

40. Duivenvoorden R, van Wijk D, Klimas M, et al. Detection of liquid phase cholesteryl ester in carotid atherosclerosis by 1H-MR spectroscopy in humans. JACC Cardiovasc Imaging 2013;6(12):1277–84.

41. Bhattacharya P, Chekmenev EY, Reynolds WF, et al. Parahydrogen-induced polarization (PHIP) hyperpolarized MR receptor imaging in vivo: a pilot study of 13C imaging of atheroma in mice. NMR Biomed 2011;24(8):1023–8.

42. Ripa RS, Kjaer A. Imaging atherosclerosis with hybrid positron emission tomography/magnetic resonance imaging. Biomed Res Int 2015; 2015(12):1–8.

43. Boellaard R, Quick HH. Current image acquisition options in PET/MR. Semin Nucl Med 2015;45(3): 192–200.

44. Quick HH. Integrated PET/MR. J Magn Reson Imaging 2013;39(2):243–58.

45. Boss A, Weiger M, Wiesinger F. Future image acquisition trends for PET/MRI. Semin Nucl Med 2015; 45(3):201–11.

46. Naeger DM, Behr SC. PET/MR imaging: current and future applications for cardiovascular disease. Magn Reson Imaging Clin N Am 2015;23(1):95–103.

47. Samarin A, Burger C, Wollenweber SD, et al. PET/MR imaging of bone lesions–implications for PET quantification from imperfect attenuation correction. Eur J Nucl Med Mol Imaging 2012;39(7): 1154–60.

48. Waldman A, Rees JH, Brock CS, et al. MRI of the brain with ultra-short echo-time pulse sequences. Neuroradiology 2003;45(12):887–92.

49. Catana C, van der Kouwe A, Benner T, et al. Toward implementing an MRI-based PET attenuation-correction method for neurologic studies on the MR-PET brain prototype. J Nucl Med 2010;51(9): 1431–8.

50. Blumhagen JO, Ladebeck R, Fenchel M, et al. MR-based field-of-view extension in MR/PET: B0 homogenization using gradient enhancement (HUGE). Magn Reson Med 2013;70(4):1047–57.

51. Ripa RS, Knudsen A, Hag AMF, et al. Feasibility of simultaneous PET/MR of the carotid artery: first clinical experience and comparison to PET/CT. Am J Nucl Med Mol Imaging 2013;3(4):361–71.

52. Fernández-Ortiz A, Jiménez-Borreguero LJ, Peñalvo JL, et al. The progression and early detection of subclinical atherosclerosis (PESA) study: rationale and design. Am Heart J 2013;166(6):990–8.

53. Michalska M, Machtoub L, Manthey HD, et al. Visualization of vascular inflammation in the atherosclerotic mouse by ultrasmall superparamagnetic iron oxide vascular cell adhesion molecule-1-specific nanoparticles. Arterioscler Thromb Vasc Biol 2012; 32(10):2350–7.

54. Burtea C, Laurent S, Port M, et al. Magnetic resonance molecular imaging of vascular cell adhesion molecule-1 expression in inflammatory lesions using a peptide-vectorized paramagnetic imaging probe. J Med Chem 2009;52(15):4725–42.

55. Deddens LH, van Tilborg GAF, van der Toorn A, et al. MRI of ICAM-1 upregulation after stroke: the importance of choosing the appropriate target-specific particulate contrast agent. Mol Imaging Biol 2013;15(4):411–22.

56. Rudd JHF. Imaging atherosclerotic plaque inflammation with [18F]-fluorodeoxyglucose positron emission tomography. Circulation 2002;105(23): 2708–11.

57. Langer HF, Haubner R, Pichler BJ, et al. Radionuclide imaging: a molecular key to the atherosclerotic plaque. J Am Coll Cardiol 2008;52(1):1–12.

58. Segers FME, Adel den B, Bot I, et al. Scavenger receptor-AI-targeted iron oxide nanoparticles for in vivo MRI detection of atherosclerotic lesions. Arterioscler Thromb Vasc Biol 2013;33(8):1812–9.

59. Rominger A, Saam T, Vogl E, et al. In vivo imaging of macrophage activity in the coronary arteries using 68Ga-DOTATATE PET/CT: correlation with coronary calcium burden and risk factors. J Nucl Med 2010; 51(2):193–7.

60. Stirrat C, Vesey A, McBride O, et al. Ultra-small superparamagnetic particles of iron oxide in magnetic resonance imaging of cardiovascular disease. J Vasc Diagn 2014;2:99–112.

61. Hermann S, Starsichova A, Waschkau B, et al. Non-FDG imaging of atherosclerosis: will imaging of MMPs assess plaque vulnerability? J Nucl Cardiol 2012;19(3):609–17.

62. Amirbekian V, Aguinaldo JGS, Amirbekian S, et al. Atherosclerosis and matrix metalloproteinases: experimental molecular MR imaging in vivo. Radiology 2009;251(2):429–38.

63. Makowski MR, Wiethoff AJ, Blume U, et al. Assessment of atherosclerotic plaque burden with an elastin-specific magnetic resonance contrast agent. Nat Med 2011;17(3):383–8.

64. Lowell AN, Qiao H, Liu T, et al. Functionalized low-density lipoprotein nanoparticles for in vivo enhancement of atherosclerosis on magnetic resonance images. Bioconjug Chem 2012;23(11):2313–9.

65. Mateo J, Izquierdo-Garcia D, Badimon JJ, et al. Noninvasive assessment of hypoxia in rabbit advanced atherosclerosis using 18F-fluoromisonidazole positron emission tomographic imaging. Circ Cardiovasc Imaging 2014;7(2):312–20.

66. Folco EJ, Sheikine Y, Rocha VZ, et al. Hypoxia but not inflammation augments glucose uptake in human macrophages. J Am Coll Cardiol 2011;58(6):603–14.

67. Burtea C, Laurent S, Lancelot E, et al. Peptidic targeting of phosphatidylserine for the MRI detection of apoptosis in atherosclerotic plaques. Mol Pharm 2009;6(6):1903–19.

68. Su H, Chen G, Gangadharmath U, et al. Evaluation of [(18)F]-CP18 as a PET imaging tracer for apoptosis. Mol Imaging Biol 2013;15(6):739–47.

69. Stirrat C, Vesey A, McBride O, et al. Ultra-small superparamagnetic particles of iron oxide in magnetic resonance imaging of cardiovascular disease. JCMG 2014;7(2):178–87.

70. Winter PM, Morawski AM, Caruthers SD, et al. Molecular imaging of angiogenesis in early-stage atherosclerosis with alpha(v)beta3-integrin-targeted nanoparticles. Circulation 2003;108(18):2270–4.

71. Chu B, Kampschulte A, Ferguson MS, et al. Hemorrhage in the atherosclerotic carotid plaque: a high-resolution MRI study. Stroke 2004;35(5):1079–84.

72. Hosseini AA, Kandiyil N, MacSweeney STS, et al. Carotid plaque hemorrhage on magnetic resonance imaging strongly predicts recurrent ischemia and stroke. Ann Neurol 2013;73(6):774–84.

73. Spuentrup E, Botnar RM, Wiethoff AJ, et al. MR imaging of thrombi using EP-2104R, a fibrin-specific contrast agent: initial results in patients. Eur Radiol 2008;18(9):1995–2005.

74. Ay I, Blasi F, Rietz TA, et al. In vivo molecular imaging of thrombosis and thrombolysis using a fibrin-binding positron emission tomographic probe. Circ Cardiovasc Imaging 2014;7(4):697–705.

Three-Dimensional Ultrasound of Carotid Plaque

J. David Spence, MD, FRCPC[a],*, Grace Parraga, PhD[b]

KEYWORDS

- Carotid arteries • Atherosclerosis • Plaque • Measurement

KEY POINTS

- Carotid plaque burden can be measured by two-dimensional or 3D ultrasound.
- Measurements of carotid plaque burden are useful in risk assessment, genetic research, and evaluation of new therapies.
- Three-dimensional ultrasound of carotid plaque volume is useful for risk stratification, for evaluating effects of therapy on atherosclerosis, and for managing patients at risk of cardiovascular events, by a strategy that has been called "treating arteries instead of risk factors."

HISTORY OF THE DEVELOPMENT OF THREE-DIMENSIONAL CAROTID PLAQUE ULTRASOUND

Early applications of ultrasound in the carotid arteries focused on using the Doppler shift to evaluate blood velocity and flow disturbances; our group used implanted ultrasound probes in the carotid arteries to assess effects of antihypertensive drugs on blood velocity and pulsatility, using spectral analysis to evaluate flow patterns.[1] The primary clinical use was for diagnosing carotid stenosis[2,3]; we used a primitive device, the Dopscan, to evaluate effects of antihypertensive drugs on turbulence at sites of stenosis.[4] When the author JDS obtained a duplex scanner because it provided spectral analysis to evaluate drug effects on flow disturbances,[5,6] he realized that it was possible to image and begin to quantify carotid plaque burden. It was Maria DiCicco RVT, in the author's laboratory, who told JDS that there was

software in the scanner that could measure plaque area, and first measured carotid total plaque area (TPA), in 1990. After JDS told Jon Wikstrand about it, Wikstrand's group published a method in 1992.[7] Then in 1997, TPA was used to study effects of mental stress on atherosclerosis[8]; Fig. 1 is reproduced from that paper.

In 1994, around the time that Delcker and Diener[9] published their early work on three-dimensional (3D) ultrasound estimation of plaque volume, Dr Aaron Fenster visited JDS at Victoria Hospital in London, Ontario to ask if he would be interested in using the 3D ultrasound system that Fenster had developed for other purposes[10,11] to measure 3D carotid plaque volume. JDS visited his laboratory soon after. Fig. 2 shows perhaps the first measurement of plaque volume, in his right carotid artery in 1994 on Fenster's prototype machine. In 1995 JDS moved to University Hospital and the Robarts Research Institute to collaborate with Dr Fenster, and then later Dr Grace

Disclosure: Dr J.D. Spence has an interest in Vascularis Inc, and has received software from Philips for use in research. Dr J.D. Spence has no other conflict that is relevant to the topic of this article. Dr G. Parraga has no conflicts of interest that are relevant to the topic of this article.

a Stroke Prevention and Atherosclerosis Research Centre, Robarts Research Institute, Western University, London, Ontario N6G 2V4, Canada; b Imaging Research Laboratories, Department of Medical Biophysics, Robarts Research Institute, Western University, London, Ontario, Canada
* Corresponding author.
E-mail address: dspence@robarts.ca

1052-5149/16/$ – see front matter © 2016 Elsevier Inc. All rights reserved.

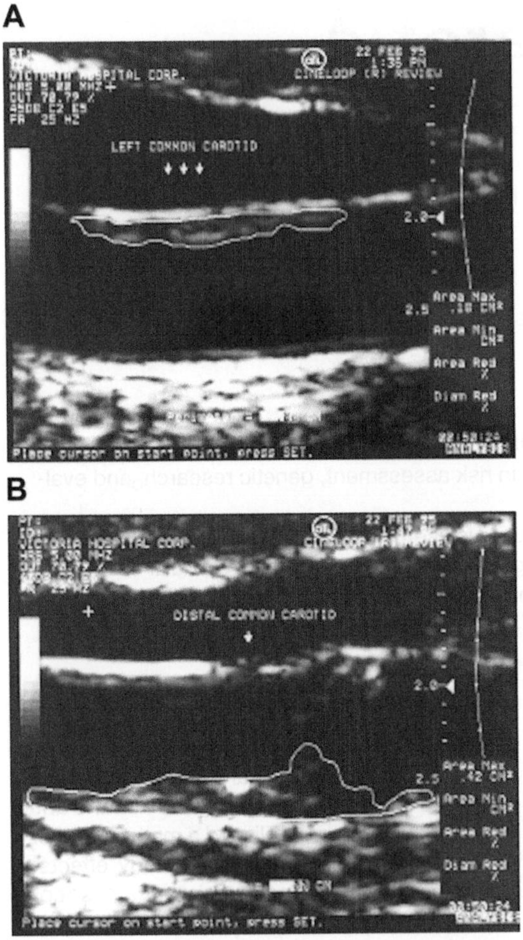

A

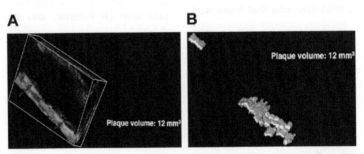

B

Fig. 1. Measurement of plaque area. B-mode ultrasound images of atherosclerotic plaques in the extracranial carotid arteries. (A) A small plaque with an area of 0.18 cm² traced by the trackball in the left common carotid artery. (B) A large plaque with an area of 0.42 cm² in the distal common carotid artery. (*From* Barnett PA, Spence JD, Manuck SB, et al. Psychological stress and the progression of carotid atherosclerosis. J Hypertension 1997;15:51; with permission.)

Parraga, to develop 3D ultrasound of carotid plaque.

Topics discussed in this article include measurement of plaque burden, ulceration, echolucency, and plaque texture.

MEASUREMENT OF PLAQUE BURDEN AND ITS PROGRESSION/REGRESSION

Measurement of carotid intima-media thickness (IMT) had begun around 1985, first in monkeys[12] and then in human subjects.[13,14] Having been taught atherosclerosis by Dr Daria Haust (for many years the Editor of *Atherosclerosis*, and a Professor of Pathology at University of Western Ontario), JDS understood early on that IMT did not truly represent atherosclerosis,[15–18] and decided to focus on quantification of plaque burden.

In 2002 his group reported[19] that TPA was a strong predictor of cardiovascular risk among patients attending cardiovascular prevention clinics. After adjusting for age, sex, blood pressure, cholesterol, smoking, diabetes, homocysteine, and treatment of blood pressure and cholesterol, patients in the top quartile of TPA had a 3.4 times higher 5-year risk of stroke, death, or myocardial infarction. By quartile of TPA, the 5-year risks were approximately 5%, 10%, 15%, and 20%. Thus TPA was much stronger than a Framingham risk profile in predicting risk. During the first year of follow-up, approximately half the patients had plaque progression, a quarter had regression, and a quarter was stable. Those with plaque progression had twice the risk of events, after adjustment for the panel of risk factors listed previously. Our findings were borne out in the Tromsø study, a population-based study in Northern Norway of more than 6000 participants who were healthy at baseline. That study showed that TPA, but not IMT in the distal common carotid, predicted myocardial infarction[20] and stroke.[21] Added to risk calculation using scores based on risk factors, TPA significantly improves risk prediction.[22] Subsequently it has

A

B

Fig. 2. (*A, B*) Measurement of carotid plaque volume, 1994. These small plaques totaling 12 mm³ were measured using disk segmentation.

become apparent in meta-analyses that IMT is only a weak predictor of cardiovascular events, adding little to a Framingham risk score,[23,24] and that progression of IMT does not predict events.[25] Brook and colleagues[26] found that TPA significantly changed risk prediction and was more predictive of coronary stenosis than IMT, coronary calcium score, or C-reactive protein.[27] Sillesen and colleagues[28] found that carotid plaque burden (an estimated plaque volume assessed by moving the probe along the carotid) was much more closely correlated with coronary calcium score than IMT.

Measurement of Three-Dimensional Plaque Volume

Perhaps the first description of estimation of plaque volume was in a study by Hennerici and Steinke in 1987.[29] Initial measurements of carotid plaque volume were laborious; the method, called disk segmentation, required acquisition of a series of two-dimensional cross-sectional slices captured by translating the ultrasound probe along the carotid artery with a mechanical device, tracing of the plaque area in serial cross-sections

of the artery, stepping through the plaque at intervals of 1 to 2 mm, and summing the slices to obtain plaque volume (**Fig. 3**). Early work specified the reproducibility, reliability, interslice distance, and other technical issues.[30–34] Ludwig and colleagues[35] in 2008 and papers in 2014 and 2015[36,37] reported good reproducibility, similar to results previously reported by Fenster's group, and also found that reproducibility was better for large plaques than for small ones.

The disk segmentation method was not only laborious; it required 2 to 3 months of training and practice to learn to do it reliably and achieve certification in its use, and some candidates (approximately a third) were not able to perform it reliably: it seemed that perfectionists struggled too much with deciding where to demarcate boundaries, and others were too careless. These issues were the impetus for development of semi-automated and automated methods that would be less operator-dependent, less laborious, and perhaps more reproducible and reliable.

Early semiautomated methods[38,39] reduced the number of slices of the plaque that required manual input to set the proximal and distal ends of each

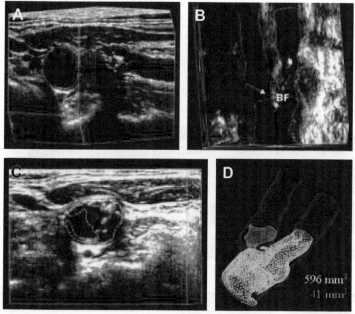

Fig. 3. Procedure for determining plaque volumes from 3D ultrasound (US) images. (*A*) An approximate axis of the vessel is selected in a longitudinal view (*purple line*) and the internal elastic lamina and lumen boundary are outlined (*yellow*). (*B*) Using the surfaces generated by the vessel contours and the 3D US image, the position of the bifurcation (BF; *yellow arrow*) is determined and marked. The axis of the vessel is selected based on the bifurcation point, and marked along the branch as far as the plaque can be measured (*purple line*). This axis is used as a reference for distance measurements. (*C*) All plaques within the measurable distance are outlined, different colors being used for each separate plaque to aid in identification. (*D*) Volumes are calculated for each plaque, and surfaces of the vessel wall and plaques are generated to better visualize the plaques in relation to the carotid arteries. (*From* Ainsworth CD, Blake CC, Tamayo A, et al. 3D ultrasound measurement of change in carotid plaque volume: a tool for rapid evaluation of new therapies. Stroke 2005;36(9):1906; with permission.)

plaque, and tracing the contour of slices at the midpoint, and 25% and 75% of the length of the plaque, with automated interpolation of the surface of the remainder of the plaque assuming uniform plaque geometry, adjustable by the operator (Fig. 4).

In 2013 an automated method was developed using mechanical movement of the probe along the artery[40] that provided good agreement with manual segmentation by experts (Fig. 5). However, the machine used to translate the ultrasound probe is large and clumsy, and difficult to use in patients with obesity or short necks. A mechanical sweep, obtained by holding the probe in one location and having the angle changed mechanically (Fig. 6), is faster and more convenient. Recently Graebe and colleagues,[36] using the Philips system used by Sillesen and colleagues[28] in the High-Risk Plaque Bioimage Study, showed that the mechanical sweep gave improved reproducibility of plaque volume quantification compared with manual translation of the probe along the artery (Fig. 7).

Progression of Carotid Plaque Volume and Cardiovascular Risk

Progression of TPA was shown to strongly predict the 5-year risk of stroke, myocardial infarction, and death after adjustment for risk factors.[19] Carotid plaques grow along the artery 2.4 times faster than they thicken,[8] so measuring plaque area is more sensitive than measuring thickness alone.

Plaques also grow and regress circumferentially, so measuring 3D plaque volume is even more sensitive than measuring area.[41] Carotid 3D plaque volume is also more sensitive to effects of therapy than coronary intravascular ultrasound (IVUS): whereas carotid plaques are focal and can change in three dimensions, coronary plaques are present along the entire length and entire circumference of the artery, so change is reduced to a change in average thickness (ie, a one-dimensional change). In a meta-analysis, Noyes and Thompson[42] concluded that using IMT or IVUS, 2 years would be required to study effects of statins on plaque progression/regression; however, change in TPA or total plaque volume can be done in 3 months.[41]

Progression of plaque volume predicted cardiovascular events in a small sample of prevention clinic patients who had plaque at baseline (N = 323), whereas progression of IMT or TPA did not significantly predict events.[43]

Regression of carotid plaque area was reported in a quarter of patients in 2002[19]; by 2010 it was observed in half of patients being followed in the same clinic,[44] probably caused by more intensive medical therapy.[45,46] In 2005, Ainsworth and colleagues[51] reported that by measuring carotid plaque volume, significant plaque regression with high-dose atorvastatin in patients with carotid stenosis could be shown in only 3 months, in a study comparing only 21 patients randomized to placebo with 17 randomized to atorvastatin. This reduced

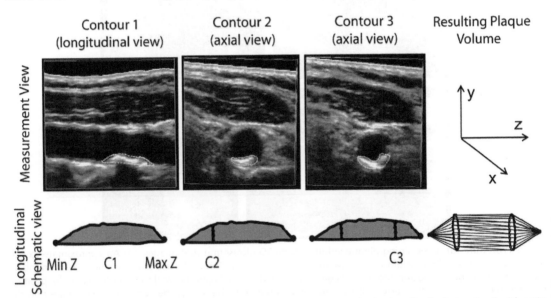

Fig. 4. User input for semiautomated total plaque volume measurement. In the longitudinal view (and with assistance from the axial view, not shown) the user identifies the maximum and minimum z-values representing the end points of the plaque (Min Z and Max Z). The user identifies the midpoint of the plaque (C1) and finally C2 and C3 are identified and generated in the axial view. Uniform plaque geometry between C2 and C3 is assumed and a final volume is generated. (*From* Buchanan D, Gyacskov I, Ukwatta E, et al. Semi-automated segmentation of carotid artery plaque volume from three-dimensional ultrasound carotid imaging. Proc SPIE 2012;8317:831701–4; with permission.)

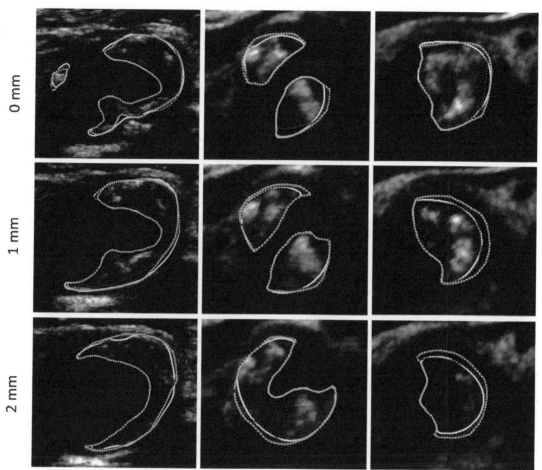

Fig. 5. Automated measurement of plaque volume. Sample results of algorithm and manual segmentations for three patients (one subject in each column). The panels in the rows were obtained at distances of 0, 1, and 2 mm from the carotid bifurcation. Yellow solid contours, algorithm results; red dashed contours, results of expert 1; green dashed contours, results of expert 2. (*From* Cheng J, Li H, Xiao F, et al. Fully automatic plaque segmentation in 3-D carotid ultrasound images. Ultrasound Med Biol 2013;39:2440; with permission.)

by two orders of magnitude the sample size and duration of studies to assess new therapies for atherosclerosis compared with IMT. Carotid plaque volume is also significantly more sensitive than IVUS, as reported by Noyes and Thompson[42] in a meta-analysis indicating that patients in studies of antiatherosclerotic therapies should be followed for 2 years to detect effects of therapy. An issue that is little understood is that because carotid plaques are focal, whereas coronary plaques extend throughout the length of the pullback, measuring progression of carotid plaque is more sensitive to effects of therapy than coronary IVUS.[41]

VESSEL WALL VOLUME

Not all patients have carotid plaque at the time they are studied. **Table 1** shows, from data in 7591 patients attending our vascular prevention clinics, the percentage with measurable plaque increased from 26.6% at age less than 35, to 50% at age 35 to 39, and 98.5% at age 70 to 74 (see **Table 1**). An issue that requires discussion is the definition of carotid plaque. The Mannheim consensus[47] defined plaque as an IMT greater than 1.5 mm. In the High Risk Plaque Study, among participants with a mean age of 68, 78% had measurable plaque. In that study, plaque was defined as local thickening of the carotid IMT of greater than 50% compared with the surrounding vessel wall, an IMT greater than 1.5 mm, or local thickening greater than 0.5 mm. However, our studies and the Tromsø study (ie, the studies that showed that TPA predicted cardiovascular events[19–21]) used a definition of a focal thickening of the intima-media complex greater than 1 mm. It is therefore suggested that the validated definition is the latter.

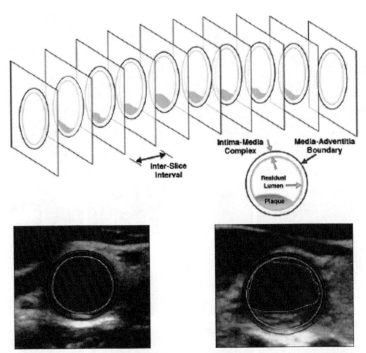

Fig. 6. Measurement of carotid plaque burden by automated software (Philips). Segment of carotid artery with a plaque (*orange*), which is scanned with a linear array transducer as a series of image slices in transverse section (*top*). Each image is analyzed with semiautomated software to quantify plaque area, plaque gray-scale statistics, percent stenosis, and other metrics of interest. Plaque areas from all images in the entire image sequence were summed as "plaque burden." (*Lower left*) Common carotid artery with no plaque. The blue border represents the lumen/intima border; the red border represents the media-adventitia boundary. (*Lower right*) Common carotid artery with plaque. The red border and blue border are the same as in previous image, but the orange border represents the boundary of the plaque. (*From* Sillesen H, Muntendam P, Adourian A, et al. Carotid plaque burden as a measure of subclinical atherosclerosis: comparison with other tests for subclinical arterial disease in the high risk plaque BioImage study. JACC Cardiovasc Imaging 2012;5:683; with permission.)

For children and healthy study participants who have no measurable plaque, it has been common to measure IMT. However, a strong alternative is measurement of vessel wall volume (VWV; the volume of the artery minus the volume of the lumen) (Fig. 8).[48] That measurement, which is conceptually equivalent to a 3D IMT, has significant advantages over IMT. Like plaque volume,[49] it has a much greater dynamic range. VWV also markedly reduces sample size and duration of therapy compared with IMT and IVUS. Atorvastatin significantly reduced VWV in 3 months[50] in the same images in which total plaque volume was measured in the study discussed previously.[51] Dietary weight loss, probably through reduction of blood pressure, significantly reduced VWV in 2 years.[52]

ULCERATION

Besides quantifying plaque burden, 3D ultrasound is being developed to identify patients with vulnerable plaque. Methods for identifying high-risk asymptomatic carotid stenosis include MR imaging characterization of plaque composition, PET/computed tomography imaging of inflammation, assessment of neovascularization in plaque, detection of microemboli by transcranial Doppler, and ultrasound imaging of echolucency and ulceration.[53,54]

Ulceration was shown in the North American Symptomatic Carotid Endarterectomy Trial to be associated with a tripling of risk[55]; however, the detection of ulceration by angiography (which provides an image of the lumen, not the wall of the artery) was unreliable.[56] Although reproducibility of ulcer detection is poor with two-dimensional ultrasound,[57] reliable detection of ulceration was shown with 3D ultrasound by Schminke and colleagues.[58]

In 2011, Madani and colleagues[59] found in patients with asymptomatic carotid stenosis that the presence of three or more ulcers in either carotid artery identified patients with 3-year risk of stroke or death of 18%, similar to the 20% risk of patients

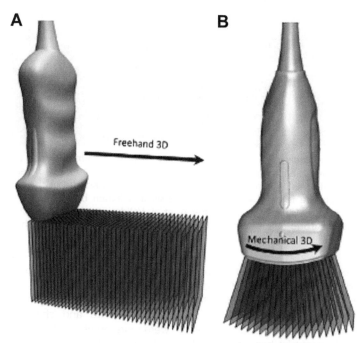

Fig. 7. Freehand scanning versus mechanical sweep. Carotid artery scanning methods. (*A*) The two-dimensional freehand sweeps were acquired using a linear array 9- to 13-MHz transducer that was moved along the neck in one direction for a 10-s acquisition. (*B*) For the 3D mechanical sweeps, the transducer was held still over the carotid bifurcation. When activated, a linear transducer inside the transducer head was mechanically propagated at a constant speed. (*From* Graebe M, Entrekin R, Collet-Billon A, et al. Reproducibility of two 3-D ultrasound carotid plaque quantification methods. Ultrasound Med Biol 2014;40:1642; with permission.)

with microemboli on transcranial Doppler, versus a 2% risk with neither ulceration nor microemboli. Importantly, and perhaps surprisingly, ulceration and microemboli identified different high-risk

Table 1
Measurable plaque area by age group

Age Group (y)	Number of Cases	Mean Total Plaque Area (mm^2)	Standard Deviation	Percent with Plaque
<35	290	7.37	29.25	26.6
35–39	218	13.48	27.16	50.0
40–44	388	28.68	47.05	71.1
45–49	594	44.07	65.27	77.8
50–54	766	69.64	101.78	86.9
55–59	861	100.97	120.44	92.5
60–64	864	133.46	138.75	96.4
65–69	910	153.20	150.87	97.6
70–74	958	175.30	146.59	98.5
75–79	797	196.10	152.17	98.9
80+	945	198.24	135.50	99.5

Data are from 7591 patients attending the Stroke Prevention and Atherosclerosis Research Centre, Robarts Research Institute, London, Canada.

patients, increasing the proportion that could benefit from endarterectomy from 5% to 10%.

In 2014, Kuk and colleagues[60] found that measurement of carotid plaque volume was useful in identifying high-risk patients among a population attending vascular prevention clinics (Fig. 9). Patients with a total ulcer volume greater than or equal to 5 mm^3 had a significantly higher risk of "stroke, transient ischemic attack, or death ($P = .009$) and of developing stroke/transient ischemic attack/death/myocardial infarction/ revascularization ($P = .017$)."

ECHOLUCENCY AND PLAQUE TEXTURE: APPROACHING PLAQUE COMPOSITION

It has long been thought that echolucent plaque represented "soft plaque" that was more likely to rupture and embolize. Several studies have shown that echolucency predicted higher risk of cardiovascular events.[61–63] Nicolaides and colleagues[64,65] discussed echolucency and "black juxtaluminal plaque," which may represent soft plaque or perhaps thrombus, as a predictor of high risk. Echolucency was shown to improve the prediction of stroke among patients in the Asymptomatic Carotid Emboli Study.[66] A combination of

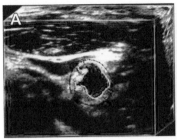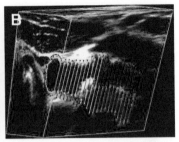

Fig. 8. Vessel wall volume segmentation. (*A*) The transverse view of the common carotid artery shows the vessel boundary outlined in red and the lumen boundary outlined in yellow. (*B*) The three-dimensional ultrasound image volume is sliced longitudinally to reveal the vessel and lumen boundaries in the common, internal, and external carotid branches. The internal carotid artery vessel and lumen boundaries are shown in blue and pink, respectively. (*From* Egger M, Spence JD, Fenster A, et al. Validation of 3d ultrasound vessel wall volume: an imaging phenotype of carotid atherosclerosis. Ultrasound Med Biol 2007;33:908; with permission.)

microemboli and echolucency identified a subgroup with a 10-fold increase in the risk of ipsilateral stroke, which remained significant after adjustment for risk factors.

More recently, radiofrequency analysis (as opposed to gray-scale analysis) has been used to study plaque "texture," a way of assessing plaque composition.[67,68] Inhomogeneity of plaque texture and some other features of plaque texture have been shown to identify patients at higher risk of events.[68,69] In 2014, van Engelen and colleagues[70] found that 2 of the 64 mathematical

algorithms, Law's spot-spot ripple and Law's edge-edge ripple (**Fig. 10**), were particularly useful, and showed that a combination of change in plaque texture and change in plaque volume were more predictive than either parameter alone.

A problem for clinicians is relating to mathematical abstractions; this is apparent from the appearance of the texture analysis images shown in **Fig. 10**. Our group has recently made some progress in comparing features of plaque texture from carotid images obtained before endarterectomy with histologic features of plaque. **Fig. 11** shows

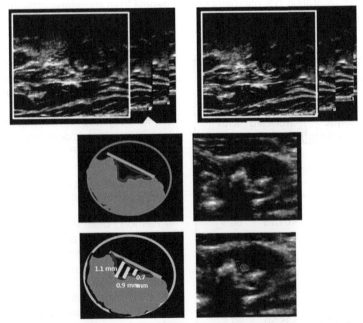

Fig. 9. Measurement of ulcer volume and ulcer depth. Contours of ulcers were traced and depth of ulcers measured in cross-sectional views. Each slice had a thickness of 1 mm; ulcer volume was computed from the sum of the volumes of all slices in which ulceration was traced. (*From* Kuk M, Wannarong T, Beletsky V, et al. Volume of carotid artery ulceration as a predictor of cardiovascular events. Stroke 2014;45:1438; with permission.)

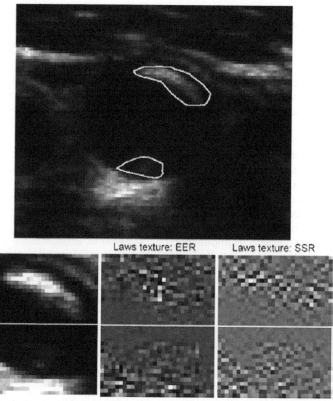

Fig. 10. Plaque texture. Texture for two plaques in the same vessel with a different appearance. In a total of 50 runs of sparse Cox regression (5 × 10-fold cross-validation) on changes in texture, Law's edge-edge ripple (EER) was selected in the model 49 times, and Law's spot-spot ripple (SSR) 48 times. (*From* van Engelen A, Wannarong T, Parraga G, et al. Three-dimensional carotid ultrasound plaque texture predicts vascular events. Stroke 2014;45:2698; with permission.)

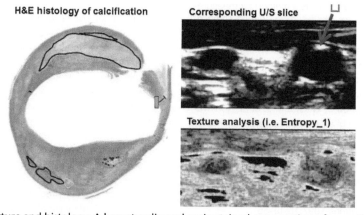

Fig. 11. Plaque texture and histology. A hematoxylin and eosin stained cross-section of a carotid endarterectomy is shown on the left, with calcification outlined in dark blue. The upper right panel shows the corresponding 3D ultrasound slice of the plaque, with the arrow pointing to the area of calcification, which is very echodense. The lower right panel shows the appearance of one of the plaque texture features, Entropy_1. (*Courtesy of* Dr Rob Hammond, Neuropathologist at University Hospital, and Lucy Chung, a medical student at the Schulich School of Medicine and Dentistry, London, Canada, who carried out a project funded by the Canadian Institutes of Health Summer Research Training Program.)

the relationship of one of the plaque texture algorithms to plaque calcification.

SUMMARY

3D ultrasound of carotid plaque volume is useful for risk stratification, for evaluating effects of therapy on atherosclerosis, and for managing patients at risk of cardiovascular events, by a strategy called "treating arteries instead of risk factors." It will also be useful for genetic research[71] and evaluation of new risk factors, such as metabolic products of the intestinal microbiome.[72] Ulceration and other features of plaque vulnerability, such as plaque texture and surface plaque roughness,[73] will probably also be useful in risk stratification, and in identifying among patients with asymptomatic carotid stenosis the small proportion that might benefit from revascularization.

REFERENCES

1. Spence JD, Pesout J, Melmon KL. Effects of antihypertensive drugs on blood velocity in rhesus monkeys. Stroke 1977;8:589–94.
2. Brinker RA, Landiss DJ, Croley TF. Detection of carotid artery bifurcation stenosis by Doppler ultrasound. Preliminary report. J Neurosurg 1968;29:143–8.
3. Keller H, Meier W, Yonekawa Y, et al. Noninavasive angiography for the diagnosis of carotid artery disease using Doppler ultrasound (carotid artery Doppler). Stroke 1976;7:354–63.
4. Spence JD. Effects of hydralazine versus propranolol on blood velocity patterns with carotid stenosis. Clin Sci 1983;65:91–3.
5. Spence JD. Quantitative spectral analysis of carotid Doppler signal: evaluation as a method for measurement of drug effects. Clin Invest Med 1989;12:82–9.
6. Spence JD. Effects of antihypertensive drugs on flow disturbances: nifedipine, captopril, and metoprolol evaluated by quantitative spectral analysis of Doppler flow patterns in patients with carotid stenosis. Clin Invest Med 1994;17:319–25.
7. Persson J, Stavenow L, Wikstrand J, et al. Noninvasive quantification of atherosclerotic lesions. Reproducibility of ultrasonographic measurement of arterial wall thickness and plaque size'. Arterioscler Thromb 1992;12:261–6.
8. Barnett PA, Spence JD, Manuck SB, et al. Psychological stress and the progression of carotid atherosclerosis. J Hypertens 1997;15:49–55.
9. Delcker A, Diener HC. Quantification of atherosclerotic plaques in carotid arteries by three-dimensional ultrasound. Br J Radiol 1994;67:672–8.
10. Picot PA, Rickey DW, Mitchell R, et al. Three-dimensional colour Doppler imaging of the carotid artery. Ultrasound Med Biol 1993;19:95–104.
11. Picot PA, Rickey DW, Mitchell R, et al. Three-dimensional colour Doppler imaging. Ultrasound Med Biol 1993;19:95–104.
12. Bond MG, Wilmoth SK, Gardin JF, et al. Noninvasive assessment of atherosclerosis in nonhuman primates. Adv Exp Med Biol 1985;183:189–95.
13. Pignoli P, Tremoli E, Poli A, et al. Intimal plus medial thickness of the arterial wall: a direct measurement with ultrasound imaging. Circulation 1986;74:1399–406.
14. Baldassarre D, Werba JP, Tremoli E, et al. Common carotid intima-media thickness measurement. A method to improve accuracy and precision. Stroke 1994;25:1588–92.
15. Spence JD. Advances in atherosclerosis: new understanding based on endothelial function. In: Fisher M, Bogousslavsky J, editors. Current review of cerebrovascular disease. 3rd edition. Philadelphia: Current Medicine; 1999. p. 1–13.
16. Spence JD, Hegele RA. Noninvasive phenotypes of atherosclerosis. Arterioscler Thromb Vasc Biol 2004; 24:e188–9.
17. Spence JD. Carotid plaque measurement is superior to IMT Invited editorial comment on: carotid plaque, compared with carotid intima-media thickness, more accurately predicts coronary artery disease events: a meta-analysis-Yoichi Inaba, M.D., Jennifer A. Chen M.D., Steven R. Bergmann M.D., Ph.D. Atherosclerosis 2011;220:34–5.
18. Finn AV, Kolodgie FD, Virmani R. Correlation between carotid intimal/medial thickness and atherosclerosis. a point of view from pathology. Arterioscler Thromb Vasc Biol 2010;30:177–81.
19. Spence JD, Eliasziw M, DiCicco M, et al. Carotid plaque area: a tool for targeting and evaluating vascular preventive therapy. Stroke 2002;33: 2916–22.
20. Johnsen SH, Mathiesen EB, Joakimsen O, et al. Carotid atherosclerosis is a stronger predictor of myocardial infarction in women than in men: a 6-year follow-up study of 6226 persons: the Tromso Study. Stroke 2007;38:2873–80.
21. Mathiesen EB, Johnsen SH, Wilsgaard T, et al. Carotid plaque area and intima-media thickness in prediction of first-ever ischemic stroke: a 10-year follow-up of 6584 men and women: the Tromso study. Stroke 2011;42:972–8.
22. Romanens M, Ackerman F, Schwenkglenks M, et al. Posterior probabilities in sequential testing improve cardiovascular risk prediction using carotid total plaque area. Cardiovasc Med 2011;14:53–7.
23. Den Ruijter HM, Peters SA, Anderson TJ, et al. Common carotid intima-media thickness measurements in cardiovascular risk prediction: a meta-analysis. JAMA 2012;308:796–803.
24. Den Ruijter HM, Peters SA, Groenewegen KA, et al. Common carotid intima-media thickness does not

add to Framingham risk score in individuals with diabetes mellitus: the USE-IMT initiative. Diabetologia 2013;56:1494–502.

25. Lorenz MW, Polak JF, Kavousi M, et al. Carotid intima-media thickness progression to predict cardiovascular events in the general population (the PROG-IMT collaborative project): a meta-analysis of individual participant data. Lancet 2012;379: 2053–62.

26. Bard RL, Kalsi H, Rubenfire M, et al. Effect of carotid atherosclerosis screening on risk stratification during primary cardiovascular disease prevention. Am J Cardiol 2004;93:1030–2.

27. Brook RD, Bard RL, Patel S, et al. A negative carotid plaque area test is superior to other non-invasive atherosclerosis studies for reducing the likelihood of having significant coronary artery disease. Arterioscler Thromb Vasc Biol 2006;26:656–62.

28. Sillesen H, Muntendam P, Adourian A, et al. Carotid plaque burden as a measure of subclinical atherosclerosis: comparison with other tests for subclinical arterial disease in the high risk plaque BioImage study. JACC Cardiovasc Imaging 2012;5:681–9.

29. Hennerici M, Steinke W. [Morphology and biochemical parameters of the regression of carotid artery lesions]. Vasa Suppl 1987;20:77–84 [in German].

30. Landry A, Fenster A. Theoretical and experimental quantification of carotid plaque volume measurements made by three-dimensional ultrasound using test phantoms. Med Phys 2002;29:2319–27.

31. Landry AM, Spence JD, Fenster A. Measurement of carotid plaque volume by 3-dimensional ultrasound. Stroke 2004;35:864–9.

32. Landry A, Spence JD, Fenster A. Quantification of carotid plaque volume measurements using 3D ultrasound imaging. Ultrasound Med Biol 2005;31: 751–62.

33. Landry A, Ainsworth C, Blake C, et al. Manual planimetric measurement of carotid plaque volume using three-dimensional ultrasound imaging. Med Phys 2007;34:1496–505.

34. Mallett C, House AA, Spence JD, et al. Longitudinal ultrasound evaluation of carotid atherosclerosis in one, two and three dimensions. Ultrasound Med Biol 2009;35:367–75.

35. Ludwig M, Zielinski T, Schremmer D, et al. Reproducibility of 3-dimensional ultrasound readings of volume of carotid atherosclerotic plaque. Cardiovasc Ultrasound 2008;6:42.

36. Graebe M, Entrekin R, Collet-Billon A, et al. Reproducibility of two 3-D ultrasound carotid plaque quantification methods. Ultrasound Med Biol 2014;40: 1641–9.

37. AlMuhanna K, Hossain MM, Zhao L, et al. Carotid plaque morphometric assessment with three-dimensional ultrasound imaging. J Vasc Surg 2015;61:690–7.

38. Ukwatta E, Awad J, Ward AD, et al. Three-dimensional ultrasound of carotid atherosclerosis: semiautomated segmentation using a level set-based method. Med Phys 2011;38:2479–93.

39. Buchanan D, Gyacskov I, Ukwatta E, et al. Semiautomated segmentation of carotid artery plaque volume from three-dimensional ultrasound carotid imaging. Proc SPIE 2012;8317.

40. Cheng J, Li H, Xiao F, et al. Fully automatic plaque segmentation in 3-D carotid ultrasound images. Ultrasound Med Biol 2013;39:2431–46.

41. Spence JD. Time course of atherosclerosis regression. Atherosclerosis 2014;235:347–8.

42. Noyes AM, Thompson PD. A systematic review of the time course of atherosclerotic plaque regression. Atherosclerosis 2014;234:75–84.

43. Wannarong T, Parraga G, Buchanan D, et al. Progression of carotid plaque volume predicts cardiovascular events. Stroke 2013;44:1859–65.

44. Spence JD, Hackam DG. Treating arteries instead of risk factors. A paradigm change in management of atherosclerosis. Stroke 2010;41:1193–9.

45. Spence JD, Coates V, Li H, et al. Effects of Intensive medical therapy on microemboli and cardiovascular risk in asymptomatic carotid stenosis. Arch Neurol 2010;67:180–6.

46. Spence JD. Technology insight: ultrasound measurement of carotid plaque–patient management, genetic research, and therapy evaluation. Nat Clin Pract Neurol 2006;2:611–9.

47. Touboul PJ, Hennerici MG, Meairs S, et al. Mannheim carotid intima-media thickness consensus (2004-2006). An update on behalf of the Advisory Board of the 3rd and 4th Watching the Risk Symposium, 13th and 15th European Stroke Conferences, Mannheim, Germany, 2004, and Brussels, Belgium, 2006. Cerebrovasc Dis 2007;23:75–80.

48. Egger M, Spence JD, Fenster A, et al. Validation of 3d ultrasound vessel wall volume: an imaging phenotype of carotid atherosclerosis. Ultrasound Med Biol 2007;33:905–14.

49. Pollex RL, Spence JD, House AA, et al. A comparison of ultrasound measurements to assess carotid atherosclerosis development in subjects with and without type 2 diabetes. Cardiovasc Ultrasound 2005;3:15.

50. Krasinski A, Chiu B, Spence JD, et al. Three-dimensional ultrasound quantification of intensive statin treatment of carotid atherosclerosis. Ultrasound Med Biol 2009;35:1763–72.

51. Ainsworth CD, Blake CC, Tamayo A, et al. 3D ultrasound measurement of change in carotid plaque volume: a tool for rapid evaluation of new therapies. Stroke 2005;36:1904–9.

52. Shai I, Spence JD, Schwarzfuchs D, et al. Dietary intervention to reverse carotid atherosclerosis. Circulation 2010;121:1200–8.

53. Bogiatzi C, Cocker MS, Beanlands R, et al. Identifying high-risk asymptomatic carotids stenosis. Expert Opin Med Diagn 2012;6:139–51.

54. Paraskevas KI, Spence JD, Veith FJ, et al. Identifying which patients with asymptomatic carotid stenosis could benefit from intervention. Stroke 2014;45(12):3720–4.

55. Eliasziw M, Streifler JY, Fox AJ, et al. Significance of plaque ulceration in symptomatic patients with high-grade carotid stenosis. North American Symptomatic Carotid Endarterectomy Trial. Stroke 1994;25:304–8.

56. Streifler JY, Eliasziw M, Fox AJ, et al. Angiographic detection of carotid plaque ulceration. Comparison with surgical observations in a multicenter study. North American Symptomatic Carotid Endarterectomy Trial. Stroke 1994;25:1130–2.

57. de Bray JM, Baud JM, Delanoy P, et al. Reproducibility in ultrasonic characterization of carotid plaques. Cerebrovasc Dis 1998;8:273–7.

58. Schminke U, Motsch L, Hilker L, et al. Three-dimensional ultrasound observation of carotid artery plaque ulceration. Stroke 2000;31:1651–5.

59. Madani A, Beletsky V, Tamayo A, et al. High-risk asymptomatic carotid stenosis: ulceration on 3D ultrasound versus TCD microemboli. Neurology 2011;77:744–50.

60. Kuk M, Wannarong T, Beletsky V, et al. Volume of carotid artery ulceration as a predictor of cardiovascular events. Stroke 2014;45:1437–41.

61. Polak JF, Shemanski L, O'Leary DH, et al. Hypoechoic plaque at US of the carotid artery: an independent risk factor for incident stroke in adults aged 65 years or older. Cardiovascular Health Study. Radiology 1998;208:649–54.

62. Mathiesen EB, Bonaa KH, Joakimsen O. Echolucent plaques are associated with high risk of ischemic cerebrovascular events in carotid stenosis: the Tromso study. Circulation 2001;103:2171–5.

63. Gronholdt ML, Nordestgaard BG, Schroeder TV, et al. Ultrasonic echolucent carotid plaques predict future strokes. Circulation 2001;104:68–73.

64. Griffin MB, Kyriacou E, Pattichis C, et al. Juxtaluminal hypoechoic area in ultrasonic images of carotid plaques and hemispheric symptoms. J Vasc Surg 2010;52:69–76.

65. Kakkos SK, Griffin MB, Nicolaides AN, et al. The size of juxtaluminal hypoechoic area in ultrasound images of asymptomatic carotid plaques predicts the occurrence of stroke. J Vasc Surg 2013;57:609–18.

66. Topakian R, King A, Kwon SU, et al. Ultrasonic plaque echolucency and emboli signals predict stroke in asymptomatic carotid stenosis. Neurology 2011;77:751–8.

67. Christodoulou CI, Pattichis CS, Pantziaris M, et al. Texture-based classification of atherosclerotic carotid plaques. IEEE Trans Med Imaging 2003;22:902–12.

68. Kakkos SK, Nicolaides AN, Kyriacou E, et al. Computerized texture analysis of carotid plaque ultrasonic images can identify unstable plaques associated with ipsilateral neurological symptoms. Angiology 2011;62:317–28.

69. Kakkos SK, Stevens JM, Nicolaides AN, et al. Texture analysis of ultrasonic images of symptomatic carotid plaques can identify those plaques associated with ipsilateral embolic brain infarction. Eur J Vasc Endovasc Surg 2007;33:422–9.

70. van Engelen A, Wannarong T, Parraga G, et al. Three-dimensional carotid ultrasound plaque texture predicts vascular events. Stroke 2014;45:2695–701.

71. Spence JD. Genetics of atherosclerosis: the power of plaque burden and progression. Invited Commentary on Dong C, Beecham A, Wang L, Blanton SH, Rundek T, Sacco RL. Follow-up association study of linkage regions reveals multiple candidate genes for carotid plaque in Dominicans. Atherosclerosis 2012;223:98–101.

72. Spence JD. Effects of the intestinal microbiome on constituents of red meat and egg yolks: a new window opens on nutrition and cardiovascular disease. Can J Cardiol 2014;30:150–1.

73. Chiu B, Beletsky V, Spence JD, et al. Analysis of carotid lumen surface morphology using three-dimensional ultrasound imaging. Phys Med Biol 2009;54:1149–67.

The Use of Contrast-enhanced Ultrasonography for Imaging of Carotid Atherosclerotic Plaques
Current Evidence, Future Directions

Sandeep A. Saha, MD*, Venu Gourineni, MD,
Steven B. Feinstein, MD, FESC

KEYWORDS

- Echo-contrast agents • Microbubbles • Carotid endarterectomy • Plaque neovascularization
- Plaque neoangiogenesis • Contrast enhancement • Safety

KEY POINTS

- Current treatment guidelines recommend treatment of symptomatic patients with carotid stenosis with low or average surgical risk based on occurrence of symptoms and the degree of ipsilateral carotid stenosis. Data related to the optimal management of asymptomatic patients or those with moderate carotid stenosis (50%–69% by duplex ultrasonography) remain limited.
- Contrast-enhanced ultrasonography (CEUS) imaging of carotid arteries provides an accurate quantification of stenosis, and permits novel, real-time access to intraplaque neovascularization (IPN); a distinct marker of plaque vulnerability notwithstanding the presence of stenosis.
- IPN correlates with localized intraplaque inflammation presaging a higher risk of plaque hemorrhage and rupture.
- Two-dimensional CEUS imaging of IPN has been shown to directly correlate with the extent of neovascularization observed in histopathologic examinations of surgically excised carotid plaques.
- Detection of IPN using CEUS carotid artery imaging may be predictive of adverse cardiovascular events in patients with known coronary artery disease. If confirmed in larger clinical trials, CEUS carotid imaging may be useful for cardiovascular risk stratification by providing a marker of subclinical atherosclerosis.

INTRODUCTION

Carotid atherosclerotic disease leading to carotid stenosis is an important cause of ischemic strokes. Pivotal clinical trials performed in the United States (NASCET [North American Symptomatic Carotid Endarterectomy Trial])[1] and Europe (ESCT [European Carotid Surgery Trial])[2] provided a clear correlation between the degree of carotid stenosis and the risk of stroke in symptomatic patients. Current treatment guidelines in the United States advocate treatment with carotid endarterectomy (CEA) for symptomatic patients (defined as those who have a transient ischemic

Financial disclosures: S.A. Saha, V. Gourineni, none. S.B. Feinstein, research support from GE Life Sciences (11111606) (IIT grant) and consultant for GE Healthcare.
Division of Cardiology, Department of Medicine, Rush University Medical Center, Chicago, IL, USA
* Corresponding author. Rush University Medical Center, Division of Cardiology, 1717 West Congress Parkway, Kellogg 321, Chicago, IL 60612.
E-mail address: sandeep_a_saha@rush.edu

1052-5149/16/$ – see front matter © 2016 Elsevier Inc. All rights reserved.

attack [TIA] or a nondisabling stroke) considered as low or average surgical risk with ipsilateral carotid stenosis of greater than or equal to 70% on noninvasive imaging or greater than or equal to 50% by angiography with the caveat that the preoperative risk is less than 6%. This guideline was consistent with the clinical data that recognized that symptomatic patients who underwent CEA had an incidence of stroke-free survival of 93% at 5 years.[3] However, in patients with moderate carotid stenosis (defined as 50%–69% stenosis) and asymptomatic patients with high-grade stenosis (>70%), the role of revascularization with CEA or carotid artery stunting (CAS) remains unclear. Current treatment decisions rely solely on the severity of anatomic stenosis associated with the presence or absence of neurologic symptoms. A notable pitfall of using luminal stenosis to detect the presence of carotid atherosclerosis is highlighted in (Fig. 1). Essentially, luminal characteristics may not fully represent the presence of a carotid plaque because of effects associated with positive arterial wall remodeling. The current guidelines also do not account for other characteristics of the atherosclerotic plaque, including presence of intraplaque neovascularization (IPN). It may now be possible to develop a more comprehensive and predictive model of plaque vulnerability by incorporating the contrast-enhanced ultrasonography (CEUS) identification of IPN coupled with preexisting anatomic descriptors of stenosis. Thus, the addition of CEUS may afford an opportunity to provide a risk assessment beyond the standards of luminal stenosis, especially in asymptomatic patients and in symptomatic patients with lower degrees of carotid stenosis.

Unenhanced duplex ultrasonography remains the principal modality for diagnosing and monitoring the progression of carotid artery stenosis. In general, diagnosticians rely on the NASCET criteria[1] to estimate the degree of stenosis within the internal carotid artery based on blood flow velocity measurements using Doppler ultrasonography. However, substantial errors limit the success of Doppler imaging technology and include individual variation in vascular anatomy, body habitus, or vessel wall calcification. Optimal two-dimensional (2D) ultrasonography imaging of carotid plaques requires controlling for tangential imaging planes caused by variations in carotid artery anatomy, and as such depends on the operator's skill. The quality of the examination is also reliant on the sonographer's ability to ensure that serially acquired carotid luminal surfaces remain within the image plane. In addition, Doppler flow measurements are angle dependent, and misalignment may lead to significant error in estimating the severity of luminal stenosis using the NASCET criteria. Comparative noninvasive imaging modalities used for carotid artery imaging include magnetic resonance (MR) imaging, computed tomography (CT), and PET/CT imaging. These related modalities provide an assessment of carotid artery stenosis albeit at increased costs, exposure to ionizing radiation, and prolonged image acquisition and processing times. Three-dimensional (3D) carotid ultrasonography imaging may circumvent the associated limitations of 2D ultrasonography, as is more fully discussed elsewhere in this issue. In a comparison of multiple imaging modalities for preoperative imaging in patients with carotid stenosis, Pfister and colleagues[4] noted that contrast-enhanced 3D B-flow ultrasonography had the highest correlation with surgical evaluation of internal carotid artery stenosis, with a Spearman correlation coefficient of 0.93. There are no reported studies to date using 3D CEUS imaging of carotid IPN. Importantly, only CEUS can directly image the IPN in real time and at the bedside. Overall, ultrasonography and CEUS provide a readily accessible imaging strategy for rapid assessment of carotid atherosclerotic disease.

Gas-filled microbubbles serve as excellent intravascular ultrasonography contrast agents based

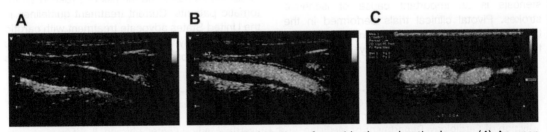

Fig. 1. Contrast-enhanced ultrasonography (CEUS) detection of carotid atherosclerotic plaques. (*A*) An unenhanced ultrasonography image of the common carotid artery, in which the plaque is faintly visible. (*B*) CEUS image of the same vessel, highlighting the presence of the plaque without significant luminal stenosis (positive remodeling). (*C*) CEUS image of the internal carotid artery showing intrusion of the vessel lumen of the plaque resulting in luminal narrowing (negative remodeling).

on a profound acoustic mismatch generated from circulating microbubbles. The diameter of microbubbles nominally ranges between 2 to 8 μm, ensuring that they remain within the intravascular space once intravenously injected. To accentuate the signal-to-noise acoustic differences between circulating microbubbles and target organs, contemporary ultrasonography machines use specific pulse sequences (eg, amplitude modulation, pulse inversion).[5] The resonance frequency (the frequency at which compression and expansion of microbubbles occurs most readily) is within the range used for clinical uses. The acoustic energy uses a transmitted frequency that is consistent with that of the microbubble resonance frequency, thus generating harmonic signals from the intravascular microbubbles. In contrast, native tissue does not generate marked harmonic acoustic responses from transmitted acoustic energy. Because of the enhanced signal/noise ratio generated from harmonic imaging, it is possible to use low mechanical indices (MIs). MI is defined as the peak negative pressure divided by the square root of the frequency of the ultrasonography transducer. Ultimately, the interaction of the interrogating ultrasonography energy coupled with the interplay of intravascular microbubbles provides unparalleled assessment of the spatial and temporal heterogeneity of microvascular perfusion within the targeted organ system. However, CT and MR angiography use contrast agents that are not exclusively intravascular, and hence require specific timing sequences for accurate visualization of vascular structures.

CEUS of the carotid arteries combines excellent spatial and temporal resolution of luminal plaques, as well as quantifying the degree of luminal stenosis. Studies by Ferrer and colleagues[6] and Droste and colleagues[7] have shown the diagnostic accuracy of CEUS for the assessment of carotid artery stenosis. Using CEUS, it is possible to identify additional characteristics of the plaque, including presence of microvessels within the plaque; a phenomenon termed IPN. There is increasing evidence to suggest that IPN plays a central role in the initiation, progression, and rupture of carotid plaques, and may therefore be a useful predictor of plaque instability and stroke risk. In addition, CEUS enables visualization of plaque ulceration, often not well visualized with unenhanced ultrasonography images (**Fig. 2**).

PATHOPHYSIOLOGIC BASIS FOR THE USE OF CONTRAST-ENHANCED ULTRASONOGRAPHY IN CAROTID DISEASE

Normal large blood vessels (including the carotid artery) contain smaller blood vessels termed vasa vasorum (VV) confined to the adventitial layer and the outer layers of the muscular medial layer that supply nutrient-rich blood to the vessel wall. Extension of the VV into atherosclerotic plaques was described in the late 1870s.[8] In addition to providing oxygen and nutrients to the developing plaque, the VV provide a milieu for leukocyte trafficking, and release of adhesion molecules and associated growth factors. This complex association contributes to the progression and expansion of the plaque. Because of the rapid recruitment of VV, the vessels often lack pericytes that provide structural support. Without pericyte development, the VV are increasingly prone to rupture, leading to intraplaque hemorrhage. An intraplaque hemorrhage results in increased release of inflammatory mediators, angiogenic factors, and growth factors, resulting in smooth muscle proliferation, accumulation of extracellular matrix components, and weakening of the fibrous cap. Intraplaque hemorrhage is thought to be an important factor in the progression of plaques leading to high-risk,

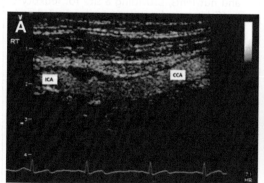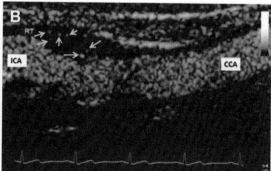

Fig. 2. CEUS image of the internal carotid artery showing plaque ulceration (*red arrow, A*). Note the presence of microbubbles within the intraplaque neovessels (*beige arrows*) of the ulcerated plaque in (*B*). CCA, common carotid artery.

unstable lesions through a myriad of molecular mechanisms.[9] Tissue hypoxia remains an important stimulus for microvessel invasion into the plaque by induction of hypoxia inducible factors (such as HIF-1a) leading to release of vascular endothelial growth factor (VEGF) by macrophages, T lymphocytes, and mast cells. VEGF is an important chemotactic and growth factor that promotes migration and proliferation of endothelial cells, resulting in progression of neovascularization within the plaque.[10,11]

Since the earliest observations, investigators reported on a direct relationship between increased arterial VV and increased cardiovascular events. Barger and Beeuwkes[12] performed cinemicrographic studies and noted the enhanced presence of neovascularization in the region of atherosclerotic plaques in coronary arteries. The investigators suggested an important role for the VV in the pathogenesis of coronary atherosclerosis and its sequelae, including intramural hemorrhage and vascular spasm.[12] An autopsy study reported that patients whose deaths were attributable to cardiovascular causes revealed a denser network of VV in the carotid, renal, and iliac vessels than was observed in patients who died of noncardiovascular causes. Further, the investigators stated that hyperplasia of the VV was an early sign of symptomatic atherosclerotic disease.[13] Dunmore and colleagues[14] reported that carotid plaques from patients with symptomatic carotid stenosis contained a higher proportion of dysmorphic, immature microvessels; similar to those found in tumors and healing wounds. The presence of these vessels seemed to contribute to plaque instability by acting as sites of vascular leakage and inflammatory cell recruitment. Carotid specimens obtained post-CEA from 91 patients, primarily in patients with symptomatic carotid stenosis, showed a high prevalence of plaque neovascularization (78%) and intraplaque hemorrhage involving more than 50% of the plaque (47%), and suggested that the angiomatoid nature of these intraplaque vessels, poor structural support from surrounding stromal tissue, and fibrinoid degeneration of the walls of these vessels provide a nexus for rupture.[15] Mofidi and colleagues[16] also reported significantly higher intraplaque microvessel density, as well as plaques with greater than 50% intraplaque hemorrhage, and unstable atherosclerotic lesions in carotid plaques obtained post-CEA from 73 symptomatic patients. Moreno and colleagues[17] performed bicolor immunohistochemistry in 269 advanced human atherosclerotic plaques and found that total intraplaque microvessel density was significantly higher in ruptured plaques, plaques with severe macrophage infiltration, and plaques with intraplaque hemorrhage and thin-cap fibroatheromas. Plaque base microvessel density was an independent predictor of plaque rupture on logistic regression analysis.

In another recent study, Hellings and colleagues[18] examined carotid artery specimens after CEA from 818 patients. The investigators prospectively followed these patients and determined the clinical cardiovascular event rates over a mean duration of 2.3 years. Intraplaque blood vessel density and plaque hemorrhage were independently associated with adverse cardiovascular events (which included death from cardiovascular causes, myocardial infarction, and cerebrovascular events), whereas, contrary to traditional beliefs, other plaque features such as lipid content, presence of smooth muscle cells, collagen, and plaque calcification were not associated with untoward clinical events. Similarly, in another recent analysis of 1640 carotid plaques (obtained by pooling 2 biobank studies) from symptomatic patients, the investigators noted a relationship between histologic plaque characteristics and 1-year and 5-year stroke risk using a validated risk prediction model. High intraplaque microvessel density significantly correlated with predicted 5-year stroke risk (odds ratio, 1.49; $P = .03$).[19] Therefore, the presence of intraplaque microvessels is associated with high-risk plaque characteristics such as intraplaque hemorrhage, and is associated with a higher risk of adverse cardiovascular events (**Box 1**).

Box 1
The role of VV in the pathophysiology of carotid artery disease

- Proliferation of VV into atherosclerotic plaques is associated with expansion and progression of the plaque through several mechanisms, including delivery of oxygen and nutrients, providing a site for leukocyte trafficking, and promoting release of chemical mediators such as adhesion molecules, cytokines, and growth factors.

- Infiltration of VV into plaques also increases the risk for microvessel rupture, leading to intraplaque hemorrhage. Plaque hemorrhage is a pathologic hallmark of unstable plaques, and is strongly associated with plaque rupture and thrombosis.

- Clinical studies have shown that increased intraplaque microvessel density significantly correlates with other high-risk characteristics of atherosclerotic plaques, and is associated with higher risk of adverse cardiovascular events.

IMAGING OF CAROTID ARTERY DISEASE USING CONTRAST-ENHANCED ULTRASONOGRAPHY

As noted, several studies[6,7] have shown that CEUS revealed enhanced diagnostic accuracy for the assessment of carotid luminal stenosis as correlated with conventional angiography,[20] cerebral CT,[21] and contrast-enhanced MR angiography.[22] Further, CEUS imaging provides additional information on focal nonobstructive carotid lesions that may be overlooked with other modalities, including nonenhanced ultrasonography imaging.[23]

Feasibility of Using Contrast-enhanced Ultrasonography for Imaging of Intraplaque Neovascularization

Feinstein[24] first reported the use of CEUS for direct visualization the carotid artery IPN and adventitial VV in 2004. This initial observation lead to the published report of regression of the adventitial carotid VV following statin therapy in a 53-year-old diabetic man with carotid stenosis.[25] Subsequently, Vicenzini and colleagues[26] performed carotid duplex ultrasonography and CEUS studies in 23 asymptomatic patients with varying degrees of carotid stenosis referred to the ultrasonography laboratory and detected the presence of microvessels within the fibrous and fibrofatty tissue around the carotid plaques regardless of the degree of luminal stenosis. Similarly, Coli and colleagues[27] studied 32 patients admitted to the coronary care unit or vascular surgery unit who underwent standard and CEUS carotid ultrasonography examinations. Of the 52 plaques analyzed, there was neovascularization that was considered extensive and/or reached the inner regions of the plaque in nearly one-third of patients, with similar results in surgical-grade lesions (symptomatic plaques or severe carotid stenosis). Van den Oord and colleagues[28] studied a novel method of quantifying the severity of IPN using CEUS in a sample of 45 carotid arteries obtained from 25 patients, and found that the IPN area, IPN area ratio, and neovessel count had good correlations with the visual IPN score ($\rho = 0.719$, $\rho = 0.538$, and $\rho = 0.474$ respectively, all $P<.01$), with excellent intraobserver and interobserver agreement. Saito and colleagues[29] performed carotid CEUS studies in 50 patients who underwent CEA, and showed that increased echo-contrast intensity of the plaque shoulder was associated with higher neovessel density ($P<.01$; $\rho = 0.43$), and enhanced intensity of the plaque shoulder was significantly higher in ruptured plaques in symptomatic patients.

Ventura and colleagues[30] recently showed that CEUS was significantly more effective than conventional Doppler ultrasonography and equally effective as CT angiography to differentiate between occlusion and pseudo-occlusion of carotid arteries in 72 patients referred for vascular surgery. In addition, CEUS provides enhanced detection of plaque ulceration, as shown in a study of 39 carotid artery specimens from 20 symptomatic patients with carotid stenosis, which reported that the sensitivity, specificity, accuracy, positive predictive value (PPV), and negative predictive value (NPV) of CEUS for detection of plaque ulceration were 88%, 59%, 72%, 63%, and 87%, respectively, using CT angiography as the reference.[31] Hjelmgren and colleagues[32] reported that plaque neovascularization measured using CEUS showed a significant, positive correlation with a tissue-based index measured by fluorodeoxyglucose PET/CT of carotid plaques, ($r = 0.67$; $P<.02$) in a cohort of 13 patients. A proposed visual system of grading IPN using CEUS is summarized in (Box 2) and illustrated in (Fig. 3).

Correlation of Intraplaque Neovascularization Imaging Using CEUS with Histopathology

There exists a significant correlation between visualization of IPN by CEUS and direct visualization of IPN by histology. Shah and colleagues[33] performed standard and CEUS examinations in 15 patients before CEA surgery and noted that the degree of IPN detected by CEUS correlated with the presence of neovascularization by histologic examination using CD31 staining. Among the 17 patients who underwent CEA in the study reported by Coli and colleagues,[27] carotid plaques with intense contrast enhancement (grade 2) showed significantly higher VV density on histologic examination (median VV density, 3.24 per mm^2; range, 1.75–4.09 per mm^2) than plaques with less intense contrast enhancement (grade 1) (median VV density, 1.82 per mm^2; range, 0.96–2.36 per mm^2;

Box 2

A proposed system of grading the severity of IPN using CEUS of the carotid artery

- Mild (grade 1) IPN: presence of moving microbubbles on the adventitial side of the plaque

- Moderate (grade 2) IPN: presence of moving microbubbles in the plaque shoulder and within the plaque but not extending to the plaque core or to the apex

- Severe (grade 3) IPN: presence of moving microbubbles within the plaque core and apex

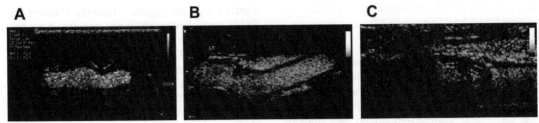

Fig. 3. A proposed system of grading the severity of IPN. (*A*) Mild (grade 1) IPN showing presence of moving microbubbles (*arrows*) on the adventitial side of the plaque; (*B*) moderate (grade 2) IPN showing presence of moving microbubbles (*arrows*) in the plaque shoulder and within the plaque but not extending to the plaque core or to the apex; (*C*) severe (grade 3) IPN showing presence of moving microbubbles within the plaque core and apex. Note the linear arrangement of microbubbles (*arrows on the right*), which suggests the presence of a large neovessel within the body of the plaque.

$P = .005$). Giannoni and colleagues[34] performed standard carotid ultrasonography and CEUS studies in 73 patients, all of whom underwent CEA. Among the 64 asymptomatic patients who underwent elective CEA, CEUS revealed weak, discrete contrast enhancement with individually identifiable microvessels emanating from the adventitial layer to the vessel lumen (type I pattern). In contrast, carotid plaques obtained from 9 acutely symptomatic patients showed more intense, diffuse contrast enhancement from multiple small-caliber microvessels along the base of the plaques (type II pattern). Histologic examination of plaques from the symptomatic patients revealed an increased number of small (20–30 μm diameter) immature microvessels along the base of the plaque associated with high-intensity staining for VEGF and matrix metalloproteinase (MMP-3); consistent with strong neoangiogenic activity. Varetto and colleagues[35] showed that, in a cohort of 51 patients (12 symptomatic, 39 asymptomatic) who underwent CEA, plaques with greater contrast enhancement on CEUS had increased numbers of newly formed capillaries on histopathologic examination and plaques with lower gray-scale median values correlated with greater vascularization. Shalhoub and colleagues[36] performed late-phase CEUS carotid studies in 31 patients with symptomatic carotid stenosis who underwent CEA, and noted that plaques that showed a normalized late-phase CEUS signal greater than or equal to 0 were associated with significantly greater immunopositivity for inflammatory (CD68, interleukin-6), angiogenic (CD31), and matrix degradation (MMP-1, MMP-3) mediators compared with plaques with a late-phase CEUS signal less than 0. Hoogi and colleagues[37] used harmonic imaging with pulse inversion and a low MI to perform CEUS studies in 27 patients with severe carotid stenosis before CEA and developed an image processing algorithm to automatically quantify the extent of IPN within the plaques. Excluding the 5 patients with heavy calcification that precluded adequate visualization, the IPN area ratio (IPN area/total plaque area) on CEUS highly correlated with the histopathologic IPN ratio (determined by CD31 immunostaining) as well as the number of inflammatory cells (determined by CD3 and CD68 immunostaining) within the plaques. Vavuranakis and colleagues[36] reported that enhancement of plaque brightness on CEUS was significant for both stable and unstable plaque subgroups in a sample of 14 patients with carotid stenosis ($P = 0.018$ for both), but the number of microvessels as assessed by CD34 antibody was significantly higher in unstable plaques compared to stable plaques (36.6 ± 17.4 vs. 13.0 ± 7.2 respectively, $P = 0.002$). Li and colleagues[39] reported that, in a sample of 17 patients having CEA, a semiquantitative CEUS analysis correlated with neovascularization by histology ($r = 0.70$; $P = .002$). Furthermore, semiquantitative and quantitative measurements were highly correlated with each other, suggesting that either can be used to detect IPN. Müller and colleagues[40] performed CEUS studies in 33 patients with moderate-to-severe carotid stenosis undergoing CEA and noted the presence of IPN by using a visual grading scale (0–2). The results correlated significantly with quantification of IPN using intensity-over-time curve (ITC) analysis ($P = .03$) and histopathologic examination (n = 19) revealed a larger CD34+ area in patients with grade 1/2 IPN versus grade 0 ($P = .03$). Iezzi and colleagues[41] also reported that plaque enhancement on preoperative CEUS had significant correlations with immunohistologic detection of plaque neovascularization with increased sensitivity, specificity, PPV, NPV, and diagnostic accuracy of 94%, 68%, 87%, 85%, and 86%, respectively, in a cohort of 50 patients referred for CEA. A higher NPV of 91% was noted when the analysis was confined to asymptomatic patients. A summary of the studies exploring the correlation between IPN seen on carotid CEUS imaging with histopathologic examination of the plaques is presented in **Table 1**.

CLINICAL UTILITY OF CONTRAST-ENHANCED ULTRASONOGRAPHY IN PATIENTS WITH CAROTID ARTERY DISEASE
Role of Contrast-enhanced Ultrasonography in the Treatment of Carotid Stenosis

Zhou and colleagues[42] reported on a cohort of 46 patients with carotid stenosis (>50%) and compared the abilities of CEUS and color Doppler ultrasonography (CDUS) for the assessment of plaque vulnerability using transcranial color Doppler monitoring of microembolic signals (MES). Using CEUS, MES were identified in 2 patients (12.5%) within class 1 (nonneovascularization) as opposed to 15 patients (50.0%) within class 2 (neovascularization) (P = .023), but plaque echogenicity on traditional CDUS could not differentiate between those with MES and those without. Shao and colleagues[43] studied the use of CEUS to determine the choice of CEA or CAS as treatment of severe carotid stenosis. The results indicated that a higher grade of plaque enhancement correlated with a higher risk of adverse events and restenosis after CAS. In patients with grade 4 plaque using CEUS, the incidence of adverse events in the CAS group was significantly higher than that in the CEA group (7.14% vs 55.56%; $P<.05$). Varetto and colleagues[44] recently studied the correlation between contrast enhancement of the plaque (with CEUS) and cerebral microembolization (with MR imaging) in a cohort of 35 patients who underwent carotid stent placement. Contrast enhancement of the carotid plaque was associated with postprocedural microembolization as noted on MR imaging poststenting. These studies suggested that plaques with a higher density of IPN may be more vulnerable to rupture and embolization of atheromatous debris to the cerebral circulation compared with patients with little or no IPN. These data support the hypothesis that patients with vulnerable carotid plaque may be surgical candidates rather than candidates for carotid stents. However, larger, randomized controlled studies are required to test this hypothesis. As a means for monitoring postprocedure results, CEUS seems to be a reliable, noninvasive method for evaluation of in-stent restenosis after internal CAS compared with color-coded duplex ultrasonography and power Doppler.[45]

Contrast-enhanced Ultrasonography in Patients Without Prior Stroke (Primary Prevention)

We recently evaluated the relationship between measures of carotid VV by CEUS and carotid intima-media thickness (CIMT) in a cohort of 465 patients (324 with diabetes mellitus [DM] and 141 nondiabetics) without a prior history of stroke who were enrolled in 2 separate clinical trials. Patients with DM had a significantly higher median VV ratio compared with nondiabetics (median VV ratio 1.21 ± 0.26 vs 0.80 ± 0.19; $P<.0001$). The presence of DM was associated with a 36% higher VV ratio (95% confidence interval, 24.3–48.0; $P<.001$) and there was no association between VV ratio and CIMT, low-density lipoprotein cholesterol, or systolic blood pressure in the combined analysis.[46] In a cohort of 104 patients with carotid plaques greater than 2 mm seen on conventional 2D ultrasonography, the use of CEUS showed that enhanced intensity in patients with DM was greater than that in their counterparts without DM, suggesting that carotid plaque in patients with DM may have more neovessels and may therefore be more vulnerable.[47] CEUS techniques were used to identify evidence of subclinical carotid atherosclerosis in nearly 90% of asymptomatic individuals with DM as reported in another study.[48] The same investigators noted that carotid CEUS showed atherosclerotic plaques in 90% of asymptomatic patients with familial hypercholesterolemia and without known atherosclerosis. IPN was present in 86% of these patients, and plaques with irregular or ulcerated surface had significantly more IPN than plaques with a smooth surface ($P<.05$).[49]

Arcidiacono and colleagues[50] performed B-mode carotid ultrasonography for CIMT measurement and used carotid CEUS for visualization of adventitial VV in 65 healthy individuals with no associated cardiovascular risk factors. Only the left CIMT was weakly correlated with left adventitial VV (Spearman rank correlation coefficient, $r = 0.37$; $P = .004$) but not the right. Furthermore, age but no other anthropometric or biochemical factor correlated with the left carotid VV ratio ($r = 0.313$; $P = .015$). The investigators hypothesized that atherosclerosis may manifest in the left carotid artery earlier than in the right, and that measurement of left carotid adventitial VV may be a sensitive marker of subclinical atherosclerosis in low-risk populations. In a study of 100 consecutive asymptomatic patients with greater than or equal to 1 cardiovascular risk factor for atherosclerosis, cardiovascular risk was estimated by calculating the Prospective Cardiovascular

Table 1
Summary of published studies of the correlation of IPN seen by carotid CEUS and histopathologic examination of carotid plaques after carotid endarterectomy

First Author (Ref.), Year of Publication	Number of Subjects	Main Inclusion Criteria	Number of Subjects with Symptomatic Stroke, n (%)	Quantification of Plaque Neovascularization on CEUS	Quantification of Plaque Neovascularization on Histology	Summary of Main Findings
Vicenzini et al,[26] 2007	23	Asymptomatic patients with carotid stenosis (varying severity)	None	Visualization of microbubbles (no quantification reported)	No scoring system used (only 1 patient underwent histologic examination of plaque)	• Microvessels seen by visualization of microbubbles penetrating in the isohyperechoic fibrous and fibrofatty tissue regardless of the severity of stenosis • Histology confirmed the presence of the microvessel seen within the plaque on CEUS
Shah et al,[33] 2007	17	Patients referred for carotid ultrasonography testing based on clinical indications (symptomatic cerebrovascular disease, preventive examinations)	5 (29)	Visual scoring: Grades 0–3 (ranging from no neovascularization to presence of pulsating, arterial vessel within the plaque suggesting arteriogenesis)	Numerical values (0–3) assigned based on number of vessels present in each slide	• Correlation between neovascularization seen on CEUS and neovascularization seen using histology (CD31 staining): Spearman rank coefficient was 0.68 • When CEUS results were correlated with the other histologic markers (CD34, von Willebrand factor, and hemosiderin), a correlation of 0.50 was obtained

Coli et al,[27] 2008	32	Patients (>18 y) with at least 1 carotid atherosclerotic stenosis >30%	6 (19)	Visual scoring: Grades 0–2 (ranging from no bubbles within the plaque to bubbles reaching plaque core and/or extensive contrast-agent enhancement throughout the plaque)	Vessel number ratio (first-order and second-order VV identified, and vessel area compared with the cross-sectional plaque area, expressed as the total number of VV per square millimeter)	• In the series of 52 lesions, echolucent plaques showed a higher degree of contrast-agent enhancement ($P<.001$) • In the surgical subgroup, plaques with higher contrast-agent enhancement showed a greater neovascularization at histology (grade 2 vs grade 1 contrast-agent enhancement: median VV density: 3.24/mm² vs 1.82/mm², respectively, $P = .005$)
Giannoni et al,[34] 2009	77	Patients referred for carotid endarterectomy	9 (11)	Qualitative assessment of echo-contrast enhancement of plaques (patterns of enhancement between asymptomatic and symptomatic patients)	Qualitative assessment of microvessel diameter and distribution within the plaque	• In asymptomatic patients, CEUS revealed weak, discrete contrast enhancement with individually identifiable microvessels running from the adventitial layer toward the vessel lumen (type I pattern), and histologic examination showed less evident neovascularization with microvessel diameters of >50 μm • Plaques from symptomatic patients showed more intense, diffuse contrast enhancement and multiple small-caliber microvessels along the base (type II pattern), and histologic examination revealed an increased number of small (diameter 20–30 μm), immature microvessels with immunohistochemical evidence of strong neoangiogenic activity

(continued on next page)

Table 1
(continued)

First Author (Ref.), Year of Publication	Number of Subjects	Main Inclusion Criteria	Number of Subjects with Symptomatic Stroke, n (%)	Quantification of Plaque Neovascularization on CEUS	Quantification of Plaque Neovascularization on Histology	Summary of Main Findings
Shalhoub et al,[36] 2011	31	Patients awaiting carotid endarterectomy	16 (52)	Normalized late-phase CEUS signal using receiver operating characteristic curve analysis	Percentage of plaque area positive for the macrophage marker CD68 and the endothelial cell marker CD31 by immunohistochemistry	Percentage area immunopositivity was significantly higher in subjects in whom normalized plaque late-phase intensity was ≥ 0 vs <0 (CD68, mean 11.8 vs 6.68, $P = .004$; CD31, mean 9.45 vs 4.82; $P = .025$)
Hoogi et al,[37] 2011	27	Patients with severe carotid stenosis scheduled for carotid endarterectomy	8 (30)	Ratio of neovascularization area to the total plaque area (calculated by dividing the neovascularization areas by the mean area of the plaque on every cardiac cycle)	Ratio of neovessel area to the total plaque area	• The ratio of the neovascularization area to the total plaque area on CEUS images was well correlated with the same histopathologic ratio ($R^2 = 0.7905$) and with the number of inflammatory cells present in the plaque ($R^2 = 0.6109$) • The histopathologic ratio and the number of intraplaque inflammatory cells also were well correlated ($R^2 = 0.7034$)
Varreto et al,[35] 2012	51	Patients with indications for carotid endarterectomy	12 (23)	Contrast enhancement of the plaque measured by SI_{max} and SI_{mean}	Neovessel density	Significant differences between symptomatic and asymptomatic patients for: • SI_{max} 30 (29–35.5) vs 24 (19.7–27) ($P<.001$) • SI_{mean} 23 (20.5–27) vs 15 (8–18.25) ($P<.001$) • Vessel density (vessels/mm^2) 41.5 (30–70) vs 12.6 (7–18.6) ($P<.001$)

Study	N	Population		CEUS method	Histology	Findings
Vavuranakis et al,[38] 2013	14	Patients with carotid plaque scheduled for carotid endarterectomy	Not available	Qualitative assessment using echo-contrast enhancement of plaque	Immunohistochemistry (CD34, VEGF, CD68, and CD3)	• Enhancement of plaque brightness on CEUS was significant for both stable and unstable plaque subgroups ($P = .018$ for both) • Immunochemistry showed that microvessels, as assessed by CD34 antibody, were more dense in unstable vs stable plaques (36.6 ± 17.4 vs 13.0 ± 7.2 respectively, $P = .002$) • Correlation between plaque brightness enhancement on CEUS and microvessel density was significant only for stable plaques ($r = 0.800$, $P = .031$)
Li et al,[39] 2014	17	Consecutive patients who underwent carotid endarterectomy	13 (76)	• Visual scoring: Grade 0–4 (ranging from no bubbles within the plaque to extensive intraplaque enhancement) • Enhancement intensity (dB) at the plaque	• Neovessel count (number of vessels/mm²). • Immunohistochemistry (CD34 and CD68)	• Semiquantitative CEUS analyses were correlated with neovascularization at histology ($r = 0.70$, $P = .002$) • Quantitative analysis was also correlated with neovascularization at histology (enhancement intensity [plaque] $r = 0.81$, $P<.001$) • Enhancement intensity (plaque) ($r = 0.64$, $P = .01$) was correlated with the degree of enhancement as assessed visually

(continued on next page)

Table 1
(continued)

First Author (Ref.), Year of Publication	Number of Subjects	Main Inclusion Criteria	Number of Subjects with Symptomatic Stroke, n (%)	Quantification of Plaque Neovascularization on CEUS	Quantification of Plaque Neovascularization on Histology	Summary of Main Findings
Müller et al,[40] 2014	33	Patients with ≥50% symptomatic or ≥60% asymptomatic stenosis (according to European Carotid Surgery Trial criteria)	17 (51)	• Visual scoring: Grades 0–2 (ranging from no enhancement to extensive enhancement)	Microvessel density with immunohistochemistry (CD34+ staining)	• Visual grading (33 patients, interobserver agreement = 94%) correlated significantly with ITC analysis (P = .03) • Histopathology (n = 19) revealed a larger CD34+ area in patients with grade 1/2 vs grade 0 (P = .03)
Iezzi et al,[41] 2015	50	Patients undergoing carotid endarterectomy	18 (36)	• Contrast enhancement ratio (ratio of the enhanced intensity in the plaque to that in the lumen of the carotid artery) • Visual scoring on a 3-point scale for dynamic CEUS imaging, 2-point scale for late-phase imaging	• Semiquantitative assessment for lipid core component, macrophages, smooth muscle cells, and collagen components • The percentage of lipid core component expressed as a percentage of the total plaque area	Qualitative CEUS evaluation obtained high statistical results compared with immunohistologic results, with values of sensitivity, specificity, PPV, NPV, and diagnostic accuracy of 94%, 68%, 87%, 85%, and 86%, respectively, which became higher if considering only asymptomatic patients, with an NPV of 91%

Abbreviations: SI$_{max}$, maximum signal intensity; SI$_{mean}$, mean signal intensity.

Münster Heart Study (PROCAM) risk score. A total of 21 patients (21%) had abnormal CIMT, 77% had plaques on conventional carotid ultrasonography, and 88% had plaques on standard carotid ultrasonography combined with CEUS. CEUS changed the PROCAM risk category in most asymptomatic patients, with a total of 79 patients (79%) reclassified as high cardiovascular risk (P<.001).[51] However, larger studies are needed to further explore the relationships between IPN and other risk factor indices in low-risk populations, and the implications of CEUS findings on the management of cardiovascular risk in these individuals.

Intraplaque Neovascularization Imaging by Carotid Contrast-enhanced Ultrasonography and Risk of Cardiovascular Disease

Identification of IPN using CEUS of the carotid arteries has been correlated with adverse clinical cardiovascular events. In a retrospective cohort of 147 consecutive patients referred for carotid duplex ultrasonography examination, we observed the presence of grade 2 IPN (clear visible appearance of bubbles within the plaque moving from the adventitial side or shoulder reaching plaque core) in carotid plaques was significantly associated with a history of cardiovascular events (myocardial infarction, TIA, or stroke) using multivariate logistic regression.[52] Huang and colleagues[53] compared plaque morphology and neovascularization by standard ultrasonography and CEUS carotid studies in 81 patients with recent ischemic strokes with 95 control subjects. The investigators noted a significantly higher risk of stroke in patients with plaques showing contrast enhancement caused by the presence of arterial VV and plaque shoulder enhancement (grade III) and extensive and internal plaque enhancement (grade IV). Patients with ischemic stroke had significantly higher signal intensity caused by contrast enhancement compared with controls. Zhu and colleagues[54] performed carotid CEUS in a cohort of 312 patients with coronary artery disease (CAD) and at least 1 carotid plaque larger than 2 mm on B-mode carotid ultrasonography. They noted that contrast enhancement of plaque was more common in patients with an acute coronary syndrome (ACS) than in those with stable CAD, and was an independent predictor of future coronary events in patients with stable CAD (odds ratio, 3.90; 95% confidence interval, 1.60–9.46; P = .003). Coronary events occurred during the follow-up period in 24 of 111 patients (21.6%) with contrast enhancement of plaque and in only 7 of 137 patients (5.1%) without enhancement (P<.001). Recently, Deyama and

colleagues[55] performed a prospective study of 304 patients with CAD who underwent coronary angiography and carotid duplex and CEUS studies at a single center in Japan. In the 270 patients without prior percutaneous coronary intervention, IPN as assessed by carotid CEUS significantly correlated with the number of diseased coronary arteries and the number of complex lesions as seen on coronary angiography. In addition, among the 84 patients who had ACS at enrollment, multivariate logistic regression analysis showed that the presence of grade 2 IPN on carotid CEUS remained a significant predictor of ACS even after adjustment for age, DM, LDL-cholesterol, C-reactive protein, and statin use at admission (odds ratio, 1.91; P = .005). In a subgroup analysis of 40 patients who underwent repeat duplex ultrasonography and CEUS after 6 months, IPN as seen on CEUS regressed in association with reduction in LDL-cholesterol levels in 46% of patients taking statins versus 14% among those not on statin therapy (**Box 3**).

LIMITATIONS IN THE USE OF CONTRAST-ENHANCED ULTRASONOGRAPHY FOR CAROTID ARTERY DISEASE

Although the application of CEUS for the detection and characterization of carotid artery disease has great utility, limitations exist. Although unlikely

---

Box 3
Clinical use of CEUS in carotid artery disease

- CEUS imaging of carotid plaques enables visualization of subclinical carotid atherosclerosis in high-risk patients, such as those with DM and familial hypercholesterolemia.

- CEUS imaging of carotid plaques enables identification of plaque characteristics not visible using conventional vascular ultrasonography, such as plaque surface irregularity, plaque ulceration, and the presence and density of IPN.

- Presence of IPN within carotid plaques has been associated with a significantly higher risk of adverse cardiovascular events in observational studies, and IPN has been shown to be an independent predictor of future coronary and cerebrovascular events even after adjustment for multiple cardiovascular risk factors.

- Small observational studies suggest that detection of IPN using carotid CEUS imaging in asymptomatic individuals may be useful as a marker of subclinical atherosclerosis.

because of low MI imaging, potentially, a small number of microbubbles may be disrupted by the incoming ultrasonography wave, resulting in possible damage to endothelial cells with recruitment of VEGF-producing inflammatory cells and stimulation of neovascularization.[56] Another limitation of CEUS imaging is the pseudoenhancement artifact caused by the nonlinear response of the microbubbles leading to enhancement of the distal vessel wall.[57] Newer ultrasonography pulse sequences are used to suppress this phenomenon. Initially in 2007, the safety of ultrasonography contrast agents was questioned by the US Food and Drug Administration (FDA). However, after review of the safety data and clinical utility of echocontrast agents, the FDA subsequently modified its warnings because of lack of proven risk as identified in a large number of prospective and retrospective analyses. The most common adverse reactions reported included headache, nausea and/or vomiting, dizziness, and flushing.[58,59] The risk of anaphylactoid reaction or serious cardiac or pulmonary events remains exceedingly small. The present use of echocontrast agents for carotid artery imaging remains an off-label indication in the United States. There is ongoing research for identifying the contrast effect within the adventitial VV and intraplaque angiogenesis. In addition, several investigators have used visual grading schemes for estimating the severity of IPN, although no uniform scale for the grading of IPN exists. Clearly, the development of a standardized, volumetric analysis is required for uniform, reliable reporting. In addition, there are no published cost-effectiveness analyses that address CEUS utility for carotid plaque imaging compared with other imaging methods.

SUMMARY

CEUS is a rapidly evolving imaging modality for accurate estimation of carotid artery stenosis. In addition, the use of CEUS identifies important luminal plaque characteristics and, uniquely, presence of IPN. IPN has been associated with increased inflammation, intraplaque hemorrhage, and matrix degradation, all of which are associated with increased plaque vulnerability. Furthermore, IPN noted within the carotid plaque portends a higher risk of cardiovascular events not limited to the cerebrovascular system. In addition, the identification of IPN with CEUS provides a mechanism to detect subclinical atherosclerosis in patients initially stratified as low risk for cardiovascular events. Most CEUS studies performed to date have used 2D ultrasonography technology; however, with 3D image reconstruction algorithms and dedicated 3D transducers, the advanced technologies presage a new era for noninvasive imaging of carotid artery disease. Current and future research will remain focused on the utility of 3D CEUS for the quantification of plaque burden and IPN, and as a predictor of cardiovascular risk.

REFERENCES

1. North American Symptomatic Carotid Endarterectomy Trial Collaborators. Beneficial effect of carotid endarterectomy in symptomatic patients with high-grade carotid stenosis. N Engl J Med 1991;325(7):445–53.
2. MRC European Carotid Surgery Trial: interim results for symptomatic patients with severe (70-99%) or with mild (0-29%) carotid stenosis. European Carotid Surgery Trialists' Collaborative Group. Lancet 1991;337(8752):1235–43.
3. Brott TG, Halperin JL, Abbara S, et al. 2011 ASA/ACCF/AHA/AANN/AANS/ACR/ASNR/CNS/SAIP/SCAI/SIR/SNIS/SVM/SVS guideline on the management of patients with extracranial carotid and vertebral artery disease: a report of the American College of Cardiology Foundation/American Heart Association Task Force on Practice Guidelines, and the American Stroke Association, American Association of Neuroscience Nurses, American Association of Neurological Surgeons, American College of Radiology, American Society of Neuroradiology, Congress of Neurological Surgeons, Society of Atherosclerosis Imaging and Prevention, Society for Cardiovascular Angiography and Interventions, Society of Interventional Radiology, Society of NeuroInterventional Surgery, Society for Vascular Medicine, and Society for Vascular Surgery. J Am Coll Cardiol 2011;57(8):e16–94.
4. Pfister K, Rennert J, Greiner B, et al. Pre-surgical evaluation of ICA-stenosis using 3D power Doppler, 3D color coded Doppler sonography, 3D B-flow and contrast enhanced B-flow in correlation to CTA/MRA: first clinical results. Clin Hemorheol Microcirc 2009;41(2):103–16.
5. Cosgrove D. Ultrasound contrast agents: an overview. Eur J Radiol 2006;60(3):324–30.
6. Ferrer JM, Samso JJ, Serrando JR, et al. Use of ultrasound contrast in the diagnosis of carotid artery occlusion. J Vasc Surg 2000;31(4):736–41.
7. Droste DW, Jurgens R, Nabavi DG, et al. Echocontrast-enhanced ultrasound of extracranial internal carotid artery high-grade stenosis and occlusion. Stroke 1999;30(11):2302–6.
8. Köster W. Endarteritis and arteritis. Berl Klin Wochenschr 1876;13:454–5.
9. Michel JB, Martin-Ventura JL, Nicoletti A, et al. Pathology of human plaque vulnerability: mechanisms and consequences of intraplaque haemorrhages. Atherosclerosis 2014;234(2):311–9.

10. Moulton KS. Plaque angiogenesis and atherosclerosis. Curr Atheroscler Rep 2001;3(3):225–33.

11. Shemirani B, Crowe DL. Hypoxic induction of HIF-1alpha and VEGF expression in head and neck squamous cell carcinoma lines is mediated by stress activated protein kinases. Oral Oncol 2002; 38(3):251–7.

12. Barger AC, Beeuwkes R 3rd. Rupture of coronary vasa vasorum as a trigger of acute myocardial infarction. Am J Cardiol 1990;66(16):41G–3G.

13. Fleiner M, Kummer M, Mirlacher M, et al. Arterial neovascularization and inflammation in vulnerable patients: early and late signs of symptomatic atherosclerosis. Circulation 2004;110(18):2843–50.

14. Dunmore BJ, McCarthy MJ, Naylor AR, et al. Carotid plaque instability and ischemic symptoms are linked to immaturity of microvessels within plaques. J Vasc Surg 2007;45(1):155–9.

15. Fryer JA, Myers PC, Appleberg M. Carotid intraplaque hemorrhage: the significance of neovascularity. J Vasc Surg 1987;6(4):341–9.

16. Mofidi R, Crotty TB, McCarthy P, et al. Association between plaque instability, angiogenesis and symptomatic carotid occlusive disease. Br J Surg 2001; 88(7):945–50.

17. Moreno PR, Purushothaman KR, Fuster V, et al. Plaque neovascularization is increased in ruptured atherosclerotic lesions of human aorta: implications for plaque vulnerability. Circulation 2004;110(14): 2032–8.

18. Hellings WE, Peeters W, Moll FL, et al. Composition of carotid atherosclerotic plaque is associated with cardiovascular outcome: a prognostic study. Circulation 2010;121(17):1941–50.

19. Howard DP, van Lammeren GW, Rothwell PM, et al. Symptomatic carotid atherosclerotic disease: correlations between plaque composition and ipsilateral stroke risk. Stroke 2015;46(1):182–9.

20. Kono Y, Pinnell SP, Sirlin CB, et al. Carotid arteries: contrast-enhanced US angiography–preliminary clinical experience. Radiology 2004;230(2): 561–8.

21. Faggioli GL, Pini R, Mauro R, et al. Identification of carotid 'vulnerable plaque' by contrast-enhanced ultrasonography: correlation with plaque histology, symptoms and cerebral computed tomography. Eur J Vasc Endovasc Surg 2011;41(2):238–48.

22. Hammond CJ, McPherson SJ, Patel JV, et al. Assessment of apparent internal carotid occlusion on ultrasound: prospective comparison of contrast-enhanced ultrasound, magnetic resonance angiography and digital subtraction angiography. Eur J Vasc Endovasc Surg 2008;35(4):405–12.

23. Baud JM, Becker F, Maurizot A, et al. Contrast enhanced ultrasound can show symptomatic carotid lesions not visualized with magnetic resonance angiography. J Mal Vasc 2013;38(6):385–91.

24. Feinstein SB. The powerful microbubble: from bench to bedside, from intravascular indicator to therapeutic delivery system, and beyond. Am J Physiol Heart Circ Physiol 2004;287(2):H450–7.

25. Feinstein SB. Contrast ultrasound imaging of the carotid artery vasa vasorum and atherosclerotic plaque neovascularization. J Am Coll Cardiol 2006; 48(2):236–43.

26. Vicenzini E, Giannoni MF, Puccinelli F, et al. Detection of carotid adventitial vasa vasorum and plaque vascularization with ultrasound cadence contrast pulse sequencing technique and echo-contrast agent. Stroke 2007;38(10):2841–3.

27. Coli S, Magnoni M, Sangiorgi G, et al. Contrast-enhanced ultrasound imaging of intraplaque neovascularization in carotid arteries: correlation with histology and plaque echogenicity. J Am Coll Cardiol 2008;52(3):223–30.

28. van den Oord SC, Akkus Z, Bosch JG, et al. Quantitative contrast-enhanced ultrasound of intraplaque neovascularization in patients with carotid atherosclerosis. Ultraschall Med 2015;36(2):154–61.

29. Saito K, Nagatsuka K, Ishibashi-Ueda H, et al. Contrast-enhanced ultrasound for the evaluation of neovascularization in atherosclerotic carotid artery plaques. Stroke 2014;45(10):3073–5.

30. Ventura CA, da Silva ES, Cerri GG, et al. Can contrast-enhanced ultrasound with second-generation contrast agents replace computed tomography angiography for distinguishing between occlusion and pseudo-occlusion of the internal carotid artery? Clinics (Sao Paulo) 2015;70(1):1–6.

31. ten Kate GL, van Dijk AC, van den Oord SC, et al. Usefulness of contrast-enhanced ultrasound for detection of carotid plaque ulceration in patients with symptomatic carotid atherosclerosis. Am J Cardiol 2013;112(2):292–8.

32. Hjelmgren O, Johansson L, Prahl U, et al. A study of plaque vascularization and inflammation using quantitative contrast-enhanced US and PET/CT. Eur J Radiol 2014;83(7):1184–9.

33. Shah F, Balan P, Weinberg M, et al. Contrast-enhanced ultrasound imaging of atherosclerotic carotid plaque neovascularization: a new surrogate marker of atherosclerosis? Vasc Med 2007;12(4): 291–7.

34. Giannoni MF, Vicenzini E, Citone M, et al. Contrast carotid ultrasound for the detection of unstable plaques with neoangiogenesis: a pilot study. Eur J Vasc Endovasc Surg 2009;37(6):722–7.

35. Varetto G, Gibello L, Bergamasco L, et al. Contrast enhanced ultrasound in atherosclerotic carotid artery disease. Int Angiol 2012;31(6):565–71.

36. Shalhoub J, Monaco C, Owen DR, et al. Late-phase contrast-enhanced ultrasound reflects biological features of instability in human carotid atherosclerosis. Stroke 2011;42(12):3634–6.

37. Hoogi A, Adam D, Hoffman A, et al. Carotid plaque vulnerability: quantification of neovascularization on contrast-enhanced ultrasound with histopathologic correlation. AJR Am J Roentgenol 2011;196(2):431–6.

38. Vavuranakis M, Sigala F, Vrachatis DA, et al. Quantitative analysis of carotid plaque vasa vasorum by CEUS and correlation with histology after endarterectomy. Vasa 2013;42(3):184–95.

39. Li C, He W, Guo D, et al. Quantification of carotid plaque neovascularization using contrast-enhanced ultrasound with histopathologic validation. Ultrasound Med Biol 2014;40(8):1827–33.

40. Müller HF, Viaccoz A, Kuzmanovic I, et al. Contrast-enhanced ultrasound imaging of carotid plaque neo-vascularization: accuracy of visual analysis. Ultrasound Med Biol 2014;40(1):18–24.

41. Iezzi R, Petrone G, Ferrante A, et al. The role of contrast-enhanced ultrasound (CEUS) in visualizing atherosclerotic carotid plaque vulnerability: Which injection protocol? Which scanning technique? Eur J Radiol 2015;84(5):865–71.

42. Zhou Y, Xing Y, Li Y, et al. An assessment of the vulnerability of carotid plaques: a comparative study between intraplaque neovascularization and plaque echogenicity. BMC Med Imaging 2013;13:13.

43. Shao A, Dong X, Zhou J, et al. Comparison of carotid artery endarterectomy and carotid artery stenting in patients with atherosclerotic carotid stenosis. J Craniofac Surg 2014;25(4):1441–7.

44. Varetto G, Gibello L, Faletti R, et al. Contrast-enhanced ultrasound to predict the risk of microembolization during carotid artery stenting. Radiol Med 2015. [Epub ahead of print].

45. Clevert DA, Sommer WH, Helck A, et al. Duplex and contrast enhanced ultrasound (CEUS) in evaluation of in-stent restenosis after carotid stenting. Clin Hemorheol Microcirc 2011;48(1):199–208.

46. Sampson UK, Harrell FE Jr, Fazio S, et al. Carotid adventitial vasa vasorum and intima-media thickness in a primary prevention population. Echocardiography 2015;32(2):264–70.

47. Xiong L, Li P, Zhao BW. Evaluation of carotid plaque neovascularization in patients with diabetes mellitus by contrast-enhanced ultrasonography. J Huazhong Univ Sci Technolog Med Sci 2014;34(1):29–32.

48. van den Oord SC, Akkus Z, Renaud G, et al. Assessment of carotid atherosclerosis, intraplaque neovascularization, and plaque ulceration using quantitative contrast-enhanced ultrasound in asymptomatic patients with diabetes mellitus. Eur Heart J Cardiovasc Imaging 2014;15(11):1213–8.

49. van den Oord SC, Akkus Z, Roeters van Lennep JE, et al. Assessment of subclinical atherosclerosis and intraplaque neovascularization using quantitative contrast-enhanced ultrasound in patients with familial hypercholesterolemia. Atherosclerosis 2013;231(1):107–13.

50. Arcidiacono MV, Rubinat E, Borras M, et al. Left carotid adventitial vasa vasorum signal correlates directly with age and with left carotid intima-media thickness in individuals without atheromatous risk factors. Cardiovasc Ultrasound 2015;13(1):20.

51. van den Oord SC, ten Kate GL, Sijbrands EJ, et al. Effect of carotid plaque screening using contrast-enhanced ultrasound on cardiovascular risk stratification. Am J Cardiol 2013;111(5):754–9.

52. Staub D, Patel MB, Tibrewala A, et al. Vasa vasorum and plaque neovascularization on contrast-enhanced carotid ultrasound imaging correlates with cardiovascular disease and past cardiovascular events. Stroke 2010;41(1):41–7.

53. Huang PT, Chen CC, Aronow WS, et al. Assessment of neovascularization within carotid plaques in patients with ischemic stroke. World J Cardiol 2010; 2(4):89–97.

54. Zhu Y, Deng YB, Liu YN, et al. Use of carotid plaque neovascularization at contrast-enhanced US to predict coronary events in patients with coronary artery disease. Radiology 2013;268(1):54–60.

55. Deyama J, Nakamura T, Takishima I, et al. Contrast-enhanced ultrasound imaging of carotid plaque neovascularization is useful for identifying high-risk patients with coronary artery disease. Circ J 2013; 77(6):1499–507.

56. Yoshida J, Ohmori K, Takeuchi H, et al. Treatment of ischemic limbs based on local recruitment of vascular endothelial growth factor-producing inflammatory cells with ultrasonic microbubble destruction. J Am Coll Cardiol 2005;46(5):899–905.

57. ten Kate GL, Renaud GG, Akkus Z, et al. Far-wall pseudoenhancement during contrast-enhanced ultrasound of the carotid arteries: clinical description and in vitro reproduction. Ultrasound Med Biol 2012;38(4):593–600.

58. Lantheus Medical Imaging. Definity (perflutren lipid microsphere) full prescribing information (product insert). Lantheus Medical Imaging website (US). Available at: http://www.definityimaging.com/pdf/DEFINITY%20Prescribing%20Information%205515987-0413.pdf 2013;515987-0413. Accessed May 1, 2015.

59. GE Healthcare. Optison (perflutren protein type-A microspheres injectable suspension, USP) full prescribing information (product insert). GE Healthcare website (US). Available at: http://www.optisonimaging.com/us/wp-content/uploads/2014/10/Updated-Optison-PI-10-21-14.pdf 2013;OPT-1F-OSLO. Accessed May 1, 2015.

Detection of Vulnerable Plaque in Patients with Cryptogenic Stroke

Anna Bayer-Karpinska, MD[a],*, Andreas Schindler, MD[b],
Tobias Saam, MD[b]

KEYWORDS

- Cryptogenic stroke • Carotid artery plaque • Carotid MR angiography • Intraplaque hemorrhage
- Lipid-rich necrotic core • Fibrous cap rupture • Echogenicity • Plaque inflammation

KEY POINTS

- Cryptogenic stroke accounts for up to 40% of ischemic stroke cases with a recurrence rate of 3% to 6%.
- Mild and nonstenosing carotid artery plaques represent a possible but underestimated embolic source in patients with cryptogenic stroke.
- Ultrasonography, computed angiography, high-resolution carotid magnetic resonance angiography, and PET with fluorodeoxyglucose allow noninvasive imaging of carotid artery plaques and characteristic features of plaque vulnerability.
- In patients with mild and nonstenosing plaques, high-resolution carotid MR imaging might be the most promising tool to assess the correlation of vulnerable plaques and cryptogenic stroke, stroke recurrence, and plaque progression.

INTRODUCTION

Stroke is still one of the leading causes of death and disability in industrialized countries.[1] Currently used stroke classification systems consider atherosclerotic lesions of the carotid bifurcation only as causative, if they are associated with substantial luminal narrowing of at least 50%.[2] Patients with mild or nonstenosing carotid artery plaques do not fulfill these criteria and, thus, are often diagnosed as stroke of unknown cause, so-called cryptogenic stroke. It has been shown in the coronary arteries that most myocardial infarctions occur in arteries with 50% or less stenosis.[3] Similarly it is commonly assumed that most macroangiopathic ischemic strokes are caused by arterio-arterial embolism from ruptured atherosclerotic plaques and not from high-grade stenosis. In fact, several studies demonstrated an association of vulnerable plaques in stenosed vessels with previous or subsequent stroke and stroke recurrence, respectively.[4] Data regarding arterio-arterial embolism from nonstenosing plaques in patients with a cryptogenic stroke are rare. Nevertheless, in this article, the authors present several plaque imaging techniques, including ultrasonography with and without contrast medium, micro-emboli signal (MES) detection, computed tomography angiography (CTA), 18F-fluorodeoxy-glucose (FDG)–PET, as well as high-resolution MR imaging, and discuss their role in the diagnostic work-up of patients with cryptogenic stroke.

Disclosure Statement: The authors have nothing to disclose.
[a] Institute for Stroke and Dementia Research, Ludwig-Maximilians-University Hospital Munich, Feodor-Lynen-Str. 17, Munich 81377, Germany; [b] Institute for Clinical Radiology, Ludwig-Maximilians-University Hospital Munich, Pettenkoferstr. 8a, Munich 81377, Germany
* Corresponding author.
E-mail address: anna.bayer@med.uni-muenchen.de

1052-5149/16/$ – see front matter © 2016 Elsevier Inc. All rights reserved.

Furthermore, the focus is on studies regarding the progression of plaque burden after stroke, the influence of medical therapy on plaque progression, and the association of vulnerable plaques and stroke recurrence. Finally, the authors highlight ongoing studies in this field.

CRYPTOGENIC STROKE

Current etiologic classification systems try to assign ischemic stroke causes into one of 4 major categories: occlusive large artery atherosclerosis, cardioembolism, small vessel disease, and other rare causes, such as arterial dissection or vasculitis. However, despite intense clinical work-up in 23% to 40% of all ischemic strokes, no definite cause can be established; they are, thus, classified as cryptogenic strokes.[5]

The definition of a cryptogenic stroke is slightly different depending on the classification system used. According to the widely used Trial of Org 10172 in Acute Stroke Treatment (TOAST) classification system, which was established in 1993, an ischemic stroke is considered to be cryptogenic if the stroke cause remains unknown, if more than one cause seems causative, or if the diagnostic assessment is incomplete.[6] Newer classification systems, such as the ASCOD classification, which was established in 2009, define cryptogenic stroke as ischemic stroke with unknown cause.[7] Thus, in this newer classification system, strokes with more than one potential source or strokes with incomplete diagnostic assessment are no longer classified as cryptogenic.

Identification of the potential cause of the ischemic stroke is of utmost importance because therapy and the risk of a recurrent event vary across different stroke subtypes.[8] Thus, the diagnosis of cryptogenic stroke is unsatisfying for the clinician as well as for patients given that recurrence rates of ischemic stroke of up to 30% within 1 year have been reported.[9] To date, standardized diagnostic criteria for cryptogenic stroke are still missing and no consensus exists on the appropriate diagnostic work-up. In the authors' opinion, the minimal diagnostic work-up should include imaging of the extracranial and intracranial vessels, brain imaging by MR imaging, and cardiac tests including 24-hour electrocardiogram (ECG) monitoring and transthoracic echocardiography (Box 1). In some cases, especially in young patients, further blood and cerebrospinal fluid investigations may be necessary.[10] With the diagnostic approach mentioned earlier, high-risk cardioembolic sources like atrial fibrillation or intraventricular thrombus, occlusive or stenosing atherosclerotic disease, vasculitis, arterial dissection, and lacunar infarcts due to cerebral small vessel disease can be diagnosed or excluded.

Recently a new clinical construct termed embolic stroke of undetermined source (ESUS) was introduced to describe stroke entities with a presumed embolic cause.[11] ESUS comprises a subset of patients with signs of embolic stroke on MR imaging and sufficient diagnostic work-up to exclude the major-risk causes of embolic stroke mentioned earlier. The rationale for this new clinical construct is the hypothesis that oral

---

Box 1
Minimal diagnostic requirements for cryptogenic stroke

Diagnostic Assessment	Stroke Cause
Imaging of the extracranial and intracranial vessels by ultrasound, CTA, or MRA	Occlusive atherosclerotic disease Artery dissection
Brain imaging by MR imaging	Small vessel disease with lacunar infarct
12-lead ECG and 24-hour or greater ECG monitoring	Major risk cardioembolic source
	• For example, atrial fibrillation
Transthoracic echocardiography	For example, thrombus from the aortic or mitral valve, the left cardiac chamber
Optional, according to age and medical history: Imaging of the aorta by CTA or TEE	Arteriogenic embolism from aortic arch atheroma
Blood tests for prothrombotic factors and inflammatory diseases	Paradoxic embolism (in combination with patent foramen ovale) Vasculitis Endocarditis
Lumbar puncture (CSF)	Vasculitis

Abbreviations: CSF, cerebrospinal fluid; MRA, magnetic resonance angiography; TEE, transesophageal echocardiography.

anticoagulation therapy will reduce the risk of stroke recurrence in patients with presumed embolic stroke, in particular in the emerging era of new oral anticoagulants, such as dabigatran, rivaroxaban, apixaban, and edoxaban, and their lower risk for intracranial bleedings compared with warfarin.[12] Until now the therapeutic recommendation for patients with cryptogenic stroke is acetylsalicylic acid, statin, and antihypertensive medication as secondary stroke prevention.[2] Randomized controlled trials (eg, Respect-ESUS, Navigate-ESUS) are currently on the way to answer the question whether patients with ESUS could profit from oral anticoagulation therapy instead of acetylsalicylic acid.

This approach seems plausible because recent studies have shown that a significant proportion of patients with ESUS might have covert intermittent atrial fibrillation.[13] With common 24-hour ECG the detection rate of atrial fibrillation is approximately 7% in patients with cryptogenic stroke.[14] However, the Cryptogenic Stroke and Underlying Atrial Fibrillation (CRYSTAL AF) study showed that continuous cardiac monitoring with an insertable cardiac monitor over a period of up to 3 years increased the detection rate of atrial fibrillation to 30% in patients with cryptogenic stroke.[13]

Nevertheless, with advances in diagnostic techniques, other covert or ambiguous stroke causes can be evaluated and have to be discussed in the context of cryptogenic stroke. The role of patent foramen ovale (PFO) and atrial septum aneurysm (ASA) in ischemic stroke is still under debate. Transesophageal echocardiographic evaluations in patients with cryptogenic stroke detected a higher prevalence of PFO and ASA in this group of patients.[15] On the other hand, prospective studies on healthy subjects with PFO and ASA showed no increased stroke risk compared with patients without PFO and ASA, indicating that the PFO is likely to be incidental.[16]

Another potentially underestimated stroke cause is arterio-arterial embolism from aortic atheromas. Atherosclerotic plaques 4 mm or greater of the ascending aorta and the aortic arch, especially with ulceration or mobile fraction, are a known potential source of thrombotic emboli.[17] Furthermore, 4-dimensional flow MR imaging studies of the aorta suggested that retrograde embolization from the atheroma of the proximal descending aorta into the brain-supplying arteries is another potential source of cryptogenic strokes.[18]

Finally cryptogenic stroke may be due to non-stenosing atherosclerotic plaques or low-grade carotid artery stenosis not fulfilling the common criteria for large artery stroke (eg, >50% stenosis according to TOAST or 70%–99% stenosis according to ASCOD). Current treatment algorithms are based mainly on the degree of stenosis rather than plaque morphology as decision criterion.[2] However, histopathologic and radiological data showed that knowledge of the degree of stenosis alone is insufficient to predict a plaque's vulnerability.[4] Plaques with a thin fibrous cap, a large lipid-rich necrotic core, or intraplaque hemorrhage are considered vulnerable and have a high risk for thrombotic complications.[3] To date, several imaging techniques allow noninvasive characterization of plaque vulnerability. Their implementation and significance in the diagnostic work-up of patients with cryptogenic stroke is presented and discussed in the next paragraphs.

METHODS OF VULNERABLE PLAQUE DETECTION IN CRYPTOGENIC STROKE
Ultrasonography

Carotid ultrasonography allows the measurement of intima-media thickness (IMT), detection of plaque formation, description of plaque morphology, especially differentiation between smooth and irregular surface, homogeneous and heterogeneous structure, as well as determination of plaque echogenicity. It is relatively cheap, widely available, has a low risk, and is, therefore, commonly used in clinical routine.

B-Mode Ultrasonography

With B-mode ultrasonography, plaques can be characterized into 5 categories according to their echogenicity (I uniformly echolucent, II predominantly echolucent, III predominantly echogenic, IV uniformly echogenic, V heavily calcified).[19] Classification can be performed either by a subjective visual rating scale, which takes qualitative aspects into account, or in a semiautomated manner. Measurement of gray-scale median (GSM) levels with adjustment of overall plaque brightness to the signal of blood and adventitia assesses global echogenicity quantitatively.[20] Echolucent plaques, with heterogeneous content and irregular surface, are considered to be unstable and to cause thromboembolic ischemic events.[21] Topakian and colleagues[22] demonstrated in a study including 435 patients with asymptomatic high-grade stenosis that plaque echolucency was associated with ipsilateral stroke during the 2-year follow-up with a hazard ratio (HR) of 6.43. The investigators found no recent data on patients with stroke with low-grade stenosis. However, a decade ago a study by Hallerstam and colleagues[23] on 81 symptomatic patients with predominantly less than 50% stenosis negated a relation of echolucent plaques with ipsilateral ischemic events and showed no differences on plaque presence or IMT thickness. Other investigators have shown that changes of GSM levels over time, in particular the decrease of GSM levels, are associated with cardiovascular and cerebrovascular events.[24]

Thus, plaque heterogeneity is not sufficiently heeded by GSM measurement; further quantitative texture analyses, like spatial gray level dependence matrices (SGLDM), obtain more information on plaque morphology. Kakkos and colleagues[25] used visual evaluation and automated software for plaque texture analyses to study plaque heterogeneity of asymptomatic and symptomatic plaques. Echolucent type 1 and 2 plaques as well as juxtaluminal echolucent areas were more frequent in symptomatic patients. In addition automatically derived textural features, especially SGLDM, were even better independent predictors for ischemic events compared with visual evaluation of plaque echolucency and measure of plaque echodensity. A further interesting parameter is the juxtaluminal black area (JBA) of the plaque. In a study on 185 symptomatic patients with varying degrees of stenosis, JBA was shown to have a strong association with ipsilateral ischemic events independent of stenosis degree and GSM levels. In addition a combination of low GSM and JBA greater than 8 mm^2 was also associated with high prevalence of symptomatic plaques.[26]

Three-Dimensional B-Mode Ultrasonography

Three-dimensional (3D) ultrasonography was developed for the measurement of plaque volume and vessel wall volume change over time.[27] Several developmental and validation studies in carotid arteries are currently ongoing.[28] However, studies examining plaque morphology in patients with cryptogenic stroke by 3D ultrasonography or low-grade stenosis have not been published, yet.

Microemboli Signal Detection

Microemboli, detected by transcranial Doppler ultrasound, are regarded as a marker of embolic activity in carotid artery stenosis. A predictive value of MES for subsequent stroke or transient ischemic attack (TIA) in patients with carotid artery stenosis was shown in several studies.[29] It is also known that MES decreases over time after an ischemic event.[30] A systematic review by Ritter and colleagues[31] stated that MES occurs predominantly in high-grade stenosis in symptomatic patients with a prevalence of 48%. In vessels with 30% to 69% stenosis, MES was detected in 19% of cases, whereas no MES was detected in patients with stroke with nonstenosing plaques.

Three studies on recurrence of ischemic events showed more recurrent events during follow-up in patients with detected MES. A limitation of this method is that the detection of MES and the evaluation of this procedure are time consuming.

Contrast-Enhanced Ultrasound

Intravenously injected contrast agent microbubbles of 1 to 10 μm remain within the vascular space and are used as contrast agents for contrast-enhanced ultrasound (CEUS). With this method, plaque angiogenesis and neovascularization can be visualized (**Fig. 1**).[32] Contrast enhancement is usually graded on a 4-point scale (0 = absent, 3 = strong).[33] So far quantification of contrast uptake within a plaque remains challenging, and methods for quantification are still under development.[34] Several studies demonstrated a good correlation of neovascularization detected by CEUS with neovascularization, microvessel density, and amount of inflammatory cells in carotid endarterectomy specimens of highly stenosed vessels.[35] However, only a few CEUS studies, which correlated contrast enhancement with ischemic events, exist. One study on 104 patients with nonstenosing carotid artery plaques showed a significantly higher percentage of echolucent plaques and a higher prevalence of contrast enhancement in plaques of symptomatic patients than those of asymptomatic patients. Furthermore, echolucent plaques had a significantly higher contrast enhancement compared with mixed, echogenic, and calcified plaques.[36] Ritter and colleagues[37]

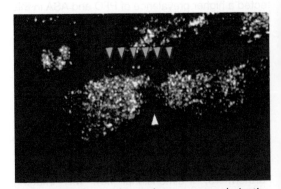

Fig. 1. CEUS of carotid intraplaque neovascularization in longitudinal section; the microbubbles are seen both within the internal carotid artery lumen and within the carotid atheromatous plaque (*green arrowheads*). Furthermore, there is a region of plaque that is not perfused by microbubble contrast (*white arrowhead*). (*From* Shalhoub J, Owen DR, Gauthier T, et al. The use of contrast enhanced ultrasound in carotid arterial disease. Eur J Vasc Endovasc Surg 2010;39(4):381–7; with permission.)

demonstrated an association of MES and the presence of plaque neovascularization in patients with TIA or stroke. Hence, the investigators reasoned that plaque neovascularization might also be a surrogate marker of stroke risk.

Another potential application of CEUS is late-phase CEUS, which visualizes retained microbubbles, indicating plaque inflammation.[38] Data of Owen and colleagues[39] demonstrated a greater normalized late-phase plaque echogenicity after contrast injection in symptomatic patients than in asymptomatic patients. The results were obtained in patients with moderate to high-grade stenosis. It remains unclear if they can be directly transferred to patients with nonstenosing plaques.

Multi-Detector Row Computed Tomography Angiography

Multi-detector row CTA (MDCTA) is an easy and fast imaging method, which is widely available. MDCTA can differentiate between hard, soft, and mixed plaques. Absolute tissue density can be measured, and plaque ulceration can be detected. Furthermore, quantification of plaque calcification and fibrous tissue with a good correlation to histopathology is possible.[40] Calcification is represented by a hard plaque component, whereas a soft plaque component can contain fibrous tissue, lipids, thrombus, or intraplaque hemorrhage. For the differentiation

of hard versus soft plaque components, multiple studies showed a sensitivity and specificity of more than 80%. However, a distinct graduation of the soft plaque component into a lipid-rich necrotic core or intraplaque hemorrhage and the identification of fibrous cap rupture, important criteria for plaque vulnerability, hardly succeeded.[41] This is due to the overlap of Hounsfield unit values of different plaque components, artifacts from calcification, and enhanced arterial lumen, which makes it impossible to identify the fibrous cap.

Most MDCTA studies on the association of plaque components and cerebrovascular events were performed in patients with high-grade carotid artery stenosis. In a study by Gupta and colleagues[42] in 76 patients with 70% to 99% carotid artery stenosis, higher soft plaque thickness and lower hard plaque thickness were associated with prior ipsilateral stroke or TIA. Also in patients with 50% to 69% stenosis, an increase of soft plaque thickness was associated with prior cerebral ischemic events, whereas an increase in hard plaque thickness decreased the odds ratio for stroke.[43]

A study by Trelles and colleagues[41] in patients with ischemic stroke with varying degrees of stenosis showed that plaques with the highest maximum soft plaque thickness on MDCTA were significantly associated with complicated lesion type VI plaques on high-resolution MR imaging (Fig. 2). At last one study associated high soft

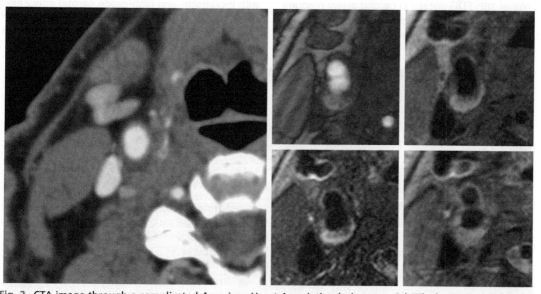

Fig. 2. CTA image through a complicated American Heart Association lesion type 6 (LT6) plaque in the right carotid artery at the carotid bifurcation shows a soft plaque with a mean attenuation of 16 Hounsfield units (range, −7 to 46) and a thickness of the soft plaque component of 6 mm. time of flight, T1, T2, and T1 postgadolinium images at the same level show a hyperintense plaque on all 4 weightings, which suggests the presence of type II intraplaque hemorrhage (IPH). (*From* Trelles M, Eberhardt KM, Buchholz M, et al. CTA for screening of complicated atherosclerotic carotid plaque–American Heart Association type VI lesions as defined by MRI. AJNR Am J Neuroradiol 2013;34(12):2331–7; with permission.)

plaque thickness with recent ipsilateral ischemic events independent of stenosis degree.[44]

Another application of MDCTA is the evaluation of plaque enhancement after injection of contrast medium. Plaque enhancement is considered to represent neovascularization of the plaque. It is stronger and more frequent in noncalcified plaques and can be associated with cerebrovascular events.[45] Plaque enhancement depends on blood flow and image acquisition, and findings regarding its significance are inconsistent.[46]

Because of the limited discrimination of the major criteria of plaque vulnerability, plaque characterization by MDCTA in patients with cryptogenic stroke with nonstenosing plaques is difficult and representative studies in this patient group are missing.

Combination of Computed Tomography or MR Imaging with 18F-Fluorodeoxyglucose–PET

18F-FDG accumulates in carotid lesions with high inflammatory activity, in particular in inflammatory cells.[47] Inflammation is suspected to mediate plaque rupture and, thus, might help to differentiate vulnerable or instable plaques. 18F-FDG uptake is quantified by mean or maximum standardized uptake value or target to background ratio and fused with anatomic structures by additional CT or MR imaging.[48] Some studies, mainly including patients with 50% to 99% stenosis, demonstrated a higher 18F-FDG uptake in carotid artery plaques ipsilateral to a prior ischemic event.[47] Marnane and colleagues[49] showed an association of

18F-FDG uptake and stroke recurrence within 90 days independently of the degree of stenosis (**Fig. 3**). Müller and colleagues[50] demonstrated that 18F-FDG uptake discriminates between symptomatic and asymptomatic high-grade stenosis and that inflammation was mainly found in the soft plaque component measured by MDCTA. In vessels with 30% to 69% stenosis, only weak correlation between 18F-FDG uptake and vulnerable plaque features, like intraplaque hemorrhage and lipid-rich necrotic core, were observed.[51] Studies with 18F-FDG–PET CT or MR imaging on patients with cryptogenic stroke or low-grade carotid artery stenosis are missing.

High-Resolution Carotid MR Imaging

More than a decade ago several studies proved the ability of high-resolution carotid MR imaging to reliably characterize plaque features essential to determine a plaque's vulnerability.[52] MR imaging can identify and quantify the lipid-rich necrotic core, fibrous tissue, calcification, and intraplaque hemorrhage with good correlation to histopathology. In addition, fibrous cap thickness and rupture can be visualized.[53] Intraplaque hemorrhage, fibrous cap rupture, and luminal thrombosis characterize complicated American Heart Association (AHA) lesion type VI plaques, which are thought to cause cerebral thromboembolic events. These associations have been described in patients with moderate- and high-grade carotid artery stenosis.[54] Interestingly, lesion type VI features are also frequent in low- and nonstenosing carotid

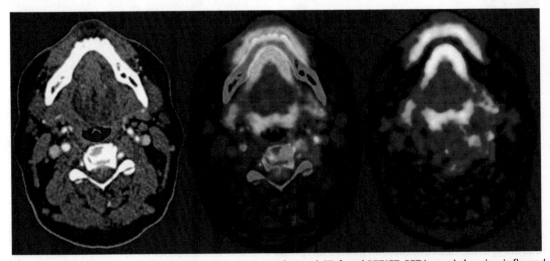

Fig. 3. Carotid PET/CT (from left to right, axial contrast-enhanced CT, fused PET/CT, PET image) showing inflamed left carotid plaque (*red arrow*) in a patient with transient dysphasia and right-arm clumsiness who subsequently had stroke recurrence in the same vascular territory. (*From* Marnane M, Merwick A, Sheehan OC, et al. Carotid plaque inflammation on 18F-fluorodeoxyglucose positron emission tomography predicts early stroke recurrence. Ann Neurol 2012;71(5):709–18; with permission.)

artery plaques,[55] demonstrating that features of vulnerable plaque are not necessarily associated with high-grade stenosis. Reviews and meta-analyses of magnetic resonance plaque imaging studies underlined that the presence of intraplaque hemorrhage, lipid-rich necrotic core, and thinning/rupture of the fibrous cap are strong predictors of subsequent cerebrovascular events in patients with carotid artery stenosis with HRs of intraplaque hemorrhage in symptomatic patients of 11.60 (95% confidence interval: 2.88–46.63; $P = .0006$) compared with an HR of 4.44 (95% confidence interval: 2.54–7.76; $P<.0001$) in asymptomatic subjects.[56]

For clarity purposes, the authors discuss the impact of MR imaging findings in low-grade carotid artery stenosis in patients with cryptogenic stroke and its clinical implications in the following section.

CLINICAL IMPLICATIONS OF MR IMAGING PLAQUE DETECTION IN PATIENTS WITH CRYPTOGENIC STROKE
Prevalence and Characterization of Vulnerable Plaques in Patients with Low-Grade Stenosis

The prevalence of lesion type VI plaques in low-grade carotid artery stenosis and cryptogenic stroke differs across literature. The main differences among plaque imaging studies are heterogeneous study cohorts regarding the index event, different degrees of stenosis, and variable time points for carotid MR imaging, reaching from 48 hours to 3 months after symptom onset. In a study by Parmar and colleagues[57] including 78 patients with suspected ischemic event in the last 48 hours, the prevalence of ipsilateral lesion type VI plaques was 15%. Lesion type VI plaques were associated with ipsilateral ischemic events with an odds ratio of 11.66 ($P<.0001$). However, the study cohort comprised patients with stroke, TIA, and amaurosis fugax; patients with and without stenosis were also included. In a study of 114 symptomatic patients with varying degrees of stenosis intraplaque hemorrhage was found in 59%, 27%, and 0% of symptomatic arteries with greater than 50%, 30% to 49%, and less than 30% stenosis, respectively. In the last group a lipid-rich necrotic core was present in 45% of symptomatic arteries.[58] In a study by Freilinger and colleagues[59] 32 patients with cryptogenic stroke and nonstenosing (<50%) eccentric carotid plaques were recruited from a single stroke unit. In this cohort, lesion type VI plaques were found in 38% of arteries ipsilateral to the stroke, whereas no lesion type VI plaques were found contralateral to the stroke ($P = .001$). The most common diagnostic feature of lesion type VI plaques was intraplaque hemorrhage (75%), followed by fibrous cap rupture (50%) and luminal thrombus (33%) (Fig. 4). Lindsay and colleagues[60] demonstrated that in carotid

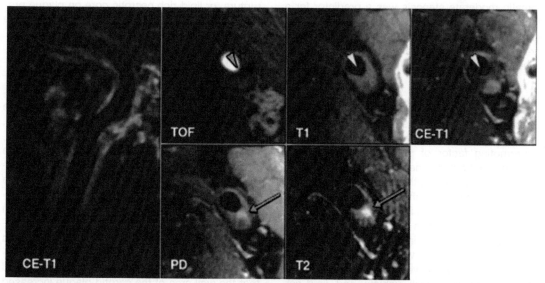

Fig. 4. This nonobstructive AHA type VI plaque was detected in a 78-year-old man with a cryptogenic stroke ipsilateral to the lesion 5 days before the MR imaging scan. The arrow points to a hyperintense area on PD-weighted (PDW) and T2-weighted images, which indicates juxtaluminal hemorrhage/thrombus. The arrowheads on the time of flight (TOF), T1-weighted (TW1), and contrast enhanced (CE-T1W) images point to the site of possible plaque rupture. The lesion consists of a large necrotic core, which does not cause substantial luminal narrowing (see coronal CE-T1W images on the left). PD, proton density. (*From* Freilinger TM, Schindler A, Schmidt C, et al. Prevalence of nonstenosing, complicated atherosclerotic plaques in cryptogenic stroke. JACC Cardiovasc Imaging 2012;5(4):397–405; with permission.)

arteries with at least 30% degree of stenosis, the prevalence of lesion type VI plaques was 54% in symptomatic patients compared with 20% in asymptomatic controls. Interestingly, 55% of lesion type VI plaques were found in vessels with stenosis less than 70%.

As one might expect, the prevalence of certain plaque features, such as lipid-rich necrotic core or intraplaque hemorrhage, is higher in symptomatic arteries and associated with ischemic events.[58,60,61] A study by Kwee and colleagues[62] in 61 patients after an ischemic event within the last 3 months showed a prevalence of 19.7% for intraplaque hemorrhage, 36.1% for thin or ruptured fibrous cap, and 6.8% for lipid-rich necrotic core in mild stenosis. In a retrospective study of patients with stroke with a mean degree of stenosis of 36% McNally and colleagues[61] found a prevalence of 18% for intraluminal thrombus and of 48% for intraplaque hemorrhage. In the control group the prevalence of these plaque features was significantly lower. However, to some extent, this might also be explained by the lower degree of stenosis in this group of 7.4%.[61] Cheung and colleagues[63] showed, in patients with bilateral carotid plaques with 50% or less lumen narrowing, a prevalence of intraplaque hemorrhage of 13% in symptomatic plaques compared with 7% in contralateral plaques.

Furthermore, in one retrospective study the presence of intraplaque hemorrhage in asymptomatic moderate stenosis was a predictor for a future ischemic event.[64] However, attention has to be paid because AHA lesion type VI plaques are also detected in up to 15% of asymptomatic low-grade stenosis.[55]

Plaque Remodeling after Cryptogenic Stroke

Previous studies in patients with high-grade stenosis have suggested that intraplaque hemorrhage is a promoting factor of plaque progression and disruption. Intraplaque hemorrhage may stimulate atherogenic activity within the plaque by free cholesterol and macrophage activation and promote lipid accumulation in the plaque.[65]

One of the first studies on plaque progression in moderate stenosis was in a cohort of asymptomatic patients. Plaques with intraplaque hemorrhage at baseline showed a significantly higher percent change in wall volume and lipid-rich necrotic core volume after 18 months compared with plaques of comparable size without intraplaque hemorrhage. Furthermore, plaques with intraplaque hemorrhage at baseline more often presented with new intraplaque hemorrhage at follow-up.[66] Another study in a similar study cohort

confirmed that in the group of patients with intraplaque hemorrhage, a decrease in lumen volume and a larger increase in wall volume were observed after 18 months. In addition, plaques of patients without statin therapy, equatable with natural plaque development, demonstrated outward remodeling, with an increase in wall volume and total vessel volume.[67]

It is tempting to hypothesize that these findings from asymptomatic patients might be transferred to patients with cryptogenic stroke with mild carotid stenosis, but data on the effect of intraplaque hemorrhage regarding stroke recurrence and plaque progression in cryptogenic stroke are lacking. The authors only found one study in symptomatic patients with TIA or stroke and less than 70% carotid artery stenosis with a follow-up period of 1 year. In this study, mean carotid wall volume increased by 11.2% and carotid lumen volume decreased by 4.8% indicating inward plaque remodeling after the ischemic event. The investigators stated that this could be a sign of plaque stabilization. Intraplaque hemorrhage, fibrous cap rupture, and lipid-rich necrotic core were not associated with plaque progression and remained stable after 12 months.[68] A proposed explanation of the investigators for this discrepant result to previous studies was that plaques in symptomatic patients are already ruptured, culprit plaques, which are healing over time and are not further disrupting. Effects of luminal thrombus, fibrous cap rupture, or lipid-rich necrotic core on plaque progression in mild and nonstenosing plaques have not been reported so far.

Influence of Secondary Stroke Prevention Medication on Plaque Remodeling

Every patient who suffered from ischemic stroke receives secondary stroke prevention medication, mostly consisting of platelet inhibitors and statins, as they were shown to significantly reduce the overall rate of stroke.[2] Statins alter plaque progression and, thus, make it difficult to investigate the natural history of plaque remodeling or progression after an ischemic stroke. However, with carotid MR imaging, the positive effect of antiatherosclerotic medication can be demonstrated by plaque regression. First, studies in asymptomatic subjects with 50% or greater stenosis showed that the wall area of the carotid plaque increased by 2.2% per year. In contrast, statin therapy and a normalized wall index greater than 0.64 were associated with a significantly reduced rate of progression in mean wall area.[69] Also in symptomatic patients with 50% or greater stenosis, newly initiated statin therapy and an increase of statin dose resulted in regression of wall volume, vessel wall thickness, and vessel wall area as well as in a decrease of plaque thickness.[70] Another study demonstrated an overall mean vessel wall volume change of 2.3% ±10.88% per year in moderate stenosis, with a faster increase of vessel wall volume in patients without statin therapy.[71] Finally, one large study in 100 patients with cryptogenic stroke and mild to moderate stenosis showed that statin use before the ischemic event was negatively correlated with the presence of intraplaque hemorrhage, thin/ruptured fibrous cap, and percentage of lipid-rich necrotic core but positively correlated with the percentage of fibrous tissue.[61]

Other studies have suggested that plaque composition is more sensitive to lipid-lowering therapy than the overall plaque burden. Especially lipid-rich necrotic core seems to be a promising candidate to demonstrate the positive effect of lipid-lowering therapy. A possible explanation is that statins might reduce the content of lipid and the inflammatory activity in the plaque and, therefore, stabilize the lesion and minimize the risk of surface rupture or intraplaque hemorrhage.[72] Hence, the measurement of lipid-rich necrotic core volume could be used to monitor the treatment effect. Indeed there are several lipid-lowering trials in patients with carotid atherosclerosis showing a reduction of lipid-rich necrotic core volume and relative content in the plaque.[72] For example, Underhill and colleagues[73] demonstrated in asymptomatic patients with mild and moderate stenosis receiving rosuvastatin a decrease of the lipid-rich necrotic core by 41% and an increase of fibrous tissue after 24 months. The overall plaque volume did not change over time. Whether these data can be reproduced in patients with cryptogenic stroke and can be used for detailed monitoring of the medical therapy has to be evaluated in future studies.

Another interesting aspect is the influence of antiplatelet therapy on plaque progression and regression, in particular the effect on intraplaque hemorrhage. So far, for moderate symptomatic stenosis only one study on the effect of cilostazol, an antiplatelet agent, has been published. After admission of 200 mg cilostazol for 12 months, contrast ratio of the carotid plaque decreased in T1-weighted images, the fibrous component in the plaque increased, and the lipid-rich necrotic core size decreased.[74]

Stroke Recurrence in Patients with Vulnerable Plaques

There are only few follow-up data on patients with cryptogenic stroke and lesion type VI plaques regarding stroke recurrence. One very promising marker to predict stroke recurrence is the presence of intraplaque hemorrhage. Altaf and colleagues[75] concluded in their study that intraplaque hemorrhage in combination with former events better predicted recurrent events during a 2-year follow-up than the degree of luminal stenosis alone. One limitation of the study was the very small number of patients (n = 22) in the low-grade stenosis group. Another study on patients with TIA with carotid stenosis of 30% to 69% showed that 52.4% of patients with juxtaluminal thrombus or hemorrhage experienced recurrent events during 2 years of follow-up.[76] On the other hand, healing of fibrous cap rupture after an ischemic event was shown to reduce the risk of future events.[77]

OUTLOOK

In summary, data on plaque vulnerability in mild and nonstenosing plaques and on the role of vulnerable plaques in patients with cryptogenic stroke are rare. Currently, 3 multicenter studies with large patient cohorts in patients with cryptogenic stroke using high-resolution carotid MR imaging are ongoing.

The Chinese Atherosclerosis Risk Evaluation-Phase II (CARE-II) study focuses on the characterization of vulnerable carotid arteries plaques in 1000 Chinese patients with ischemic events. The outcomes of the study include carotid wall and brain infarct measurements, which will be used to determine the relationship of carotid wall features with the volume of cerebral white matter lesions or infarcts. Furthermore, the association of the volume and incidence of carotid plaque calcification, lipid core, and intraplaque hemorrhage with vascular risk factors will be evaluated; the incidence and volume of carotid plaque features will be compared with geographic regions of subjects (clinicaltrials.gov identifier NCT02017756).

The Assessment of the Plaque At RISK by Noninvasive (Molecular) Imaging and Modeling (PARISK) study aims to include 300 patients with ischemic events in the last 3 months and 30% to 69% carotid artery stenosis. The combined primary end point implies ipsilateral recurrent stroke or TIA or new ischemic brain lesions after 2 years of follow-up.[78] The first results of 105 patients showed a high prevalence of ipsilateral intraplaque hemorrhage of 42% and thin or ruptured fibrous cap of 39%. Furthermore, in this substudy Truijman and colleagues[79] analyzed microembolic signal in these patients but found no differences between patients with and without intraplaque hemorrhage.

The Carotid Plaque Imaging in Acute Stroke (CAPIAS) study aims to include 300 patients with unilateral diffusion-weighted-imaging positive lesions in the anterior circulation on brain MR imaging, carotid artery stenosis less than 70%, and the presence of carotid artery plaques in the ipsilateral or contralateral carotid artery of greater than 2-mm plaque thickness. The primary outcome is the prevalence of vulnerable plaques in patients with cryptogenic stroke ipsilateral to the ischemic infarct compared with the contralateral side and compared with patients with a defined stroke cause. In the baseline data of 79 patients in which carotid MR imaging was performed within 10 days after stroke, the prevalence of complicated AHA type VI plaques in patients with cryptogenic stroke was 37% ipsilateral to the ischemic stroke and 3% on the asymptomatic side.[80] Furthermore, the study focuses on the association of vulnerable plaques with recurrent ischemic events and the influence of specific plaque features on plaque progression.

Follow-up results of these studies have not been reported yet, but one interesting follow-up case of the CAPIAS study has been published recently. A patient with a cryptogenic stroke and ipsilateral lesion type VI plaque with a large lipid-rich necrotic core and intraplaque hemorrhage presented during follow-up with a new ipsilateral amaurosis fugax. The repeated carotid MR imaging 11 months after baseline MR imaging demonstrated that large parts of the former lipid core were missing and a new ulceration had occurred. The investigators hypothesized an arterio-arterial embolization from the plaque into the right retinal artery (Figs. 5 and 6).[81]

The results of these ongoing studies might offer important implications for stratification of patients at high risk for arterio-arterial embolism with nonstenosing or moderate stenosing plaques. There is hope that from these studies one can learn more about the progression of atherosclerotic disease after an ischemic event and about the rates and mechanisms of stroke recurrence in patients

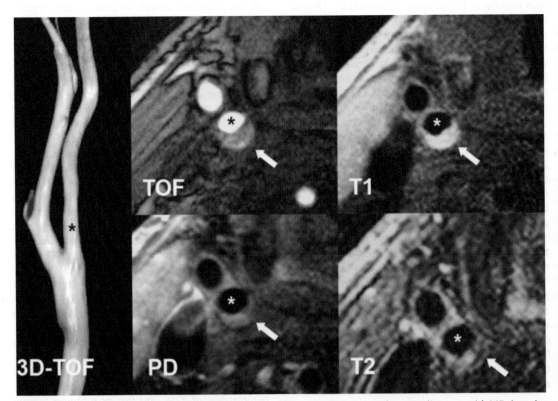

Fig. 5. Baseline high-resolution carotid MR imaging after cryptogenic stroke. Baseline carotid MR imaging demonstrating a complicated AHA type-VI plaque of the right internal carotid artery (*asterisk*). High signal on time-of-flight (TOF) and T1-weighted images (*arrow*) corresponding to intraplaque hemorrhage within a large lipid/necrotic core. PD, proton density; 3D, 3-dimensional. (*From* Schwarz F, Bayer-Karpinska A, Poppert H, et al. Serial carotid MRI identifies rupture of a vulnerable plaque resulting in amaurosis fugax. Neurology 2013;80(12):1171–2; with permission.)

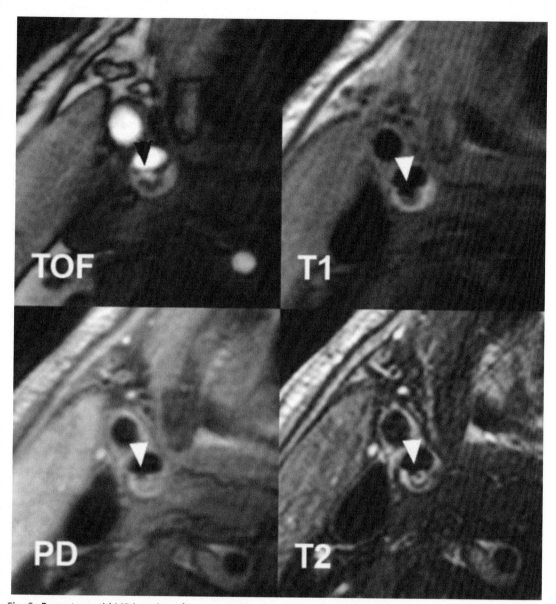

Fig. 6. Repeat carotid MR imaging after an episode of amaurosis fugax (11 months later). At repeat MR imaging, this plaque showed profound superficial irregularities, with a new ulceration and parts of the former lipid/necrotic core missing (*arrowhead*). PD, proton density; TOF, time of flight. (*From* Schwarz F, Bayer-Karpinska A, Poppert H, et al. Serial carotid MRI identifies rupture of a vulnerable plaque resulting in amaurosis fugax. Neurology 2013;80(12):1171–2; with permission.)

with cryptogenic stroke and atherosclerosis. Furthermore, they will provide the basis for targeted studies to answer the question of whether cryptogenic patients with vulnerable plaques should receive a more aggressive treatment.

REFERENCES

1. Rosamond W, Flegal K, Furie K, et al. Heart disease and stroke statistics–2008 update: a report from the American Heart Association Statistics Committee and Stroke Statistics Subcommittee. Circulation 2008;117(4):e25–146.

2. Brott TG, Halperin JL, Abbara S, et al. 2011 ASA/ACCF/AHA/AANN/AANS/ACR/ASNR/CNS/SAIP/SCAI/SIR/SNIS/SVM/SVS guideline on the management of patients with extracranial carotid and vertebral artery disease: executive summary: a report of the American College of Cardiology Foundation/American Heart Association Task Force on

Practice Guidelines, and the American Stroke Association, American Association of Neuroscience Nurses, American Association of Neurological Surgeons, American College of Radiology, American Society of Neuroradiology, Congress of Neurological Surgeons, Society of Atherosclerosis Imaging and Prevention, Society for Cardiovascular Angiography and Interventions, Society of Interventional Radiology, Society of NeuroInterventional Surgery, Society for Vascular Medicine, and Society for Vascular Surgery. J Am Coll Cardiol 2011;57(8): 1002–44.

3. Falk E, Shah PK, Fuster V. Coronary plaque disruption. Circulation 1995;92(3):657–71.

4. Spagnoli LG, Mauriello A, Sangiorgi G, et al. Extracranial thrombotically active carotid plaque as a risk factor for ischemic stroke. JAMA 2004;292(15): 1845–52.

5. Putaala J, Curtze S, Hiltunen S, et al. Causes of death and predictors of 5-year mortality in young adults after first-ever ischemic stroke: the Helsinki Young Stroke Registry. Stroke 2009;40(8):2698–703.

6. Adams HP Jr, Bendixen BH, Kappelle LJ, et al. Classification of subtype of acute ischemic stroke. Definitions for use in a multicenter clinical trial. TOAST. Trial of Org 10172 in Acute Stroke Treatment. Stroke 1993;24(1):35–41.

7. Amarenco P, Bogousslavsky J, Caplan LR, et al. New approach to stroke subtyping: the A-S-C-O (phenotypic) classification of stroke. Cerebrovasc Dis 2009;27(5):502–8.

8. Eriksson SE, Olsson JE. Survival and recurrent strokes in patients with different subtypes of stroke: a fourteen-year follow-up study. Cerebrovasc Dis 2001;12(3):171–80.

9. Bang OY, Lee PH, Joo SY, et al. Frequency and mechanisms of stroke recurrence after cryptogenic stroke. Ann Neurol 2003;54(2):227–34.

10. Yaghi S, Elkind MS. Cryptogenic stroke: a diagnostic challenge. Neurol Clin Pract 2014;4(5):386–93.

11. Hart RG, Diener HC, Coutts SB, et al. Embolic strokes of undetermined source: the case for a new clinical construct. Lancet Neurol 2014;13(4): 429–38.

12. Ruff CT, Giugliano RP, Braunwald E, et al. Comparison of the efficacy and safety of new oral anticoagulants with warfarin in patients with atrial fibrillation: a meta-analysis of randomised trials. Lancet 2014; 383(9921):955–62.

13. Sanna T, Diener HC, Passman RS, et al. Cryptogenic stroke and underlying atrial fibrillation. N Engl J Med 2014;370(26):2478–86.

14. Rizos T, Guntner J, Jenetzky E, et al. Continuous stroke unit electrocardiographic monitoring versus 24-hour Holter electrocardiography for detection of paroxysmal atrial fibrillation after stroke. Stroke 2012;43(10):2689–94.

15. Handke M, Harloff A, Olschewski M, et al. Patent foramen ovale and cryptogenic stroke in older patients. N Engl J Med 2007;357(22):2262–8.

16. Di Tullio MR, Sacco RL, Sciacca RR, et al. Patent foramen ovale and the risk of ischemic stroke in a multiethnic population. J Am Coll Cardiol 2007; 49(7):797–802.

17. Kronzon I, Tunick PA. Aortic atherosclerotic disease and stroke. Circulation 2006;114(1):63–75.

18. Wehrum T, Kams M, Strecker C, et al. Prevalence of potential retrograde embolization pathways in the proximal descending aorta in stroke patients and controls. Cerebrovasc Dis 2014;38(6):410–7.

19. Geroulakos G, Ramaswami G, Nicolaides A, et al. Characterization of symptomatic and asymptomatic carotid plaques using high-resolution real-time ultrasonography. Br J Surg 1993;80(10):1274–7.

20. Sztajzel R, Momjian S, Momjian-Mayor I, et al. Stratified gray-scale median analysis and color mapping of the carotid plaque: correlation with endarterectomy specimen histology of 28 patients. Stroke 2005;36(4):741–5.

21. Russell DA, Wijeyaratne SM, Gough MJ. Relationship of carotid plaque echomorphology to presenting symptom. Eur J Vasc Endovasc Surg 2010; 39(2):134–8.

22. Topakian R, King A, Kwon SU, et al. Ultrasonic plaque echolucency and emboli signals predict stroke in asymptomatic carotid stenosis. Neurology 2011; 77(8):751–8.

23. Hallerstam S, Carlstrom C, Zetterling M, et al. Carotid atherosclerosis in relation to symptoms from the territory supplied by the carotid artery. Eur J Vasc Endovasc Surg 2000;19(4):356–61.

24. Reiter M, Effenberger I, Sabeti S, et al. Increasing carotid plaque echolucency is predictive of cardiovascular events in high-risk patients. Radiology 2008;248(3):1050–5.

25. Kakkos SK, Nicolaides AN, Kyriacou E, et al. Computerized texture analysis of carotid plaque ultrasonic images can identify unstable plaques associated with ipsilateral neurological symptoms. Angiology 2011;62(4):317–28.

26. Griffin MB, Kyriacou E, Pattichis C, et al. Juxtaluminal hypoechoic area in ultrasonic images of carotid plaques and hemispheric symptoms. J Vasc Surg 2010;52(1):69–76.

27. Ainsworth CD, Blake CC, Tamayo A, et al. 3D ultrasound measurement of change in carotid plaque volume: a tool for rapid evaluation of new therapies. Stroke 2005;36(9):1904–9.

28. AlMuhanna K, Hossain MM, Zhao L, et al. Carotid plaque morphometric assessment with three-dimensional ultrasound imaging. J Vasc Surg 2015;61(3):690–7.

29. Markus HS, MacKinnon A. Asymptomatic embolization detected by Doppler ultrasound predicts stroke

risk in symptomatic carotid artery stenosis. Stroke 2005;36(5):971–5.

30. Markus HS, Droste DW, Kaps M, et al. Dual anti-platelet therapy with clopidogrel and aspirin in symptomatic carotid stenosis evaluated using Doppler embolic signal detection: the Clopidogrel and Aspirin for Reduction of Emboli in Symptomatic Carotid Stenosis (CARESS) trial. Circulation 2005; 111(17):2233–40.

31. Ritter MA, Dittrich R, Thoenissen N, et al. Prevalence and prognostic impact of microembolic signals in arterial sources of embolism. A systematic review of the literature. J Neurol 2008;255(7):953–61.

32. Shalhoub J, Owen DR, Gauthier T, et al. The use of contrast enhanced ultrasound in carotid arterial disease. Eur J Vasc Endovasc Surg 2010;39(4):381–7.

33. Shah F, Balan P, Weinberg M, et al. Contrast-enhanced ultrasound imaging of atherosclerotic carotid plaque neovascularization: a new surrogate marker of atherosclerosis? Vasc Med 2007;12(4):291–7.

34. Li C, He W, Guo D, et al. Quantification of carotid plaque neovascularization using contrast-enhanced ultrasound with histopathologic validation. Ultrasound Med Biol 2014;40(8):1827–33.

35. Hoogi A, Adam D, Hoffman A, et al. Carotid plaque vulnerability: quantification of neovascularization on contrast-enhanced ultrasound with histopathologic correlation. AJR Am J Roentgenol 2011;196(2):431–6.

36. Xiong L, Deng YB, Zhu Y, et al. Correlation of carotid plaque neovascularization detected by using contrast-enhanced US with clinical symptoms. Radiology 2009;251(2):583–9.

37. Ritter MA, Theismann K, Schmiedel M, et al. Vascularization of carotid plaque in recently symptomatic patients is associated with the occurrence of transcranial microembolic signals. Eur J Neurol 2013; 20(8):1218–21.

38. Shalhoub J, Monaco C, Owen DR, et al. Late-phase contrast-enhanced ultrasound reflects biological features of instability in human carotid atherosclerosis. Stroke 2011;42(12):3634–6.

39. Owen DR, Shalhoub J, Miller S, et al. Inflammation within carotid atherosclerotic plaque: assessment with late-phase contrast-enhanced US. Radiology 2010;255(2):638–44.

40. Serfaty JM, Nonent M, Nighoghossian N, et al. Plaque density on CT, a potential marker of ischemic stroke. Neurology 2006;66(1):118–20.

41. Trelles M, Eberhardt KM, Buchholz M, et al. CTA for screening of complicated atherosclerotic carotid plaque–American Heart Association type VI lesions as defined by MRI. AJNR Am J Neuroradiol 2013; 34(12):2331–7.

42. Gupta A, Baradaran H, Kamel H, et al. Evaluation of computed tomography angiography plaque thickness measurements in high-grade carotid artery stenosis. Stroke 2014;45(3):740–5.

43. Gupta A, Mtui EE, Baradaran H, et al. CT angiographic features of symptom-producing plaque in moderate-grade carotid artery stenosis. AJNR Am J Neuroradiol 2015;36(2):349–54.

44. Gupta A, Baradaran H, Mtui EE, et al. Detection of symptomatic carotid plaque using source data from MR and CT angiography: a correlative study. Cerebrovasc Dis 2015;39(3–4):151–61.

45. Saba L, Mallarini G. Carotid plaque enhancement and symptom correlations: an evaluation by using multidetector row CT angiography. AJNR Am J Neuroradiol 2011;32(10):1919–25.

46. Saba L, Piga M, Raz E, et al. Carotid artery plaque classification: does contrast enhancement play a significant role? AJNR Am J Neuroradiol 2012; 33(9):1814–7.

47. Rudd JH, Warburton EA, Fryer TD, et al. Imaging atherosclerotic plaque inflammation with [18F]-fluorodeoxyglucose positron emission tomography. Circulation 2002;105(23):2708–11.

48. Judenhofer MS, Wehrl HF, Newport DF, et al. Simultaneous PET-MRI: a new approach for functional and morphological imaging. Nat Med 2008; 14(4):459–65.

49. Marnane M, Merwick A, Sheehan OC, et al. Carotid plaque inflammation on 18F-fluorodeoxyglucose positron emission tomography predicts early stroke recurrence. Ann Neurol 2012;71(5):709–18.

50. Müller HF, Viaccoz A, Fisch L, et al. 18FDG-PET-CT: an imaging biomarker of high-risk carotid plaques. Correlation to symptoms and microembolic signals. Stroke 2014;45(12):3561–6.

51. Truijman MT, Kwee RM, van Hoof RH, et al. Combined 18F-FDG PET-CT and DCE-MRI to assess inflammation and microvascularization in atherosclerotic plaques. Stroke 2013;44(12):3568–70.

52. Yuan C, Zhang SX, Polissar NL, et al. Identification of fibrous cap rupture with magnetic resonance imaging is highly associated with recent transient ischemic attack or stroke. Circulation 2002;105(2):181–5.

53. Cai JM, Hatsukami TS, Ferguson MS, et al. Classification of human carotid atherosclerotic lesions with in vivo multicontrast magnetic resonance imaging. Circulation 2002;106(11):1368–73.

54. Takaya N, Yuan C, Chu B, et al. Association between carotid plaque characteristics and subsequent ischemic cerebrovascular events: a prospective assessment with MRI–initial results. Stroke 2006; 37(3):818–23.

55. Saam T, Underhill HR, Chu B, et al. Prevalence of American Heart Association type VI carotid atherosclerotic lesions identified by magnetic resonance imaging for different levels of stenosis as measured by duplex ultrasound. J Am Coll Cardiol 2008; 51(10):1014–21.

56. Saam T, Hetterich H, Hoffmann V, et al. Meta-analysis and systematic review of the predictive value

of carotid plaque hemorrhage on cerebrovascular events by magnetic resonance imaging. J Am Coll Cardiol 2013;62(12):1081–91.

57. Parmar JP, Rogers WJ, Mugler JP 3rd, et al. Magnetic resonance imaging of carotid atherosclerotic plaque in clinically suspected acute transient ischemic attack and acute ischemic stroke. Circulation 2010;122(20):2031–8.

58. Zhao H, Zhao X, Liu X, et al. Association of carotid atherosclerotic plaque features with acute ischemic stroke: a magnetic resonance imaging study. Eur J Radiol 2013;82(9):e465–70.

59. Freilinger TM, Schindler A, Schmidt C, et al. Prevalence of nonstenosing, complicated atherosclerotic plaques in cryptogenic stroke. JACC Cardiovasc Imaging 2012;5(4):397–405.

60. Lindsay AC, Biasiolli L, Lee JM, et al. Plaque features associated with increased cerebral infarction after minor stroke and TIA: a prospective, case-control, 3-T carotid artery MR imaging study. JACC Cardiovasc Imaging 2012;5(4):388–96.

61. McNally JS, McLaughlin MS, Hinckley PJ, et al. Intraluminal thrombus, intraplaque hemorrhage, plaque thickness, and current smoking optimally predict carotid stroke. Stroke 2015;46(1):84–90.

62. Kwee RM, van Oostenbrugge RJ, Prins MH, et al. Symptomatic patients with mild and moderate carotid stenosis: plaque features at MRI and association with cardiovascular risk factors and statin use. Stroke 2010;41(7):1389–93.

63. Cheung HM, Moody AR, Singh N, et al. Late stage complicated atheroma in low-grade stenotic carotid disease: MR imaging depiction–prevalence and risk factors. Radiology 2011;260(3):841–7.

64. Singh N, Moody AR, Gladstone DJ, et al. Moderate carotid artery stenosis: MR imaging-depicted intraplaque hemorrhage predicts risk of cerebrovascular ischemic events in asymptomatic men. Radiology 2009;252(2):502–8.

65. Kolodgie FD, Gold HK, Burke AP, et al. Intraplaque hemorrhage and progression of coronary atheroma. N Engl J Med 2003;349(24):2316–25.

66. Takaya N, Yuan C, Chu B, et al. Presence of intraplaque hemorrhage stimulates progression of carotid atherosclerotic plaques: a high-resolution magnetic resonance imaging study. Circulation 2005; 111(21):2768–75.

67. Underhill HR, Yuan C, Yarnykh VL, et al. Arterial remodeling in [corrected] subclinical carotid artery disease. JACC Cardiovasc Imaging 2009;2(12):1381–9.

68. Kwee RM, van Oostenbrugge RJ, Mess WH, et al. Carotid plaques in transient ischemic attack and stroke patients: one-year follow-up study by magnetic resonance imaging. Invest Radiol 2010; 45(12):803–9.

69. Saam T, Yuan C, Chu B, et al. Predictors of carotid atherosclerotic plaque progression as measured by noninvasive magnetic resonance imaging. Atherosclerosis 2007;194(2):e34–42.

70. Migrino RQ, Bowers M, Harmann L, et al. Carotid plaque regression following 6-month statin therapy assessed by 3T cardiovascular magnetic resonance: comparison with ultrasound intima media thickness. J Cardiovasc Magn Reson 2011;13:37.

71. Boussel L, Arora S, Rapp J, et al. Atherosclerotic plaque progression in carotid arteries: monitoring with high-spatial-resolution MR imaging–multicenter trial. Radiology 2009;252(3):789–96.

72. Zhao XQ, Dong L, Hatsukami T, et al. MR imaging of carotid plaque composition during lipid-lowering therapy a prospective assessment of effect and time course. JACC Cardiovasc Imaging 2011;4(9):977–86.

73. Underhill HR, Yuan C, Zhao XQ, et al. Effect of rosuvastatin therapy on carotid plaque morphology and composition in moderately hypercholesterolemic patients: a high-resolution magnetic resonance imaging trial. Am Heart J 2008;155(3):584.e1–8.

74. Yamaguchi Oura M, Sasaki M, Ohba H, et al. Carotid plaque characteristics on magnetic resonance plaque imaging following long-term cilostazol therapy. J Stroke Cerebrovasc Dis 2014;23(9):2425–30.

75. Altaf N, Daniels L, Morgan PS, et al. Detection of intraplaque hemorrhage by magnetic resonance imaging in symptomatic patients with mild to moderate carotid stenosis predicts recurrent neurological events. J Vasc Surg 2008;47(2):337–42.

76. Teng Z, Sadat U, Huang Y, et al. In vivo MRI-based 3D mechanical stress-strain profiles of carotid plaques with juxtaluminal plaque haemorrhage: an exploratory study for the mechanism of subsequent cerebrovascular events. Eur J Vasc Endovasc Surg 2011;42(4):427–33.

77. Teng Z, Degnan AJ, Sadat U, et al. Characterization of healing following atherosclerotic carotid plaque rupture in acutely symptomatic patients: an exploratory study using in vivo cardiovascular magnetic resonance. J Cardiovasc Magn Reson 2011;13:64.

78. Truijman MT, Kooi ME, van Dijk AC, et al. Plaque At RISK (PARISK): prospective multicenter study to improve diagnosis of high-risk carotid plaques. Int J Stroke 2014;9(6):747–54.

79. Truijman MT, de Rotte AA, Aaslid R, et al. Intraplaque hemorrhage, fibrous cap status, and microembolic signals in symptomatic patients with mild to moderate carotid artery stenosis: the Plaque at RISK study. Stroke 2014;45(11):3423–6.

80. Bayer-Karpinska A, Schwarz F, Wollenweber FA, et al. The carotid plaque imaging in acute stroke (CAPIAS) study: protocol and initial baseline data. BMC Neurol 2013;13:201.

81. Schwarz F, Bayer-Karpinska A, Poppert H, et al. Serial carotid MRI identifies rupture of a vulnerable plaque resulting in amaurosis fugax. Neurology 2013; 80(12):1171–2.

Plaque Assessment in the Management of Patients with Asymptomatic Carotid Stenosis

J. Kevin DeMarco, MD[a],*, J. David Spence, MD, FRCPC[b]

KEYWORDS

- Carotid atherosclerosis • Plaque • MR imaging • Ultrasonography • Asymptomatic carotid stenosis

KEY POINTS

- Despite current medical therapy, some patients with asymptomatic carotid stenosis go on to stroke.
- Carotid plaque imaging may identify these high-risk asymptomatic patients who could benefit from more intensive medical therapy.
- The presence of a measurable lipid-rich necrotic core may be the phenotype of asymptomatic atherosclerotic carotid plaque disease that is more responsive to intensive medical therapy.
- Direct monitoring of the necrotic core size and/or overall plaque burden in patients with asymptomatic carotid stenosis may provide a better measure of intensive medical therapy than serum markers such as low-density lipoprotein cholesterol.
- The presence of carotid intraplaque hemorrhage and/or ulceration in patients with asymptomatic carotid stenosis may require close monitoring to identify progression despite intensive medical therapy that is better treated with surgical intervention.

INTRODUCTION

Current Medical Therapy in Patients with Asymptomatic Carotid Stenosis

The identification and treatment of cardiovascular risk factors has been the hallmark of stroke prevention, starting in the 1970s and 1980s with the medical management of hypertension associated with a sharp decline in stroke mortality.[1] With the widespread use of statin therapy to lower LDL cholesterol (LDL-C) levels there was an additional, if slower, decline in stroke mortality in the 1990s.[2]

The most recent revision of the American College of Cardiology/American Heart Association (AHA) Task Force on Practice Guidelines continued the emphasis on the use of fixed doses of cholesterol level–lowering drugs to reduce cardiovascular risk based on epidemiologically defined risk factors.[3] The members of this 2013 task force did acknowledge that other treatment approaches, including the use of carotid plaque burden features to determine individual risk and modify treatment therapy based on plaque burden, have been advocated but have not yet been evaluated in randomized

Disclosures: J.K. DeMarco, speaker bureau and prior research funding from Bracco Diagnostic INC (05-IRGP-472), consultant for GE Medical Systems. J.D. Spence, interest in Vascularis Inc and has received software from Philips for use in research.

[a] Department of Radiology, Michigan State University, Radiology Building, 846 Service Road, Room 184, East Lansing, MI 48824, USA; [b] Departments of Neurology and Clinical Pharmacology, Stroke Prevention and Atherosclerosis Research Centre, Robarts Research Institute, Western University, 1400 Western Road, London, Ontario N6G 2V4, Canada
* Corresponding author.
E-mail address: jkd@rad.msu.edu

Neuroimag Clin N Am 26 (2016) 111–127
http://dx.doi.org/10.1016/j.nic.2015.09.009
1052-5149/16/$ – see front matter © 2016 Elsevier Inc. All rights reserved.

neuroimaging.theclinics.com

clinical trials. New randomized clinical trials are underway that will study carotid burden imaging in the treatment of patients with asymptomatic carotid stenosis (ACS). In addition, multiple natural history studies have confirmed the ability of carotid burden imaging to better stratify risk compared with known atherosclerotic cardiovascular disease (ASCVD) risk factors, with multiple imaging studies showing the ability to monitor therapeutic response directly.

Potential New Medical Therapy in Patients with Asymptomatic Carotid Stenosis Based on Plaque Assessment

There are 2 ongoing large randomized clinical trials evaluating medical therapy versus surgical/endovascular intervention in patients with ACS (Carotid Revascularization Endarterectomy versus Stenting Trial [CREST-2] and Asymptomatic Carotid Surgery Trial [ACST-2]). Both will include an imaging substudy to evaluate the role of vulnerable plaque imaging in asymptomatic patients with greater than 70% carotid stenosis. In addition, the Asymptomatic Carotid Stenosis and Risk of Stroke trial is a large prospective study on patients with ACS undergoing medical intervention. ACSRS showed that not all patients with ACS carry the same risk of stroke. Specifically, the severity of carotid stenosis, a history of contralateral transient ischemic attack (TIA), and several carotid plaque features on ultrasonography could stratify patients into groups of varying annual stroke risk from less than 1% to greater than 10%.[4,5] Two large prospective studies showed that microemboli on transcranial Doppler (TCD) identify high-risk patients with ACS.[6,7] More intensive medical therapy based on measurements of carotid total plaque area (TPA) calculated from high-resolution duplex ultrasonography (DUS) rather than consensus guidelines reduced the occurrence of microemboli from 12.6% to 3.7% of patients, slowed the progression of carotid TPA, and reduced the risk of stroke or myocardial infarct by more than 80%.[8] In addition, there are multiple single-center prospective trials showing the ability of multiple magnetic resonance (MR)–defined plaque characteristics to stratify risk of future juxtaluminal carotid TIA or stroke such as the size of the lipid-rich necrotic core (LRNC),[9,10] intraplaque hemorrhage (IPH),[11] and thin/ruptured fibrous cap (FC).[9]

This article reviews this growing body of literature, which suggests that carotid plaque assessment with ultrasonography and MR imaging provides superior risk stratification for individual patients compared with carotid stenosis and other epidemiologically identified cardiovascular risk factors. It also reviews current drug trials using carotid plaque imaging to assess the effectiveness of medical therapy. In addition, it reviews how certain carotid plaque features, such as a large LRNC, may represent a phenotype of ASCVD with high risk of future events that is amenable to intensive medical therapy. It also reviews other plaque features, such as IPH and ruptured FC/ulceration, that may represent vulnerable plaque that requires close monitoring to identify plaque progression or new symptoms despite intensive medical therapy and may require surgical intervention. Tables 1 and 2 summarize these important carotid plaque features on MR imaging and ultrasonography, their associated outcomes, and potential clinical utility to optimize the clinical management of patients with ACS. The potential to individualize the patients' medical therapy for ASCVD based on carotid burden imaging is stressed. Carotid burden imaging has the potential to change the treatment paradigm of patients with ACS from treating risk factors to treating arteries.[7]

IMAGING TECHNIQUES
Overview

MR imaging depiction of plaque burden is most reliably measured as percentage wall volume (PWV), which is similar to the percentage atheroma volume measured in coronary arteries during intravascular ultrasonography. Ultrasonography depiction of plaque burden includes TPA and total plaque volume (TPV). The ultrasonography and MR imaging techniques to precisely estimate plaque burden are reviewed. The progression or regression of plaque burden can be a powerful measurement of an individual's response to medical therapy.

Histologic studies have shown that coronary artery plaques with a large LRNC and an overlying thin FC are associated with sudden cardiac death.[12] This finding and additional research have led to the concept of vulnerable plaque.[13,14] From this work emerged key plaque features of the vulnerable plaque, including a large LRNC with a thin FC, active inflammation with activated macrophages, fissured plaque, superficial calcified nodules, and IPH. The AHA has proposed a detailed classification scheme of atherosclerotic plaque[15] that has now been extended to in vivo carotid plaque MR imaging.[16] Patients with ACS with LRNC are classified with an AHA type IV to V plaque and those with IPH, ruptured FC, and/or calcified protruding nodule are showing an AHA type VI plaque, which some investigators also call a vulnerable plaque. This article reviews the histologically validated research detailing the MR imaging techniques to identify LRNC, thin/ruptured FC, protruding nodule, and IPH.

Table 1
Summary of important carotid plaque MR features, associated outcomes, and possible clinical utility

Plaque Feature	AHA Type	MR Appearance	Associated Outcomes	Possible Clinical Utility
LRNC	IV–V	1. Nonenhancing region on contrast-enhanced T1W images	1. Larger LRNC associated with higher risk of future stroke/TIA	1. LRNC is optimal plaque phenotype to treat with intense statin therapy
		2. May or may not be associated with IPH	2. Carotid atherosclerotic score 3 or 4 associated with future IPH or ulcers	2. Intensive statin therapy has been shown to decrease LRNC size (delipidation theory)
		—	—	3. Stabilization of carotid plaque with decrease/resolution LRNC may decrease future stroke/TIA
IPH	VI	1. High signal on T1W images including MPRAGE, TOF, and FSE	1. Increased risk of future stroke/TIA	1. High-risk patients who require close clinical monitoring for new symptoms or stenosis progression
		2. Typically within LRNC, but may be seen adjacent to calcifications	2. IPH is proinflammatory with risk of future plaque growth or new ulcerations	2. Very intensive statin therapy may be required to arrest plaque progression
		—	—	3. May require revascularization if there is sufficient stenosis progression or new symptoms despite maximal medical therapy
Ulceration	VI	Best seen on contrast-enhanced MR angiogram	1. NASCET showed higher risk of future stroke with ulcerations	1. High-risk patients who require close clinical monitoring for new symptoms or stenosis progression
		—	2. Thin/ruptured FC has highest hazard ratio for future stroke/TIA	2. Ulcerations can resolve with intense statin therapy
		—	—	3. If new symptoms despite maximal medical therapy, may require revascularization

Abbreviations: FSE, fast spin echo; MPRAGE, magnetization-prepared rapid acquisition gradient-echo; T1W, T1 weighted; TOF, time of flight.

Recently a variety of ultrasonography-defined high-risk features have been defined, including large juxtaluminal black area (JBA)/hypoechoic area that represents a large LRNC with thin/absent FC. The detection of carotid ulcerations, including the number and total volume of carotid plaque ulcerations, has improved with the advent of three-dimensional (3D) carotid ultrasonography, as discussed by Spence and Parraga.[17] In addition, TCD detection of microemboli has been shown to characterize vulnerable carotid plaque.

Table 2
Summary of important carotid plaque ultrasonography features, associated outcomes, and possible clinical utility

Plaque Features	Ultrasonography Appearance	Associated Outcomes	Possible Clinical Utility
TPA/TPV	Automated method to measure 3D plaque volume with mechanical sweep	1. TPA was shown to predict risk well beyond Framingham Risk Score	Treating progression of TPA/TPV instead of standard guidelines leads to reduced stroke and MI (treating arteries instead of risk factors)
		2. Progression of TPA/TPV associated with higher risk of new stroke, MI, and death	—
TCD microemboli detection (TCD+)	Visual/auditory signal from posterior/middle temporal window	1. TCD+ patients are at ↑ risk of future stroke	1. TCD+ benefits from intensive medical therapy
		2. Intensive medical therapy ↓ TCD microemboli	2. Persistent TCD+ after intensive medical therapy identifies high-risk patients
Ulceration	Both number and volume of ulcers best seen on 3D US	Patients with 3 or more ulcers and/or total ulcer volume ≥5 mm³ are at higher risk stroke and death	3 or more ulcers and large ulcer volume identify high-risk patients
JBA	With critical image normalization JBA size quantification used in multicenter trial	Size of JBA in patients with ACS showed linear association with future stroke/TIA	JBA size >8 mm² identifies high-risk patients

Abbreviations: 3D, three-dimensional; JBA, juxtaluminal black area; MI, myocardial infarction; TPV, total plaque volume; US, ultrasonography.

Carotid Plaque Imaging with MR Imaging

MR imaging depiction of percentage wall volume

The intrareader and interreader as well as the interscan reproducibility of quantitative MR imaging measurements of total plaque burden as well as the volume of various plaque components have been extensively reported and recently well summarized.[18] The most reliable measure of plaque burden is PWV. The black-blood technique is critical for PWV analysis that included two-dimensional (2D) spin-echo T1 weighted (T1W) and T2 weighted (T2W). There are commercially available programs to semiautomatically detect the lumen and outer boundaries of the carotid wall to assess the PWV, which is defined as follows: PWV = 100% × wall volume/(wall volume + lumen volume). In the carotid, the interscan coefficient of variation for PWV at 1.5 and 3.0 T using dedicated carotid coils and 2D T1W has been estimated at 3.2%[19] and 3.0%,[20] respectively.

MR imaging depiction of intraplaque hemorrhage

Quantitative measures of various plaque components such as LRNC and IPH compared with histology have been less reproducible than PWV. Most advances in directly imaging plaque components have been directed toward the detection of IPH, which shows T1 hyperintensity at least 1.5 times greater than the adjacent sternocleidomastoid muscle. Identification of IPH has been shown to be field strength dependent.[21] At 1.5 T, IPH detection has sensitivities of 87% to 96% and specificities of 74% to 82%.[22–24] A 3D magnetization-prepared rapid acquisition gradient-echo (MPRAGE) sequence was shown to best depict IPH at 3 T with sensitivity of 80% and specificity of 97% with very small IPH and heavily calcified IPH excluded[25] (**Fig. 1**). Given the weak association of IPH volume quantification with histology, most longitudinal studies us IPH as a dichotomous variable.[18]

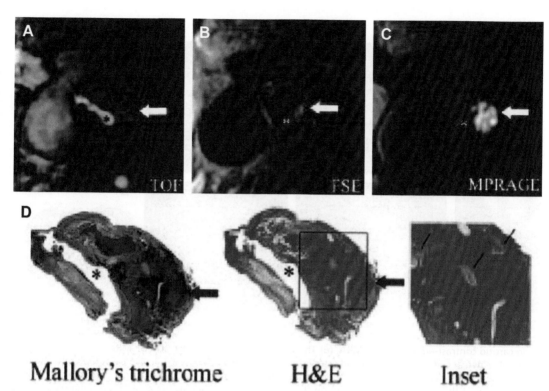

Fig. 1. Histologic validation of intraplaque hemorrhage detected with in vivo 3-T MR imaging in a 75-year-old man with moderately calcified IPH in the left internal carotid artery. (*A–C*) On T1W MR images, high-signal-intensity area (*arrows*) measures 15.8 mm^2 on time-of-flight (TOF) image (23/3.5, 20° flip angle), 8.6 mm^2 on fast spin-echo (FSE) image (800/11), and 24.8 mm^2 on MPRAGE image (13.2/3.2, 15° flip angle). (*D*) Mallory tri-chrome–stained histologic specimen shows variable red staining pattern in necrotic core (*arrow*). Adjacent section stained with hematoxylin-eosin (H&E, original magnification x10) shows large necrotic core (*arrow*) filled with IPH measuring 34.9 mm^2. The inset is a magnified region of necrotic core (*outlined in black*) showing small frag-ments of calcification (*thin arrows*, original magnification x100). * = lumen. (*From* Ota H, Yarnykh VL, Ferguson MS, et al. Carotid intraplaque hemorrhage imaging at 3.0-T MR imaging: comparison of the diagnostic perfor-mance of three T1-weighted sequences 1. Radiology 2010;254(2):557; with permission.)

MR imaging depiction of lipid-rich necrotic core and thin/ruptured fibrous cap

Multicontrast MR imaging of the carotid arteries using T1W, T2W, and 3D time-of-flight (TOF) bright blood sequences has been validated with histology and shown to identify and quantify LRNC and FC[23,26] (**Fig. 2**). Contrast-enhanced (CE) T1W images improve the differentiation be-tween the nonenhancing LRNC and the remainder of the fibrous carotid plaque tissue.[27] The LRNC without IPH is hypointense on T2W and CE-T1W images. In sections where an LRNC is seen, the overlying FC is described as intact if there is an enhanced band adjacent to the dark lumen on CE-T1W and a smooth luminal surface of TOF and CE-T1W images. Given the spatial resolution of CE-T1W images, it is likely that a thick and intact FC is 500 μm or thicker. A thin but intact FC has been described as the absence of the dark band on CE-T1W but with smooth luminal surface. A ruptured FC shows a disrupted dark band on CE-T1W with an irregular luminal surface on all images. The most relevant discrimination is whether the FC is thick or not, because thin and ruptured FCs are both associated with increased risk of future stroke/TIA. Although the differentia-tion between thick and thin/ruptured FC probably requires the use of dedicated carotid coils, ulcer-ations are well visualized as focal outpouchings on CE MR angiography (MRA) using large field of view neurovascular coils.

Translation of carotid plaque burden imaging from research to clinical MR imaging

Recently, the ability of black-blood 3D carotid pla-que MR imaging to depict carotid plaque burden and plaque components at 1.5 and 3.0 T using neurovascular (NV) coils with standard large field of view (FOV) has been shown.[28] Given the com-mercial availability of 3D fast spin-echo (FSE) T1W and 3D MRPAGE clinical sequences, it may be possible to add these to the routine clinical

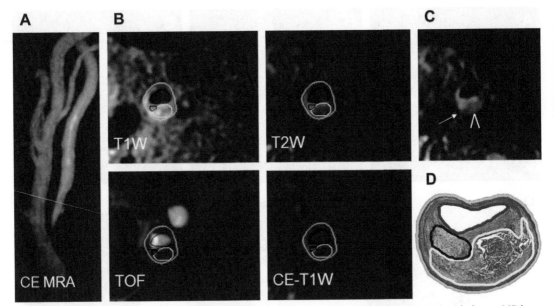

Fig. 2. Comparison of high-resolution MR angiography (MRA), multicontrast 3-T in vivo carotid plaque MR imaging, and ex vivo histologic evaluation of a CEA specimen. (*A*) There is 82% carotid stenosis on the 500-μm resolution carotid contrast-enhanced (CE) MRA. (*B*) These examples of T1W, T2W, 3D TOF MRA, and CE-T1W plaque images obtained at the level of the carotid artery stenosis (*A*) show how the 3-T in vivo carotid plaque MR imaging identifies the LRNC (*yellow outline*) and loose matrix (*purple outline*) through the right carotid artery plaque. (*C*) The region of the LRNC is dark (*chevron*) on these T2W images, whereas the area of loose matrix (*arrow*) is bright. (*D*) The percentage areas of plaque that were characterized as LRNC (*yellow outline*) and loose matrix (*blue outline*) on the histologic slide is similar to that measured on the in vivo 3-T MR images. (*From* DeMarco JK, Huston J 3rd. Imaging of high-risk carotid artery plaques: current status and future directions. Neurosurg Focus 2014;36(1):3; with permission.)

carotid MR angiogram to evaluate for carotid plaque burden and component analysis (**Fig. 3**). While the comparison of clinical and research versions of multicontrast carotid plaque MR imaging is underway, preliminary work suggests that the clinical version of 3D T1W and CE-T1W images will be able to detect moderate to large LRNC seen on 2 or more contiguous research 2-mm thick 2D CE-T1W series as well as those patients with ACS with carotid atherosclerotic score (CAS) 3 or 4 (**Fig. 4**).

Carotid Plaque Imaging with Duplex Ultrasonography

Ultrasonography depiction of plaque volume
An automated method to measure 3D plaque volume was developed using mechanical movement of the DUS probe along the artery.[29] A mechanical sweep, obtained by holding the DUS probe in 1 location and having the angle change mechanically, is faster and more convenient.[30] The acquired images can be analyzed using semiautomated planimetry.

Compared with manual cross-sectional 2D freehand sweep, the newer mechanical 3D sweep

holds the promise of reducing variability and increasing the sensitivity in quantification of plaque volume measurements. The step from manual 2D freehand sweep to an automated mechanical 3D sweep significantly increased the reliability of repeat measurements between different ultrasonographers. Intrareader offline analysis of the 3D mechanical sweep was high, but the interreader analyses revealed that one reader systematically measured larger plaque areas.[30]

Ultrasonography depiction of ulceration
Initial attempts to classify carotid plaque ulceration by 2D DUS was poor, but with the advent of 3D DUS ulcer detection became reliable.[31] Using a mechanical linear 3D scanning system, Madani and colleagues[32] defined an ulcer as a continuous contour showing focal depression, a well-defined break in the surface of 1 mm or more across, a well-defined back wall at the base of the depression, and an anechoic area within the plaque that extended to the surface and was 1 mm or more deep (**Fig. 5**). Their analysis showed that the number of DUS-detected ulcers were reliably detected (κ = 0.83) and the interobserver reliability was κ = 0.78.

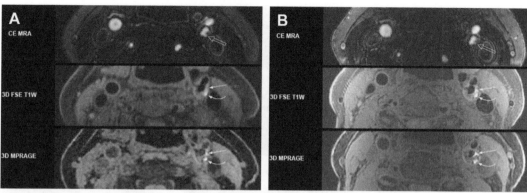

Fig. 3. Comparison of clinical and research versions of carotid plaque MR imaging to detect IPH. (*A*) Axial 2-mm thick multiplanar axial reformations of the coronal clinical 3D CE MRA, 3D FSE T1W, and 3D MPRAGE using large-FOV neurovascular coil. Note the positive remodeling and thickening of the left internal carotid artery wall, focal areas of high signal intensity greater than the sternocleidomastoid muscle consistent with plaque hemorrhage adjacent to the lumen (*straight arrow*) and deep within the plaque (*curved arrow*), as well as the focal ulceration (*open arrow*). (*B*) Similar axial 2-mm thick multiplanar axial reformations of coronal research 3D CE MRA and 3D FSE T1W series as well as axial 3D MPRAGE using dedicated carotid coils and higher spatial resolution. Note the similar appearance of the T1 hyperintense plaque hemorrhage, although the research MPRAGE images show better spatial resolution and depiction, especially where the plaque hemorrhage is small.

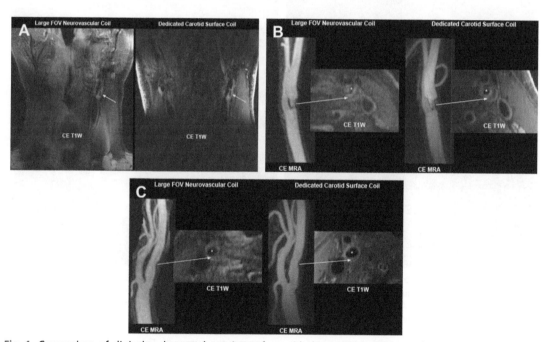

Fig. 4. Comparison of clinical and research versions of carotid plaque MR imaging to detect LRNC. (*A*) Selective coronal image from CE 3D FSE CE-T1W series using large-FOV neurovascular coil and dedicated carotid surface coils show a nonenhancing region involving the proximal left internal carotid artery consistent with an LRNC that can be appreciated despite prominent motion artifact on the series obtained with the large-FOV coil (*straight arrow*). (*B*) Selective maximum intense projection (MIP) images on the CE MRA and axial 2-mm thick multiplanar axial reformations of the coronal 3D CE-T1W series using both coils detect a large LRNC (*straight arrow*) in left internal carotid artery wall despite the motion artifact. The residual left internal carotid artery lumen is highlighted with an asterisk. This LRNC was present on more than 2 continuous 2-mm thick images from the research CE-T1W series and measured greater than 40% maximum percentage wall area consistent with a CAS of 4. (*C*) Selective MIP images of the right carotid on CE MRA reveals a small LRNC (*straight arrow*) seen on only one 2-mm thick multiplanar axial reformation of the 3D CE-T1W series. The asterisk marks the right internal carotid artery lumen. The maximum wall area of LRNC was less than 20%, representing a CAS-2 on the research carotid images.

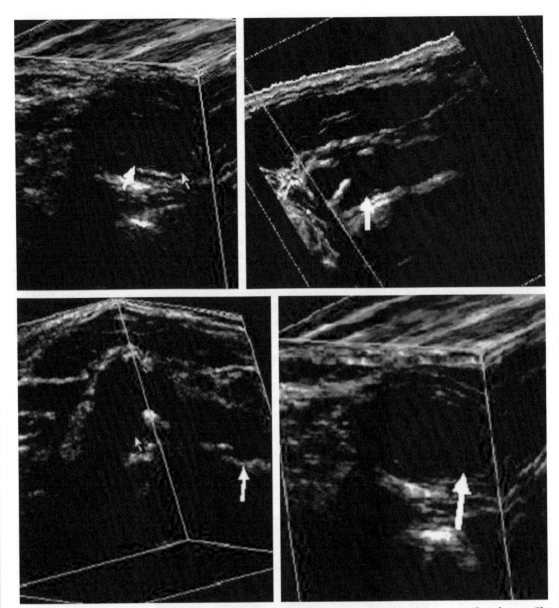

Fig. 5. Carotid plaque images obtained with 3D ultrasonography and analyzed with 3D quantify software. The carotid artery can be examined in any axis for detection of ulcers in atherosclerotic plaques. White arrows show ulcers. (*From* Madani A, Beletsky V, Tamayo A, et al. High-risk asymptomatic carotid stenosis: ulceration on 3D ultrasound vs TCD microemboli. Neurology 2011;77(8):746; with permission.)

Ultrasonography depiction of juxtaluminal black/hypoechoic area

Hypoechoic or black regions involving the carotid plaque without a visible echogenic cap are defined as JBAs. A JBA noted on DUS was associated with an LRNC close to the lumen on histologic examinations of carotid endarterectomy (CEA) specimens.[33] The JBA was defined as the largest plaque region adjacent to the lumen with pixels having a gray-scale value less than 25 without a visible echogenic cap (pixels with gray-scale value >25) and manually outlined using the computer cursor.[34] This technique has now been applied in the multicenter ACSRS study with care taken to digitize the baseline DUS video images and normalize the image data for gray-scale analysis (Fig. 6). Several prerequisites were applied during DUS acquisition to achieve consistent image normalization.[4]

Ultrasonography depiction of intracranial microembolus with transcranial Doppler

TCD is performed through a posterior or middle temporal window with monitoring of both middle

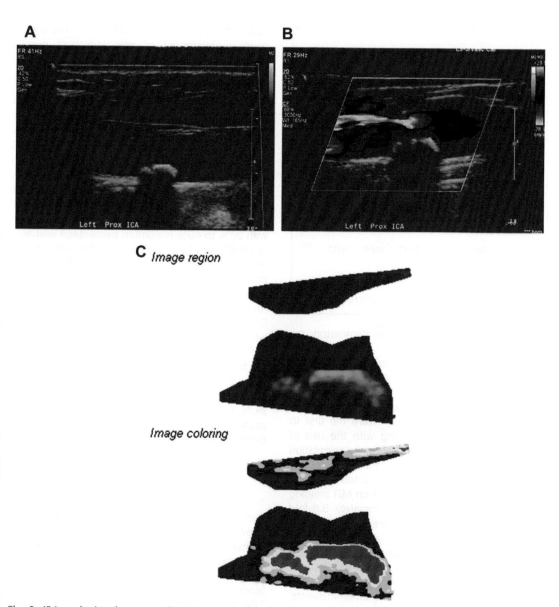

Fig. 6. JBA as depicted on carotid DUS imaging after image normalization. (*A*) Normalized gray-scale image of the origin of the internal carotid artery showing an apparently hyperechoic plaque. (*B*) Color flow image of the same plaque showing the jet of blood at the tightest part of the stenosis (90%–95% North American Symptomatic Carotid Endarterectomy Trial method) and a JBA (hypoechoic) as a filling defect on the far wall component of the plaque. (*C*) Segmented gray-scale image of the same plaque before and after color contouring according to the gray level of pixels (gray-scale: 0–25 = black; 26–50 = blue; 51–75 = green; 76–100 = yellow; 101–125 = orange; >125 = red). The larger JBA of the far wall component of the plaque measures 13.6 mm². The larger JBA of the near wall component of the plaque measures 2.7 mm². (*From* Kakkos SK, Griffin MB, Nicolaides AN, et al. The size of juxtaluminal hypoechoic area in ultrasound images of asymptomatic carotid plaques predicts the occurrence of stroke. J Vasc Surg 2013;57(3):611; with permission.)

cerebral arteries. A harness is placed on the head and the patient is monitored for a period of time. There is usually a visual and auditory signal when the embolus occurs. A decibel threshold improved reliability of microembolus detection.[35] In 1998 a consensus approach to microembolus detection was published[36] (**Box 1**).

IMAGING FINDINGS/PATHOLOGY
Predictive Value of Plaque Imaging for MR Imaging

Intraplaque hemorrhage
With IPH there is extravasation of lipid-rich membranes of the red blood cells plus iron into the

Box 1
Imaging protocol

- MR imaging
  - CE MRA depicts ulcerations
  - Black-blood T1W depicts plaque burden (PWV)
  - LRNC best seen as nonenhancing region on CE-T1W
  - IPH best seen on MPRAGE
- Ultrasonography
  - 2D and 3D ultrasonography can measure TPA/volume
  - Ulcerations are best seen with 3D ultrasonography
  - JBA correlates with LRNC close to lumen
  - TCD can detect intracranial microemboli

carotid wall, both of which are proinflammatory, resulting in plaque destabilization.[37] The presence of IPH was associated with accelerated plaque progression and new IPH deposits, suggesting that IPH is an important transition point from stable to unstable carotid plaque morphology[38] (Fig. 7). In 2003, Moody and colleagues[39] were the first to discuss tissue-specific imaging with the use of MPRAGE to identify IPH and show its correlation with cerebral ischemia. In a recent meta-analysis of 8 longitudinal studies of IPH detected on in vivo MR imaging, the presence of IPH on MR imaging was associated with an approximately 5.6-fold higher risk for stroke/TIA compared with the risk in subjects without IPH despite the large degree of detected heterogeneity in the published studies.[11] In a separate meta-analysis to summarize the association of MR imaging–determined IPH, LRNC, and thin/ruptured FC with subsequent ischemic events, Gupta and colleagues[40] noted that the prediction of future events using MPRAGE with large-FOV neck coils was not significantly different from predictions using a multisequence technique with a carotid coil. Thus, it is reasonable to conclude that clear T1 hyperintensity greater than 1.5 times the adjacent sternocleidomastoid muscle on TOF, T1W, and MPRAGE sequences using commercial MR sequences and large-FOV NV coils represents carotid plaque IPH that is associated with a higher risk of subsequent stroke/TIA. It is likely that small IPH will be missed with these clinical sequences.

Lipid-rich necrotic core and thin/ruptured fibrous cap

Numerous studies have shown the correlation between LRNC size and/or the presence of a thin/ruptured FC overlying the LRNC with the subsequent development of new ipsilateral carotid stroke/TIA. In a 3-year natural history study of 154 patients with ACS with 50% to 79% stenosis, the presence of a thin/ruptured FC (hazard ratio [HR], 17.0; $P<.001$) and larger maximum percentage of LRNC (HR for 10% increase, 1.6; $P = .004$) were predictors of future ipsilateral carotid symptoms.[9] Subsequently, a simple CAS was developed as a 4-tier grading system to describe the LRNC size.[41] Patients with a thin wall (<2 mm) and no LRNC are CAS 1. Patients with less than 20% maximum percentage wall area of LRNC are CAS 2. CAS 3 refers to patients with 20% to 40% maximum percentage wall area of LRNC, and CAS 4 is reserved for patients with greater than 40%. In a prospective study of 120 patients with ACS, increasing CAS was associated with the development of new ulceration or FC rupture and increasing plaque burden[10] (Fig. 8). Percentage carotid stenosis was not associated with either the development of new ulceration/FC rupture or increasing plaque burden, confirming the improved risk stratification of CAS compared with carotid stenosis measurements. In a recent meta-analysis of 9 studies with a total of 779 subjects, Gupta and colleagues[40] reported that the presence of LRNC and thin/ruptured FC was associated with increased risk of future stroke/TIA.

Predictive Value of Plaque Imaging for Ultrasonography

Total plaque area

Carotid plaque burden, measured as TPA, was shown to strongly predicted risk, well beyond a Framingham Risk Score: after adjustment for age, sex, blood pressure, cholesterol level, smoking, diabetes, homocysteine, and treatment of blood pressure, patients in the top quartile of TPA had a 3.4-fold higher 5-year risk of stroke, death, or myocardial infarction compared with the lowest quartile.[42] The risk was graded; by quartile of TPA, the 5-year risk of those events was approximately 5%, 10%, 15%, and 20%.

Measurement of carotid plaque progression/regression is a sensitive measurement because carotid plaques are focal and progress along the artery wall, in the axis of flow, 2.4 times faster than they thicken. Carotid plaque volume can change in 3 dimensions: length, thickness, and circumferential extent.[43]

Transcranial Doppler microemboli detection

In a prospective study of 319 patients with ACS enrolled between 2000 and 2005, 10% had a positive study with 2 or more microemboli during an hour of monitoring with a 1-year stroke risk of

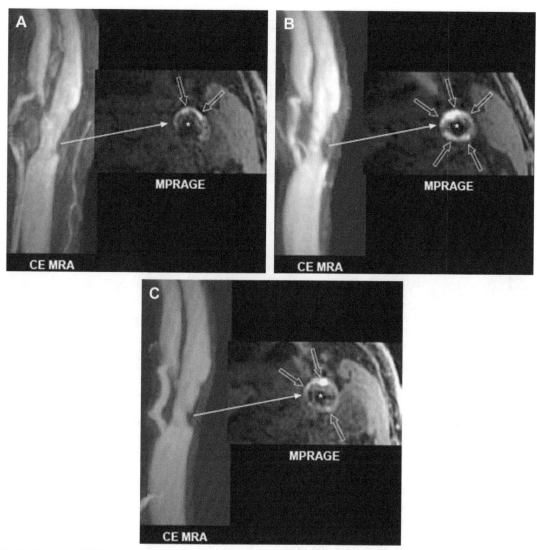

Fig. 7. Presence of IPH is associated with plaque growth and increasing stenosis on standard statin therapy that regressed with intensive statin therapy as seen on serial research carotid plaque MR studies. (A) This 76-year-old asymptomatic patient who had been on atorvastatin 10 mg for 3 years presented with a 51% stenosis of the left internal carotid artery on CE MRA. On 3D MPRAGE images, IPH was seen as the focally intense region (*open arrows*). (B) Despite increased statin therapy with atorvastatin 40 mg for 2 2 years, there was a progression in the size of the IPH (*open arrows*) and increase in carotid stenosis to 69%. (C) Based on the plaque and stenosis progression, statin therapy was increased again to 80 mg of atorvastatin. Over the next 2 to 3 years there was clear regression of the IPH (*open arrows*) with the carotid stenosis now measuring 58%. * indicates internal carotid artery lumen.

15.6%.[44] The other 90% of these patients with no microemboli had only a 1% risk of stroke. All patients with TCD microemboli detection were placed on intensive medical therapy. Serial TCD studies showed a precipitous reduction in microemboli detection with each year of treatment, so that after 2 years of intensive medical therapy only 9% of patients still had TCD microemboli detected. This finding suggested that intensive medical therapy could reduce microemboli, perhaps by stabilizing plaque.

The Asymptomatic Carotid Emboli Study confirmed the value of TCD microembolus detection to identify high-risk patients with ACS. Of the 467 patients with ACS, 77 (16.5%) had embolic signals. The absolute annual risk of ipsilateral TIA/stroke between baseline and 2 years was 7.13% in these patients with ACS with TCD microemboli detection compared with 3.04% in patients without TCD microemboli detection.[6]

In 2010 Spence and colleagues[7] reported on 468 patients with ACS; 199 had been enrolled

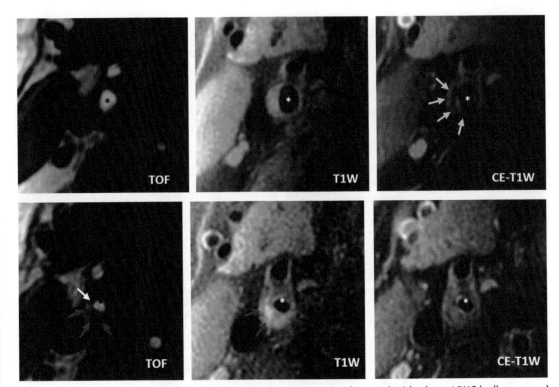

Fig. 8. Baseline large LRNC progresses to new IPH. Baseline MR imaging (*top row*) with a large LRNC (*yellow arrows*). The 3-year follow-up MR imaging (*bottom row*) of the matched cross section shows FC rupture (*white arrow*) with IPH (*red arrows*). Also note the large increase in internal carotid wall area and decrease in lumen area. The asterisk marks the lumen of the internal carotid artery. CE-T1W, contrast-enhanced T1 weighted image; TOF, time-of-flight; T1W, T1 weighted image. (*From* Xu D, Hippe DS, Underhill HR, et al. Prediction of high-risk plaque development and plaque progression with the carotid atherosclerosis score. JACC Cardiovasc Imaging 2014;7(4):369; with permission.)

before 2003, and 269 after 2003, when a more intensive approach to therapy had been implemented. Although the frequency of microemboli had declined from 12.6% of patients before 2003% to 3.7% of patients after 2003, the presence of microemboli continued to identify a high-risk group (Fig. 9).

Plaque ulceration and plaque texture on three-dimensional ultrasonography

Carotid plaque ulceration on 3D ultrasonography has been shown to be a strong predictor of risk in patients with ACS. Patients with 3 or more ulcers (on either side) were more likely to have a stroke or death during the 3-year follow-up than patients with fewer or no ulcers.[32] This risk was equivalent to that of patients with ACS with microemboli on TCD. This work was extended to quantifying carotid total ulcer volume by 3D DUS. Total ulcer volume greater than or equal to 5 mm[3] experienced a significantly higher risk of developing new stroke, TIA, or death during less than or equal to 5 years of follow-up.[45] A prospective study of 298 patients found that change in carotid plaque texture

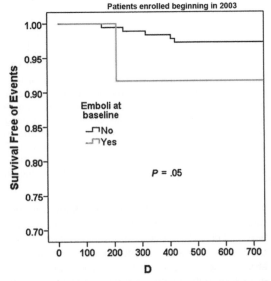

Fig. 9. Kaplan-Meier survival free of stroke, death, or TIAs after more intensive medical therapy beginning in 2003. Microemboli on TCD continued to identify high-risk ACS after more intensive medical therapy reduced the proportion of patients with microemboli from 12.6% to 3.7%[7] (n = 269).

(assessed from analysis of radiofrequency signals, as opposed to echolucency) was a strong predictor of the risk of cardiovascular events at 1 year among patients attending vascular prevention clinics.[46] Combining change in plaque texture with change in plaque volume increased the area under the curve for prediction of events compared with either alone.

Juxtaluminal black/hypoechoic area

The ACSRS study was a prospective multicenter international cohort study that evaluated several baseline clinical, biochemical, and ultrasonography determined features of patients with ACS and followed for up to 8 years. The size of JBA in carotid ultrasonography images of patients with ACS in the ACSRS study showed a linear association of future ipsilateral ischemic events (amaurosis fugax, TIA, stroke).[4] Of the 1121 patients with ACS with 50% to 99% stenosis, 706 patients had a JBA less than 4 mm^2. This large group of patients with ACS had a mean annual stroke rate of 0.4%. On the other extreme was the group of 198 patients with ACS with a JBA greater than 10 mm^2 who had a mean annual stroke rate of 5%. The JBA size (<4 mm^2, 4–8 mm^2, >8 mm^2) remained a significant predictor of new symptoms after adjusting for other imaging risk factors, including carotid stenosis.

Potential of Plaque MR Imaging to Individualize the Medical Therapy of Patients with Asymptomatic Carotid Stenosis

Lipid-rich necrotic core

Ten clinical trials using serial carotid MR imaging to determine the in vivo effects on ASCVD of cholesterol level–lowering drugs have been completed or nearing completion were recently summarized.[18] These studies show that carotid plaques with LRNC are more likely to show a measurable decrease with statin therapy (Fig. 10). Changes in plaque components such as LRNC and inflammation are more dynamic and respond before the overall PWV decreases. In addition, sufficient time of at least 1 year is needed to detect an effect of statin therapy. These observations will provide guidelines for using carotid MR imaging to identify patients for intensive statin therapy and follow them over time.

Based on prior prospective studies, decreasing LRNC should decrease future cardiovascular events.[9] Understanding LRNC progression under intensive risk factor control compared with standard of care has broader clinical implications for managing patients with subclinical atherosclerosis, not limited to ischemic stroke. In this regard, carotid artery plaques provide an easy-to-access window to study therapeutic effects on plaque lipid content. The changes to carotid LRNC may be relevant to coronary artery disease and future coronary events.

Using carotid plaque MR imaging to predict future stroke/TIA was first published in 2006.[9] These initial results were confirmed in multiple subsequent prospective trials.[40] Taken as a whole, there is ample peer-reviewed literature to suggest that the presence of an LRNC in patients with ACS represents a phenotype of atherosclerotic disease with a high risk of future cardiovascular events, that the presence and size of an LRNC provides a reasonable selection criterion to identify patients suitable for additional intensive lipid level–lowering therapy, and that in vivo MR imaging provides a reproducible technique to measure the effectiveness of lipid level–lowering therapies.[47] Using in vivo MR to identify patients with ACS with LRNC who may be amenable to more intensive lipid level–lowering therapy and noninvasively monitor therapeutic efficacy may represent the highest-yield option for reducing stroke mortality since the sharp decline that occurred with better blood pressure management in the 1970s and 1980s.[18]

Additional clinical trials randomizing patients with ACS with LRNC to standard and intensive medical therapy are being proposed. Based on recent work, approximately 50% of patients with ACS with mild to moderate stenosis show an LRNC.[48] Patients with untreated or undertreated LRNC may be at risk for future growth of the LRNC and/or development of IPH or plaque ulceration. Recently published cholesterol guidelines do not recognize ACS as an indication for high-intensity statin therapy.[3] However, this subgroup theoretically represents the group that may benefit the most from intensive lipid level–lowering and antihypertensive therapy. These initial trials are likely to use a decrease in LRNC size as a surrogate marker for improved atherosclerotic treatment, although larger multicenter trials with enough patients to test for a statistically significant improvement in hard end points, such as stroke/TIA and decreased cognition, will be needed to fully test the hypothesis.[47]

While these new randomized clinical trials are awaited, can clinical versions of carotid plaque MR imaging be used in everyday practice? Based on reproducibility studies, it has been proposed that future drug trials include patients with at least 2 contiguous 2-mm thick CE-T1W axial images showing a LRNC. Also patients with ACS with CAS of 3 to 4 are at increased risk of developing carotid plaque ulceration or ruptured FC and

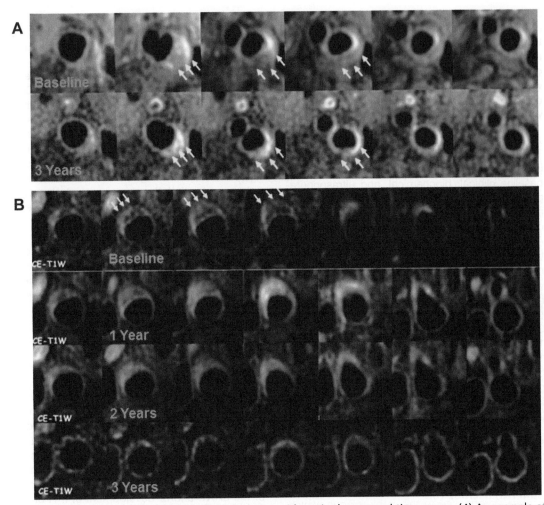

Fig. 10. MR imaging example of plaque lipid depletion with statin therapy and time course. (*A*) An example of significant lipid content reduction (*yellow arrows*) and plaque regression at 3 years compared with baseline in the left carotid artery. Overall, 11% of study subjects had completed plaque lipid depletion over 3 years. (*B*) MR imaging example of the plaque lipid depletion time course. Regression in LRNC size was notable between the baseline, 1-year, and 2-year MR imaging scans. Regression in plaque volume seemed to follow plaque lipid depletion and was most pronounced from years 1 to 3. (*From* Zhao X-Q, Dong L, Hatsukami T, et al. MR imaging of carotid plaque composition during lipid-lowering therapy a prospective assessment of effect and time course. JACC Cardiovasc Imaging 2011;4(9):982; with permission.)

may also represent a group of patients in whom intensive lipid level–lowering therapy is warranted. As discussed earlier, it is likely that 3-T MR imaging with 3D T1W and CE-T1W images will be able to identify this size of LRNC using standard large-FOV NV coils and commercially available sequences (see Fig. 4). Therefore, it may be possible to add the detection of LRNC to the routine clinical evaluation of carotid stenosis by CE MRA with the addition of these two 4-minute 3D MR sequences. Additional training to interpret carotid plaque MR images and the use of dedicated commercially available programs to analyze carotid plaque images may be warranted.

Intraplaque hemorrhage

Carotid plaques with IPH represent a later, more advanced stage of atherosclerotic disease compared with plaque showing only LRNC. Ulceration is considered as part of the AHA type VI plaque along with IPH, but is usually considered an even more advanced type of plaque atherosclerosis. The presence of juxtaluminal IPH and larger IPH are considered particularly high risk for future stroke/TIA.[9] Tissue-specific carotid plaque MR imaging of IPH seen with high contrast-to-noise ratio (CNR) on MPRAGE images has been used in multiple longitudinal studies, usually as a dichotomous variable (present or absent). A recent meta-analysis showed that the prediction of future stroke/TIA using a large-FOV NV coil was not significantly different from predictions based on carotid coils, although the small number of studies in this subset analysis resulted in borderline statistically significant heterogeneity, suggesting that further work is needed to confirm that these techniques do perform similarly.[40]

It is reasonable to conclude from these studies that patients with ACS with IPH are at increased risk of future stroke/TIA and this risk may be worse in patients with IPH and ulceration or in patients with juxtaluminal IPH. In addition, a recent prospective study showed that the IPH detected in carotid endarterectomy specimens was associated with future vascular death, nonfatal stroke, and nonfatal myocardial infarction, suggesting that carotid IPH holds prognostic information about future cardiovascular events throughout the body.[49] This subgroup of patients with ACS is likely to benefit from very intense medical therapy as well as close clinical monitoring (see Fig. 7). Simple carotid stenosis measurements and traditional risk factor analysis does not define this subgroup of patients with ACS at increased risk of future symptoms. If clear carotid plaque progression (new ulceration, increased size of IPH, increase PWV) or new ipsilateral carotid symptoms (stroke or TIA) or microemboli are detected on TCD despite very intense medical therapy, the subgroup of patients with ACS may warrant intervention with carotid endarterectomy/carotid stenting. The need for intervention in this subgroup of patients with ACS is discussed elsewhere in this issue.

Potential of Plaque Ultrasonography Imaging to Individualize the Medical Therapy of Patients with Asymptomatic Carotid Stenosis

Total plaque area

After establishing the utility of TPA to measure risk well beyond Framingham Risk Score, Spence and colleagues[42] began a prospective study of a large number of patients with serial TPA measurements. During the first year of follow-up, half the patients had plaque progression; a quarter had regression of TPA. After adjustment for the same panel of risk factors, patients with plaque progression had twice the risk of those with stable plaque or regression, which meant that treatment according to usual guidelines was failing half the patients. This finding led to development of a new strategy for vascular prevention: treating arteries instead of treating risk factors such as the serum level of LDL-C.[8] In 2010, this group reported that implementation of this strategy had reversed the

---

Box 2
What physicians need to know

- MR imaging
  - Measurable LRNC represents the carotid plaque phenotype that optimal responds to intense statin therapy
  - Untreated/undertreated moderate to large LRNC (CAS of 3–4) is at increased risk of new IPH or ulceration as well as new stroke/TIA
  - IPH and ulceration represent a very-high-risk group of patients with ACS
- Ultrasonography
  - Treat arteries instead of risk factors by following TPA/volume in response to intense medical therapy instead of serum lipid levels
  - Lack of decreasing TPA/volume with statin therapy represents a high-risk group of patients with ACS
  - Three or more ulcerations, large volume of ulcerations, large JPA, and TCD microemboli represents a very high-risk group of patients with ACS

---

proportion of patients with plaque progression versus regression.[8] Among patients with ACS, this strategy had markedly reduced the occurrence of microemboli, progression of plaque, and the occurrence of stroke or myocardial infarction.[7] It is likely that multiple DUS-defined risk factors, such as plaque progression despite intensive medical therapy, number and volume of plaque ulcerations, size of JPA, and presence of microemboli of TCD, can be combined to better define the overall risk of future cardiovascular events of individual patients with ACS. These types of analyses are being planned for the imaging substudies of CREST-2 (Box 2).

SUMMARY

The continued occurrence of stroke despite advances in medical therapy for patients with ACS strongly indicates that individual response to therapy varies widely. The current guidelines for treating patients with ACS are based on risk stratification derived from population-driven outcomes. Although treating patients with ACS based on the currently accepted risk factors has led to a decrease in stroke mortality, this decline has begun to plateau, suggesting that some patients are not responding to current recommended medical therapy. It is likely that these nonresponders are patients at increased risk of future stroke/TIA.

There is ample peer-reviewed literature to suggest that patients with ACS with measurable LRNC, or progression of carotid plaque burden, represent the phenotype of atherosclerosis that is most amenable to intensive medical therapy. There is also good evidence to suggest that directly monitoring the effect of medical therapy with plaque burden imaging is more effective than following serum markers such as LDL-C. Recent work has shown that it is beginning to be possible to identify and measure necrotic core with US Food and Drug Administration–approved coils and MR sequences. Additional radiologist training and software are needed to aid in the identification and quantification of the necrotic core.

Additional markers of carotid plaque burden imaging can identify vulnerable plaque features such as IPH, ulceration, microemboli detected by TCD, as well as the presence of large JBA on DUS plaque imaging. These features likely represent a small subset of patients with ACS who are at very high risk of future stroke/TIA and who warrant close observation for any signs of plaque burden progression or new symptoms despite maximal medical therapy.

REFERENCES

1. Bonita R, Stewart A, Beaglehole R. International trends in stroke mortality: 1970-1985. Stroke 1990; 21(7):989–92.
2. Amarenco P, Labreuche J. Lipid management in the prevention of stroke: review and updated meta-analysis of statins for stroke prevention. Lancet Neurol 2009;8(5):453–63.
3. Stone NJ, Robinson JG, Lichtenstein AH, et al. 2013 ACC/AHA guideline on the treatment of blood cholesterol to reduce atherosclerotic cardiovascular risk in adults: a report of the American College of Cardiology/American Heart Association Task Force on Practice Guidelines. Circulation 2014;129(25 Suppl 2):S1–45.
4. Kakkos SK, Griffin MB, Nicolaides AN, et al. The size of juxtaluminal hypoechoic area in ultrasound images of asymptomatic carotid plaques predicts the occurrence of stroke. J Vasc Surg 2013;57(3):609–18.e1 [discussion: 617–8].
5. Paraskevas KI, Spence JD, Veith FJ, et al. Identifying which patients with asymptomatic carotid stenosis could benefit from intervention. Stroke J Cereb Circ 2014;45(12):3720–4.
6. Markus HS, King A, Shipley M, et al. Asymptomatic embolisation for prediction of stroke in the Asymptomatic Carotid Emboli Study (ACES): a prospective observational study. Lancet Neurol 2010;9(7):663–71.
7. Spence JD, Coates V, Li H, et al. Effects of intensive medical therapy on microemboli and cardiovascular risk in asymptomatic carotid stenosis. Arch Neurol 2010;67(2):180–6.
8. Spence JD, Hackam DG. Treating arteries instead of risk factors: a paradigm change in management of atherosclerosis. Stroke J Cereb Circ 2010;41(6): 1193–9.
9. Takaya N, Yuan C, Chu B, et al. Association between carotid plaque characteristics and subsequent ischemic cerebrovascular events: a prospective assessment with MRI–initial results. Stroke 2006; 37(3):818–23.
10. Xu D, Hippe DS, Underhill HR, et al. Prediction of high-risk plaque development and plaque progression with the carotid atherosclerosis score. JACC Cardiovasc Imaging 2014;7(4):366–73.
11. Saam T, Hetterich H, Hoffmann V, et al. Meta-analysis and systematic review of the predictive value of carotid plaque hemorrhage on cerebrovascular events by magnetic resonance imaging. J Am Coll Cardiol 2013;62(12):1081–91.
12. Virmani R, Burke AP, Kolodgie FD, et al. Vulnerable plaque: the pathology of unstable coronary lesions. J Interv Cardiol 2002;15(6):439–46.
13. Naghavi M, Libby P, Falk E, et al. From vulnerable plaque to vulnerable patient: a call for new definitions and risk assessment strategies: Part I. Circulation 2003;108(14):1664–72.
14. Naghavi M, Libby P, Falk E, et al. From vulnerable plaque to vulnerable patient: a call for new definitions and risk assessment strategies: Part II. Circulation 2003;108(15):1772–8.
15. Stary HC, Chandler AB, Dinsmore RE, et al. A definition of advanced types of atherosclerotic lesions and a histological classification of atherosclerosis. A report from the Committee on Vascular Lesions of the Council on Arteriosclerosis, American Heart Association. Circulation 1995;92(5):1355–74.
16. Cai JM, Hatsukami TS, Ferguson MS, et al. Classification of human carotid atherosclerotic lesions with in vivo multicontrast magnetic resonance imaging. Circulation 2002;106(11):1368–73.
17. Spence JD, Parraga G. Three-dimensional ultrasound of carotid plaque. Neuroimag Clin N Am 2015, in press.
18. Underhill HR, Yuan C. Carotid MRI: a tool for monitoring individual response to cardiovascular therapy? Expert Rev Cardiovasc Ther 2011;9(1):63–80.
19. Saam T, Kerwin WS, Chu B, et al. Sample size calculation for clinical trials using magnetic resonance imaging for the quantitative assessment of carotid atherosclerosis. J Cardiovasc Magn Reson 2005; 7(5):799–808.
20. Li F, Yarnykh VL, Hatsukami TS, et al. Scan-rescan reproducibility of carotid atherosclerotic plaque morphology and tissue composition measurements using multicontrast MRI at 3T. J Magn Reson Imaging 2010;31(1):168–76.

21. Underhill HR, Yarnykh VL, Hatsukami TS, et al. Carotid plaque morphology and composition: initial comparison between 1.5- and 3.0-T magnetic field strengths. Radiology 2008;248(2):550–60.

22. Chu B, Kampschulte A, Ferguson MS, et al. Hemorrhage in the atherosclerotic carotid plaque: a high-resolution MRI study. Stroke 2004;35(5):1079–84.

23. Saam T, Ferguson MS, Yarnykh VL, et al. Quantitative evaluation of carotid plaque composition by in vivo MRI. Arterioscler Thromb Vasc Biol 2005; 25(1):234–9.

24. Kampschulte A, Ferguson MS, Kerwin WS, et al. Differentiation of intraplaque versus juxtaluminal hemorrhage/thrombus in advanced human carotid atherosclerotic lesions by in vivo magnetic resonance imaging. Circulation 2004;110(20):3239–44.

25. Ota H, Yarnykh VL, Ferguson MS, et al. Carotid intraplaque hemorrhage imaging at 3.0-T MR imaging: comparison of the diagnostic performance of three T1-weighted sequences 1. Radiology 2010;254(2): 551–62.

26. Cai J, Hatsukami TS, Ferguson MS, et al. In vivo quantitative measurement of intact fibrous cap and lipid-rich necrotic core size in atherosclerotic carotid plaque: comparison of high-resolution, contrast-enhanced magnetic resonance imaging and histology. Circulation 2005;112(22):3437–44.

27. Yuan C, Kerwin WS, Ferguson MS, et al. Contrast-enhanced high resolution MRI for atherosclerotic carotid artery tissue characterization. J Magn Reson Imaging 2002;15(1):62–7.

28. Narumi S, Sasaki M, Natori T, et al. Carotid plaque characterization using 3D T1-weighted MR imaging with histopathologic validation: a comparison with 2D technique. AJNR Am J Neuroradiol 2015;36(4):751–6.

29. Cheng J, Li H, Xiao F, et al. Fully automatic plaque segmentation in 3-D carotid ultrasound images. Ultrasound Med Biol 2013;39(12):2431–46.

30. Græbe M, Entrekin R, Collet-Billon A, et al. Reproducibility of two 3-D ultrasound carotid plaque quantification methods. Ultrasound Med Biol 2014;40(7):1641–9.

31. Schminke U, Motsch L, Hilker L, et al. Three-dimensional ultrasound observation of carotid artery plaque ulceration. Stroke J Cereb Circ 2000;31(7):1651–5.

32. Madani A, Beletsky V, Tamayo A, et al. High-risk asymptomatic carotid stenosis: ulceration on 3D ultrasound vs TCD microemboli. Neurology 2011; 77(8):744–50.

33. Sztajzel R, Momjian S, Momjian-Mayor I, et al. Stratified gray-scale median analysis and color mapping of the carotid plaque: correlation with endarterectomy specimen histology of 28 patients. Stroke 2005;36(4): 741–5.

34. Griffin MB, Kyriacou E, Pattichis C, et al. Juxtaluminal hypoechoic area in ultrasonic images of carotid plaques and hemispheric symptoms. J Vasc Surg 2010;52(1):69–76.

35. Markus HS, Molloy J. Use of a decibel threshold in detecting Doppler embolic signals. Stroke J Cereb Circ 1997;28(4):692–5.

36. Ringelstein EB, Droste DW, Babikian VL, et al. Consensus on microembolus detection by TCD. International Consensus Group on Microembolus Detection. Stroke J Cereb Circ 1998;29(3):725–9.

37. Kolodgie FD, Gold HK, Burke AP, et al. Intraplaque hemorrhage and progression of coronary atheroma. N Engl J Med 2003;349(24):2316–25.

38. Takaya N, Yuan C, Chu B, et al. Presence of intraplaque hemorrhage stimulates progression of carotid atherosclerotic plaques: a high-resolution magnetic resonance imaging study. Circulation 2005; 111(21):2768–75.

39. Moody AR, Murphy RE, Morgan PS, et al. Characterization of complicated carotid plaque with magnetic resonance direct thrombus imaging in patients with cerebral ischemia. Circulation 2003;107(24):3047–52.

40. Gupta A, Baradaran H, Schweitzer AD, et al. Carotid plaque MRI and stroke risk: a systematic review and meta-analysis. Stroke J Cereb Circ 2013;44(11): 3071–7.

41. Underhill HR, Hatsukami TS, Cai J, et al. A noninvasive imaging approach to assess plaque severity: the carotid atherosclerosis score. AJNR Am J Neuroradiol 2010;31(6):1068–75.

42. Spence JD, Eliasziw M, DiCicco M, et al. Carotid plaque area: a tool for targeting and evaluating vascular preventive therapy. Stroke J Cereb Circ 2002;33(12):2916–22.

43. Spence JD. Time course of atherosclerosis regression. Atherosclerosis 2014;235(2):347–8.

44. Spence JD, Tamayo A, Lownie SP, et al. Absence of microemboli on transcranial Doppler identifies low-risk patients with asymptomatic carotid stenosis. Stroke J Cereb Circ 2005;36(11):2373–8.

45. Kuk M, Wannarong T, Beletsky V, et al. Volume of carotid artery ulceration as a predictor of cardiovascular events. Stroke J Cereb Circ 2014;45(5):1437–41.

46. Van Engelen A, Wannarong T, Parraga G, et al. Three-dimensional carotid ultrasound plaque texture predicts vascular events. Stroke J Cereb Circ 2014; 45(9):2695–701.

47. Demarco JK, Huston J 3rd. Imaging of high-risk carotid artery plaques: current status and future directions. Neurosurg Focus 2014;36(1):E1.

48. Demarco JK, Ota H, Underhill HR, et al. MR carotid plaque imaging and contrast-enhanced MR angiography identifies lesions associated with recent ipsilateral thromboembolic symptoms: an in vivo study at 3T. AJNR Am J Neuroradiol 2010;31(8):1395–402.

49. Hellings WE, Peeters W, Moll FL, et al. Composition of carotid atherosclerotic plaque is associated with cardiovascular outcome: a prognostic study. Circulation 2010;121(17):1941–50.

Low-Grade Carotid Stenosis
Implications of MR Imaging

Mahmud Mossa-Basha, MD[a],*, Bruce A. Wasserman, MD[b]

KEYWORDS

• MR imaging • Carotid vessel wall imaging • Low-grade carotid stenosis • Stroke

KEY POINTS

• Luminal imaging techniques do not adequately evaluate extracranial carotid atherosclerotic plaque burden and characteristics in patients with low-grade carotid stenosis.
• Although multiple randomized controlled trials have not indicated an advantage to surgery over medical management in the low-grade stenosis population, there is an associated risk of stroke.
• Plaque features such as intraplaque hemorrhage, fibrous cap rupture, and ulceration, among others, confer an increased risk of stroke in low-grade stenosis.
• Considering that atherosclerosis is a systemic disease, vessel wall MR imaging can help determine the culprit lesion in the setting of cryptogenic stroke.
• Carotid vessel wall MR imaging can be helpful in identifying likelihood of plaque and its associated risk in other vascular beds that are not as easily imaged.

INTRODUCTION

Stroke is the second most common cause of mortality and a leading cause of morbidity worldwide. Approximately 80% of strokes are presumed to be ischemic in etiology, with 20% to 30% arising from extracranial carotid atherosclerosis.[1] In the setting of extracranial carotid artery disease, the decision to treat symptomatic patients surgically or with carotid artery stenting has traditionally relied on the degree of luminal stenosis on catheter angiography based on the results of randomized controlled trials.[2,3] Pooled data from the trials showed a 16% absolute reduced 5-year risk of future stroke events in patients with 70% or greater stenosis undergoing carotid endarterectomy in comparison with medical management.[4]

Over the past 10 years, however, investigation has placed less emphasis on the degree of stenosis and more on plaque features that confer lesion vulnerability. These vulnerable plaque features support the hypothesis, as in coronary artery disease, that many cerebral infarctions result from plaque rupture and distal embolization or acute occlusion, and not long-standing hypoperfusion.[5–9] Multiple studies have provided evidence that plaques resulting in moderate stenosis can rupture and result in acute ischemic events.[10–12] Barnett and colleagues[13] indicated a significantly increased 5-year risk of ipsilateral stroke (P = .045) in patients with 50% to 69% stenosis treated medically (22.2%) compared with those treated surgically (15.7%). For those with less than 50% stenosis in the North American Symptomatic Carotid Endarterectomy Trial (NASCET), the stroke rate was lower in the surgical group relative to the medically managed group, although

Disclosure Statement: The authors have nothing to disclose.
[a] Division of Neuroradiology, University of Washington Medical Center, University of Washington School of Medicine, 1959 Northeast Pacific Street, Box 357115, Seattle, WA 98195, USA; [b] Russell H. Morgan Department of Radiology and Radiological Sciences, Johns Hopkins School of Medicine, 367 East Park Building, 600 North Wolfe Street, Baltimore, MD 21287, USA
* Corresponding author.
E-mail address: mmossab@uw.edu

Neuroimag Clin N Am 26 (2016) 129–145
http://dx.doi.org/10.1016/j.nic.2015.09.010
1052-5149/16/$ – see front matter © 2016 Elsevier Inc. All rights reserved.

this did not reach statistical significance (14.9% vs 18.7%, P = .16). According to pooled data from the randomized control trials,[4] the 5-year reduction in ipsilateral stroke rate was 4.6% for surgical patients with moderate (50%–69%) stenosis. There was no benefit in stroke rate for patients with 30% to 49% stenosis between the surgical and medical management groups, whereas there was increased risk of stroke in the surgical group for those with less than 30% stenosis (absolute risk reduction −2.2%, P = .05).[4,14,15] The European Carotid Surgical Trial[9] reported a 1.3% rate of ipsilateral ischemic stroke lasting longer than 7 days in patients with symptomatic mild (0%–29%) stenosis during a 3-year follow-up (0.43% per year). Fritz and Levien[16] reported an 8.6% rate of ipsilateral ischemic events during a 2-year follow-up of 35 symptomatic patients with low-grade carotid stenosis or ulcerated plaque on medical management. In the setting of carotid atherosclerosis, including lesions resulting in low-grade carotid stenosis, there may be other lesions ipsilateral to the symptomatic side including aortic and intracranial plaques. Plaque-component characterization can provide important information to help stratify the likelihood that the carotid plaque is indeed the culprit lesion so that an appropriate treatment strategy can be implemented, including resection of the low-grade lesion. With moderate or severe carotid stenosis the associated plaques are presumed to be the culprits, and the randomized controlled trials have indicated the value of surgical intervention. The overestimation of stroke risk by contemporary standards in the medically managed groups for these trials that predate statin treatment suggests potential overtreatment of high-grade stenosis by surgery, and MR vessel wall imaging might also help to stratify high-grade lesions for a more appropriate balance of medical versus surgical treatments.

Although the rate of stroke in low-grade extracranial carotid stenosis differs based on the aforementioned trials, these trials have indicated that the benefit of surgery in low-grade stenosis may not improve the outcome over medical management when surgical risks are taken into consideration. However, these trials are based on narrowing to guide surgical management, which cannot stratify the risk of rupture for low-grade lesions and identify those at high enough risk to benefit from endarterectomy, and for this reason plaque characterization by MR imaging can potentially play an important role. Furthermore, despite a lower risk of stroke from low-grade carotid plaque compared with high-grade lesions, the chance for stroke from low-grade plaque cannot be discounted when considering the high prevalence of this disease. The occurrence of low-grade carotid stenosis in elderly populations is frequent, as 75% of men and 62% of women older than 64 years had carotid stenosis on ultrasonography in the Cardiovascular Health Study,[17] whereas only 7% of men and 5% of women had stenosis greater than 49%.

MODIFICATIONS IN MEDICAL MANAGEMENT

Since the publication of the trials for evaluation of disease management based on luminal stenosis, there have been significant changes to the optimal medical management regimen that have modified stroke risk in medically managed patients. 3-Hydroxy-3-methylglutaryl-coenzyme A reductase inhibitors (statins), a class of cholesterol-lowering drugs, have become a staple of atherosclerosis-related stroke management. The Stroke Prevention by Aggressive Management in Cholesterol Levels Investigators (SPARCL)[18] randomized 4731 patients with prior stroke or transient ischemic attack (TIA) (between 1 and 6 months from the event), no known coronary heart disease, and low-density lipoprotein cholesterol (LDL-C) between 100 and 190 mg/dL to 80 mg atorvastatin therapy or placebo. The 5-year absolute reduction in risk of major cardiovascular events was 3.5% (hazard ratio [HR] 0.8, 95% confidence interval [CI] 0.69–0.92; P = .002) with no significant difference in mortality rates. Of the 4731 randomized patients, 4278 were evaluated for carotid disease, and of those 1007 were found to have carotid stenosis.[19] By randomization to the atorvastatin group, the incidence of any cardiovascular events was reduced by 42% relative to placebo (HR 0.58; 95% CI 0.46–0.73; P<.00001). The risk of cerebrovascular events (TIA or stroke) was reduced by 34% in the atorvastatin group (HR 0.66, 95% CI 0.5–0.89; P = .005). The risk of undergoing carotid revascularization was reduced by 54% (HR 0.44, 95% CI 0.24–0.79; P = .006). The Heart Protective Study Collaborative Group[20] randomized 20,536 patients in the United Kingdom with coronary artery disease, other occlusive artery disease, or diabetes mellitus to 40 mg simvastatin or placebo groups, and found a significant reduction in fatal and nonfatal stroke risk in the statin group (4.3% vs 5.7%, P<.0001). For the first occurrence of major vascular events, there was a 24% reduction in the event rate (19.8% vs 25.2%, P<.0001). Hegland and colleagues[21] evaluated 230 patients with 318 carotid arteries with at least 40% carotid stenosis on carotid ultrasonography without occlusion or referral for carotid revascularization. Of these, 171 were not receiving statin therapy while 147 were treated with simvastatin. There was no significant difference in baseline stenosis but there was a significant difference in change in stenosis, as the group that did not receive statin therapy had a +4.9% change in stenosis while the simvastatin group had on average a stenosis change of −10% (P<.001). A meta-analysis[22] that included more than 90,000 patients evaluated all trials testing the effect of statin drugs on the incidence of strokes and carotid intima-media (IMT) measurements by ultrasonography according to LDL-C reduction. The relative risk reduction for stroke was 21% (odds ratio [OR] 0.79). Statin size effect was significantly associated with LDL-C reduction, as each 10% reduction in LDL-C was estimated to reduce the risk of all strokes by 15.6% and carotid IMT by 0.73% per year. Statins have become a mainstay in the management of atherosclerosis-related stroke events and, as already indicated, can significantly reduce stroke and stroke recurrence. However, there have been no recent randomized controlled trials comparing surgical and medical management with optimized medical therapy including statins to determine how their inclusion would modify surgical management algorithms.

EVALUATION OF PLAQUE BEYOND THE DEGREE OF LUMINAL STENOSIS

Coronary angiographic studies have indicated that moderate to low-grade arterial stenoses may lead to myocardial infarction, and frequently the most stenotic artery will not be upstream from the myocardial infarction.[23–25] Subsequent histopathologic studies indicated that plaque erosion and disruption were common features in symptomatic lesions.[24,26] Similar findings have been made with carotid plaques and associated cerebrovascular events.[10–12] Lovett and colleagues[10] found a significant association between carotid plaque surface irregularity on angiography and associated plaque rupture and histologic vulnerable plaque characteristics including intraplaque hemorrhage (IPH), lipid-rich necrotic core, and plaque instability. Histologic evaluation indicated that plaque erosion and rupture were frequently seen in these culprit lesions, indicating that stenosis was not the sole predictor of stroke risk. The degree of stenosis is a poor predictor of plaque volume and extent.[10,12,27]

Inflammation is thought to represent an important destabilizing factor for atherosclerosis and is considered a major component of high-risk vulnerable plaque.[28,29] Spagnoli and colleagues[12] evaluated 269 carotid endarterectomy specimens, and

found a significantly higher rate of inflammatory infiltrate and acute thrombus formation with associated fibrous cap rupture in patients with acute infarct when compared with patients with TIA or no symptoms. Seventy-four percent of infarct patients had a thrombotically active plaque (fresh clot composed of platelets and fibrin on the plaque surface) compared with 35% with TIA (P<.001) and 14% of asymptomatic (P<.001) patients. There was also a significant difference in the presence of cap rupture between stroke and TIA patients (67% vs 23%, P<.001), stroke and asymptomatic patients (67% vs 13%, P<.001) and TIA and asymptomatic patients (23% vs 13%, P = .004). The study also found that ruptured plaques in stroke patients had inflammation that was twice as dense as that seen in TIA (P = .001) and asymptomatic (P = .001) patients. Redgrave and colleagues[11] evaluated 526 consecutive endarterectomy specimens, and found that dense plaque inflammation (with macrophage infiltration) was the feature most strongly associated with fibrous cap rupture (OR 3.9, P<.001) and time since stroke (P = .001). There were significant negative associations between time since stroke and multiple plaque histologic features, including plaque macrophages (P = .007), overall plaque inflammation (P = .003), cap rupture (P = .02), and overall plaque instability (P = .001). There has been recent investigation of plaque inflammation and its correlation with plaque characteristics using PET/MR imaging.[30–33] In the evaluation of 31 patients there was progressively significantly increased ^{18}F-fluorodeoxyglucose activity on PET imaging between thick, thin, and ruptured fibrous caps.[31] Plaques with lipid-rich necrotic cores or IPH also had significantly higher metabolic activity than those predominantly composed of collagen or calcification.[31,33]

LIMITATIONS OF LUMINAL IMAGING IN EVALUATION OF PLAQUE VOLUME

Atherosclerotic lesions frequently remodel outwardly in their early development, which allows for maintenance of luminal size even for prominent lesions. Glagov and colleagues[34] showed that luminal encroachment occurs in coronary arteries once plaque occupies 40% of the area encapsulated by the internal elastic lamina. For this reason, luminal imaging is limited in its ability to detect early lesions and frequently underestimates plaque burden in more advanced disease. Underestimation of plaque burden by angiography has been confirmed by correlation with endarterectomy specimens.[15,35] Furthermore, luminal imaging evaluates disease at the point of maximum stenosis in comparison with adjacent "normal" segments. However, this does not take into account the diffuse nature of atherosclerotic disease, which further contributes to the underestimation of disease burden.[36]

Low-grade carotid lesions are often overlooked as a source of cerebral infarcts because of coexistent disease elsewhere, making it difficult to determine which lesion is the culprit and because plaque size is underestimated as a result of vascular remodeling. Identifying a plaque as having been the source of a stroke may change its risk profile for future events. Inzitari and colleagues[37] showed that stroke risk in the territory of an asymptomatic carotid artery is substantially less than stroke risk in the territory of a symptomatic artery with a similar degree of stenosis. Dennis and colleagues[38] showed that patients who experienced a TIA had a 13-fold excess stroke risk during the first year and a 7-fold excess risk over the first 7 years compared with those without TIAs. TIA might therefore be considered a warning for an impending cerebrovascular event and should warrant investigation of the culprit lesion.

There is a growing body of literature indicating that plaque features and lesion volume play an important role in the assessment of stroke risk, especially when there is little to no narrowing. Fig. 1 illustrates carotid plaque characteristics to be further discussed herein. Freilinger and colleagues[39] prospectively evaluated 32 consecutive stroke patients with less than 50% ipsilateral carotid stenosis with vessel wall MR imaging. American Heart Association (AHA) type VI plaques were found in 37.5% of plaques ipsilateral to the symptomatic side, with none on the contralateral side (P = .001). The most frequent vulnerable plaque features visualized included IPH (75%), fibrous cap rupture (50%), and intraluminal thrombus (33%). In reviewing 217 symptomatic patients with bilateral low-grade carotid stenosis, Cheung and colleagues[40] found that the symptomatic

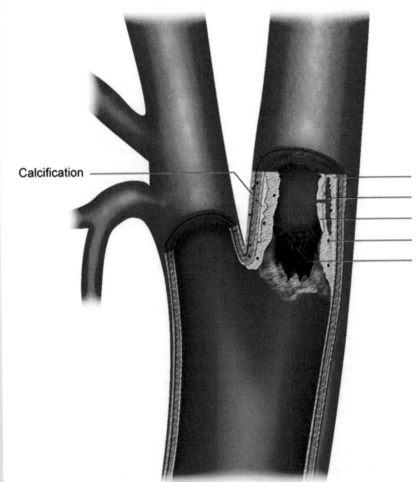

Calcification
Lipid rich necrotic core
Intraplaque hemorrhage
Ruptured fibrous cap
Neovascularity
Intraluminal thrombus

Fig. 1. Illustration of plaque characteristics.

side showed a significantly higher prevalence of IPH on T1-weighted vessel wall MR imaging than the contralateral side (13% vs 7%, P<.05). Altaf and colleagues[41] evaluated patients with symptomatic mild carotid stenosis (30%–49%) and found that recurrence rates of ipsilateral stroke differed between patients with IPH represented by T1 hyperintensity (25%) compared with those without (10%). Yoshida and colleagues[42] evaluated 25 patients with symptomatic low-grade (<50%) carotid stenosis and atherosclerotic plaque with high T1 signal and expansive remodeling on MR imaging. Eleven of the 25 patients had 30 recurrent infarcts on diffusion-weighted imaging (46% per patient-year) refractory to medical therapy, and were treated with carotid endarterectomy. Seven of the 11 patients in the recurrence group had no further stroke events in the postoperative follow-up period of 19.1 ± 14.6 months. Weinstein[43] found that IPH and plaque ulceration on ultrasonography were strongly associated with symptoms despite many lesions showing less than 50% luminal stenosis. In the review of vessel wall MR imaging of 47 patients, Qiao and colleagues[44] found that symptoms were significantly associated with IPH (OR 10.18, P = .03). There was a progressively increasing significant association between symptoms and extent of neovascularity as indicated by grades of adventitial enhancement (0 = absent, 1 = <50%, 2 = ≥50%) (P = .02). The degree of stenosis did not correlate with ischemic events. These studies indicate how in the setting of low-grade or no stenosis, vulnerable plaque characteristics can determine the likelihood of symptoms and future events. There is continued investigation with multicenter trials to determine the role of vessel wall MR imaging in plaque characterization in the setting of cryptogenic stroke.[45]

Plaque surface irregularity or ulceration has been found to be an important plaque vulnerability factor, significantly increasing the risk of stroke (Fig. 2).[46–49] In the analysis of 3007 patient angiograms from the European Carotid Surgery Trial,[49] plaque surface irregularity was an independent predictor of ipsilateral ischemic stroke on medical treatment at all degrees of stenosis (HR 1.80, 95% CI 1.14–2.83; P = .01). In the evaluation of 659 patients who were found to have severe stenosis on angiography in NASCET, the risk of ipsilateral stroke at 24 months for medically treated patients with ulcerated plaques increased incrementally from 26.3% to 73.2% as the degree of stenosis increased from 75% to 95%. For patients with no ulcer, the risk of stroke remained constant at 21.3% for all degrees of stenosis. The net result yielded relative risks of stroke (ulcer vs no ulcer)

ranging from 1.24 (95% CI 0.61–2.52) to 3.43 (95% CI 1.49–7.88).[46] Catheter angiography is not sensitive or specific for the detection of plaque ulcerations. The sensitivity and specificity of detecting ulcerated plaques were 45.9% and 74.1%, respectively. The positive predictive value of identifying an ulcer was 71.8%.[50] MR imaging/contrast-enhanced MR angiography is a sensitive technique for the detection of ulceration.[51,52]

PLAQUE PROGRESSION THROUGH REPEATED SILENT RUPTURES

Coronary plaques that may rupture will frequently be associated with only mild to moderate stenosis and have vulnerable plaque characteristics, similar to what can be seen with vulnerable carotid atheroma. The coronary plaques that rupture have a lipid-rich necrotic core and a thin fibrous cap rich in macrophage and T-cell infiltration with focal disruption.[53] Reports of the mean necrotic core size seen with plaque rupture related to sudden coronary death range from 34%[53] to 50%.[54] These plaques are highly vascularized with extensive ingrowth of the vasa vasorum.[55] Carotid atheromas follow a similar pattern of disruption, with fibrous cap foam cell infiltration, thinning, and neovascularity also influencing the likelihood of rupture.[56,57]

Morphologic studies of coronary arteries suggest that plaque progression beyond 50% cross-sectional luminal narrowing occurs secondary to repeated ruptures, which may be clinically silent.[58,59] The sites of healed plaque ruptures can be recognized by demonstrating a necrotic core with a discontinuous fibrous cap, which is rich in type I collagen, and an overlying neointima formed by smooth muscle cells in a matrix rich in proteoglycan and type III collagen.[58]

Few angiographic studies have demonstrated plaque progression, and short-term studies have suggested that thrombosis is the likely cause. Mann and Davies[59] showed that the frequency of healed plaque rupture increases along with lumen narrowing. Burke and colleagues[58] found healed plaque ruptures in 61% of hearts from victims of sudden coronary death. Multiple healed plaque ruptures with layering were common in segments with acute and healed ruptures, and the percentage of cross-sectional luminal narrowing was dependent on the number of healed repair sites. The underlying percentage of luminal narrowing for acute ruptures exceeded that for healed ruptures (79% ± 15% vs 66% ± 14%; P<.0001).[58] Therefore, the progression of atherosclerotic disease to severe stenosis is the result of repeated ruptures. At least 40% to 50% of

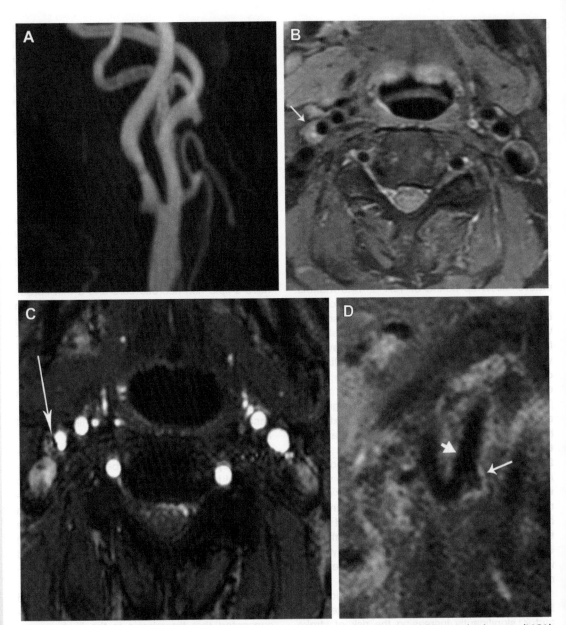

Fig. 2. A 66-year-old man with repeated TIAs referable to territory of the right middle cerebral artery (MCA). Sagittal 3-dimensional (3D) maximum-intensity projection (MIP) reformat of the right carotid bifurcation (*A*) shows eccentric narrowing of the right carotid bulb measuring less than 25%. There is a focal ulceration along the outer wall. Axial T1 postcontrast double-inversion recovery black-blood sequence of the right carotid bulb (*B*) shows an outward remodeling plaque with focal areas of plaque enhancement. On time-of-flight MR angiography at the level of the carotid bulbs (*C*), there is juxtaluminal hypointensity on the right consistent with juxtaluminal calcification (*long arrow*), and intraplaque T1 shortening compatible with IPH. Sagittal T1 postcontrast double-inversion recovery black-blood sequence (*D*) confirms the presence of a small ulceration along the outer wall (*white arrows*). Short arrow points to the proximal internal carotid artery just distal to the carotid bifurcation.

coronary rupture sites show less than 50% diameter stenosis, and the same may be true in carotid disease.[5,60] Spagnoli and colleagues[12] reported a higher incidence of carotid thrombosis in patients with recent stroke in comparison with asymptomatic individuals.

HIGH-RESOLUTION VESSEL WALL MR IMAGING FOR CAROTID PLAQUE COMPONENT ASSESSMENT

There has been increasing acceptance of noninvasive imaging for the evaluation of vulnerable plaque characteristics and their contribution to patient symptoms. Although ultrasonography has been proved to be a valuable technique for evaluation of plaque components, it is limited in its ability to differentiate IPH and lipid-rich necrotic core.[61] Ultrasonography is sensitive for detecting calcifications but does a poor job imaging calcified plaques, as the acoustic shadowing limits soft-tissue visualization deep to the calcifications.[62] Computed tomography (CT) imaging techniques can be used for plaque characterization, and provide a sensitive technique for the detection of calcifications. Some investigators have attempted to use lesion component attenuation for analysis[63,64]; however, attenuation characteristics depend on the energy level used[65] and the administration of contrast,[66,67] both of which can dramatically alter attenuation of lesion components. CT can also be of limited value in depicting some plaque components, including IPH. MR imaging has shown the ability to optimally differentiate plaque characteristics that confer plaque vulnerability, owing to its improved contrast resolution in comparison with CT and ultrasonography.[68] Although CT is considered the best imaging technique for calcium detection in plaques, Clarke and colleagues[69] reported MR imaging sensitivity of 97.6% for calcification detection compared with micro-CT and histology as the reference standard. MR imaging evaluation of calcification with histologic comparison showed MR imaging sensitivities ranging from 76% to 84% and specificity from 86% to 94%, with substantial agreement between the 2 techniques (κ = 0.65–0.75).[70–73] Saam and colleagues[73] determined the presence of calcification if there was matching plaque hypointensity on T1-weighted, T2-weighted, proton density–weighted, and time-of-flight (TOF) MR angiography sequences, with sensitivity of 76% and specificity of 86% when compared with histology. The sensitivity and specificity increased to 84% and 91% when only regions measuring greater than 2 mm^2 were considered. Puppini and colleagues[72] used these same 4 MR sequences to evaluate for calcifications, and found strong agreement with histologic evaluation. Cappendijk and colleagues[71] chose the best combination of contrast weightings from 5 different weightings to assess plaque calcifications among other plaque components, and found that on MR imaging 100% of plaque calcifications could readily be identified and differentiated from other plaque components relative to histologic evaluation.

There have been multiple reports of fibrous cap imaging on MR with histologic specimen correlation.[70,72,74–76] Hatsukami and colleagues[75] evaluated the fibrous cap on a 3-dimensional multiple overlapping thin-slab MR angiographic technique, and found good agreement on fibrous cap status (89% agreement, weighted κ = 0.87) with histologic findings. The fibrous cap was determined to be thick or thin based on the presence of a dark band between the bright lumen and gray wall. The cap was considered disrupted if the dark band was not visualized and there was bright gray signal adjacent to the lumen with or without an irregular luminal surface. Cai and colleagues[70] used TOF MR angiography to determine fibrous cap status, differentiating between thick (>0.25 mm) or disrupted with similar determination of disrupted cap as described in the aforementioned study. There was good accuracy of MR imaging in identifying AHA type VI lesion characteristics including fibrous cap disruption, with sensitivity and specificity of 82% and 91%, respectively. Trivedi and colleagues[77] defined fibrous cap as the juxtaluminal hyperintense component on short-tau inversion recovery sequences. These investigators compared MR imaging and histology-derived fibrous cap lipid-rich necrotic core thickness measurement ratios, and found strong agreement between the two, with a mean difference between the ratios of 0.02 ± 0.004. Mitsumori and colleagues[76] used a multicontrast MR protocol to evaluate fibrous cap status, with an unstable cap represented by irregularity of discontinuity of the juxtaluminal hypointense band on TOF MR angiography, absence of intimal tissue between the lumen and deeper plaque structures, or focal contour abnormalities along the lumen surface. There was good agreement between imaging and histology for the evaluation of the fibrous cap. Detection of unstable fibrous cap on the multicontrast protocol had sensitivity of 81% and specificity of 90%. Wasserman and colleagues[78,79] demonstrated improved detection of fibrous cap and outer wall boundary on MR imaging after contrast administration. Areas of increased enhancement within the cap may indicate areas of inflammatory infiltrate that may suggest impending rupture or neovascularity associated with plaque instability.[80,81]

CLINICAL IMPLICATIONS OF PLAQUE FEATURES

IPH has emerged as one of the most important atherosclerotic plaque features, contributing to plaque progression and leading to cerebrovascular ischemic events (Fig. 3).[40,41,82–87] In the setting of moderate asymptomatic carotid stenosis, Singh and colleagues[83] reported a significant association between IPH and ipsilateral future

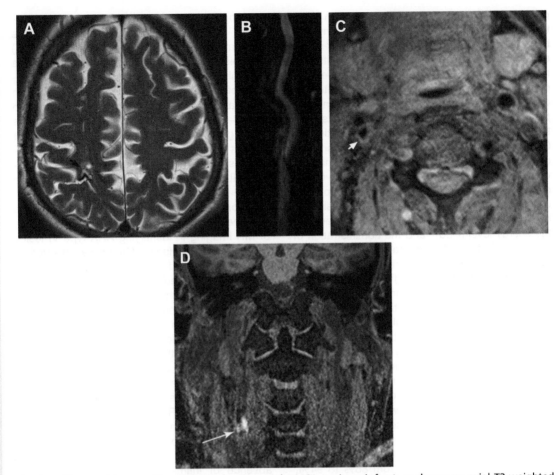

Fig. 3. A 62-year-old man with a history of remote right MCA-territory infarct, as shown on axial T2-weighted image (A) (*short black arrow*). The patient at the time of imaging presented with TIA referable to the right MCA territory. On 3D MIP reformat of the right internal carotid artery (B), there is 0% stenosis of the right carotid bulb. On axial fat-saturated proton-density imaging (C), there is wall thickening with outer wall remodeling (*short white arrow*). Hyperintense signal representing IPH involving the outer wall of the right carotid bulb (*long white arrow*) is seen on coronal T1 magnetization-prepared rapid-acquisition gradient echo sequence (D).

cerebrovascular ischemic events (HR 3.59, 95% CI 2.48–4.71; $P<.001$). The presence of carotid IPH is associated with progression of plaque volume, increased lipid-rich necrotic core volume, and development of new intraplaque hemorrhages.[84,85] During and after the development of IPH, the plaque growth rate is 18.3 ± 6.5 mm³/year, significantly higher than the plaque growth rate before IPH development (-20.5 ± 13.1 mm³, $P = .018$) and showed significant progression over baseline ($P = .008$ compared with a slope of 0).[84] Underhill and colleagues[87] longitudinally imaged 67 asymptomatic patients with 16% to 49% carotid stenosis, and found that those with IPH showed significant progressive luminal narrowing when compared with those without IPH ($P = .005$), and a progressive increase in plaque volume ($P<.001$).

In addition to the association between IPH and patient symptoms, several studies have evaluated the ability of intraplaque hemorrhage to detect future cerebrovascular ischemic events. Takaya and colleagues[86] prospectively followed 154 consecutive patients with asymptomatic moderate carotid stenosis for a mean period of 38.2 months at 3-month intervals. Among the 12 ischemic events that occurred during follow-up ipsilateral to the index carotid artery, two plaque characteristics at baseline showed a significant association with the future events: IPH (HR 5.2, $P = .005$) and larger mean intraplaque hemorrhage area (HR 2.6 for 10-mm² increase, $P = .006$). Kwee and colleagues[88] evaluated 126 TIA/stroke patients with 30% to 69% carotid stenosis using vessel wall MR imaging, and prospectively followed them for 1 year to determine the likelihood of recurrence and its relationship to plaque characteristics. The carotid stenosis grade (30%–49% vs 50%–69%) was not associated with recurrent events, whereas the presence of lipid-rich necrotic core (HR 3.2001, $P<.04$), thin/ruptured fibrous cap (HR 5.756, $P = .002$), and IPH (HR 3.542, $P = .04$) were significantly correlated with recurrence. Altaf and colleagues[41] prospectively followed 64 TIA or stroke patients with 30% to 69% carotid stenosis who had undergone a black-blood MR imaging examination for a median of 28 months after MR imaging. Sixty-one percent of patients had IPH on the ipsilateral side at baseline imaging. Fourteen stroke/TIA events occurred during follow-up, 13 of which manifested in a territory downstream from carotid plaque with IPH (HR 9.8, 95% CI 1.3–75.1; $P = .03$). The same group followed 66 symptomatic patients with high-grade carotid stenosis who underwent vessel wall MR imaging until endarterectomy or for 30 days, in whom IPH was found to significantly increase the likelihood of recurrent ischemic events (HR 4.8, 95% CI 1.1–20.9; $P<.05$).[82] These studies indicate the importance of IPH as a risk factor for future stroke events. Although carotid IPH can cause or be a result of plaque rupture, once it is detected on MR imaging it confers a poorer prognosis.

The interplay between IPH and angiogenesis is an area of investigational interest,[44,81,89–93] although their exact relationship is not yet clearly understood. One theory for the development of IPH is that it arises from leaky neovessels that grow into the plaque from the adventitial vasa vasorum.[91,93] Sluimer and colleagues[91] indicated that microvessel density was higher in advanced plaques than in early plaques. In early plaques and normal artery segments, the microvessel density was higher on the adventitial side than within the wall/plaque, whereas in advanced plaques the adventitial and intraplaque microvessel density were equivalent, suggesting inward growth of neovessels into the wall with plaque development. In autopsy evaluation, intraplaque neovessels were thin-walled with compromised endothelial integrity and basement membrane detachment, indicating increased wall permeability.[91] This supports the idea that these fragile vessels would be more likely to rupture. IPH may also develop first on the intimal surface secondary to fibrous cap fissuring or disruption,[94] and lead to intimal hypoxia and stimulate angiogenesis.[90] Autopsy studies evaluating IPH and angiogenesis have shown their coexistence within plaques.[81,89] McCarthy and colleagues[81] found a significantly higher density of neovessels within symptomatic carotid plaques in comparison with asymptomatic lesions ($P<.0001$). The neovessels within symptomatic plaques were also significantly larger and more irregular. IPH and fibrous cap rupture were significantly associated with neovessels within the plaque ($P<.017$, $P<.001$) and fibrous cap ($P<.046$, $P<.004$). Sun and colleagues[92] evaluated carotid atherosclerotic plaques with a multicontrast MR protocol and dynamic contrast-enhanced perfusion, and found a significant relationship between IPH and K^{trans}, indicating an increased endothelial surface area or increased permeability in the setting of intraplaque hemorrhage. Conversely, there was no significant difference in v_p (blood supply) between the IPH and non-IPH groups, indicating that the difference in K^{trans} reflects increased vasa vasorum ingrowth of capillaries and terminal arterioles. Qiao and colleagues[44] demonstrated carotid IPH (OR 10.18, $P = .03$) and extent of adventitial neovascularity as indicated by grade of adventitial enhancement (grade 0 none, grade 1 <50%, grade 2 $\geq$50%) (compared with grade 0: OR 14.9 for grade 1, OR 51.17 for grade 2; $P = .02$) to be independently associated with ischemic events.

The status of the fibrous cap assessed on MR imaging has proved to be an important characteristic of carotid plaque vulnerability. Yuan and colleagues[95] initially described the relationship between fibrous cap rupture and patient symptoms in a study where they scanned 53 consecutive patients scheduled for carotid endarterectomy, There was an increased likelihood of symptomatic than asymptomatic patients having ruptured caps (70% vs 9%, $P = .001$). Compared with patients with thick fibrous caps, those with ruptured caps were 23 times more likely to have had a recent cerebrovascular ischemic event. In the evaluation of 154 patients (52 symptomatic) with a carotid plaque measuring at least 3 mm on ultrasonography, Millon and colleagues[96] found a significantly higher occurrence of cap rupture in the symptomatic group (30% vs 9%; OR 2.8, $P = .001$). However, the difference between symptomatic and asymptomatic was only appreciated during the first 15 days after the ischemic event. In the longitudinal MR evaluation of asymptomatic patients with severe carotid stenosis, percent volume increase of lipid-rich necrotic core was found to be a significant predictor of future fibrous cap rupture (per 5% increase: OR 2.6, $P = .035$).[97]

HIGH-RESOLUTION MR IMAGING FOR THE EVALUATION OF LOW-GRADE CAROTID STENOSIS
Clinical Applications

In the setting of low-grade carotid stenosis, vessel wall MR imaging can have an immediate impact on assessing plaque volume, despite compensatory outer wall remodeling, and identifying plaque composition and vulnerable characteristics that can help predict rupture. Identification of carotid atherosclerotic lesions, even with little to no stenosis, can provide insight into atherosclerosis elsewhere in the body including the intracranial arteries and the aorta. Shimizu and colleagues[98] showed that increased carotid IMT measurements are associated with complex aortic atheromas that are more likely to lead to embolic events. In fact, complex descending thoracic aorta plaques are not an uncommon source for cryptogenic infarcts secondary to retrograde aortic flow.[99] Retrograde descending aortic flow from the vicinity of a complex atherosclerotic plaque reached the common carotid artery on time-resolved computational flow MR imaging in 24.5% of cases, with 24.3% of cases of cryptogenic stroke attributed to these downstream aortic plaques in a study of 94 acute stroke patients with descending aortic plaque as defined on transesophageal echo.

There has been a growing body of literature assessing carotid plaque characteristics in the setting of low-grade stenosis. Wang and colleagues[100] evaluated MR imaging features of plaque vulnerability in 114 symptomatic patients. Lipid-rich necrotic core was found in 86.7% of plaques with 30% to 49% stenosis and 45.1% of lesions with 0% to 29% narrowing. In addition, IPH and fibrous cap rupture was seen in 26.7% and 6.7% of plaques, respectively, with 30% to 49% stenosis. There was a significant association between cerebral infarct volume and lipid-rich necrotic core volume ($P<.04$), and a marginal association between infarct volume and wall thickness percentage ($P = .05$) after adjusting for carotid luminal stenosis. Saam and colleagues[101] found that 21.7% of carotid arteries with 16% to 49% stenosis and 8.1% of arteries with 0% to 15% stenosis will have complicating features on ultrasonography including IPH, fibrous cap rupture, and calcified nodules. Dong and colleagues[102] indicated an 8.7% and 4.3% incidence of IPH and surface disruption, respectively, in carotid arteries with 0% stenosis. In low-grade stenosis (<50%), there is a significantly increased prevalence of vulnerable plaque characteristics in males compared with females, including ruptured/thinned fibrous cap, IPH, AHA type VI plaques, and significantly larger lipid-rich necrotic core volumes.[103] In a separate study evaluating 181 patients, Zhao and colleagues[104] found a 4.4% prevalence of IPH in patients with 0% stenosis. These studies indicate that plaques associated with low-grade carotid stenosis can and will have vulnerable plaque features that confer an increased risk of subsequent growth and rupture that could lead to stroke.

Associations of Low-Grade Carotid Stenosis with Systemic Atherosclerosis

Atherosclerosis is a systemic process that is known to involve multiple arterial beds simultaneously. Considering that specific vulnerable plaque characteristics can increase the likelihood of plaque rupture, this, in addition to systemic features, can confer an increased likelihood of symptoms. As atherosclerosis is a chronic, systemic, inflammatory disease, there is the potential for multisystemic plaque-rupture complications such as myocardial, renal, cerebral, and mesenteric infarctions, in addition to hypoperfusion complications proceeding in the same individual.[105]

The relationship of carotid IMT on ultrasonography and severity of coronary artery disease (CAD) has also been a topic of investigation. Graner and colleagues[106] examined the association of carotid IMT on B-mode ultrasonography and the severity and extent of CAD on angiography in 108 patients with known or suspected CAD. Maximum and mean IMT were significantly correlated with CAD severity ($P = .004$ and $P = .005$, respectively), extent ($P = .022$ and $P = .016$, respectively), and atheroma burden ($P = .008$ for both). Carotid IMT was associated with disease extent in the mid and distal coronary segments, but not in proximal segments. In 558 consecutive patients who underwent carotid ultrasonography and coronary angiography, there was a significant correlation between mean IMT and advancing CAD ($P<.0001$), with a significant increase in carotid IMT in patients with 1-, 2-, and 3-vessel CAD.[107] The investigators found that with a mean IMT greater than 1.15 mm, there was a 94% probability of having CAD, with 65% sensitivity and 80% specificity in high-risk CAD patients. Whereas 16.6% of patients with 3-vessel CAD had severe stenosis of the carotid, subclavian, or vertebral arteries, none of the patients with normal coronary arteries had severe extracranial arterial stenoses. In 224 patients, Lekakis and colleagues[108] also found common carotid artery ($P = .015$) and carotid bulb ($P = .04$) IMT to be independent predictors of CAD extent.

The clinical usefulness of carotid IMT assessment on ultrasonography and its added predictive risk beyond atherosclerosis risk factors identified by the Framingham Risk Score has recently come under challenge.[109–111] A meta-analysis collating data from 14 population-based cohorts (45,828 participants) indicated that for every 0.1-mm increase in the common carotid IMT, the HR of first-time myocardial infarction or stroke was 1.09 (95% CI 1.07–1.12),[109] with minor improvement in prediction when added to the Framingham Risk Score. This finding suggests that current evidence does not support the routine use of carotid IMT in the general population to screen for cardiovascular disease because the added value is too small to result in health benefits. Carotid IMT has typically been measured in the common carotid artery because it is easily visualized perpendicular to the ultrasound beam and provides more accurate, reproducible, and quantitative measurements[112]; however, the appropriateness of carotid IMT as a marker of atherosclerosis has been questioned because the main determinants of medial hypertrophy of the common carotid artery are age and hypertension, which do not necessarily reflect atherosclerotic plaque formation. Atherosclerosis of the carotid arteries typically first develops in the carotid bulb, and rarely occurs in the common carotid artery except in advanced disease.[113] A meta-analysis of 11 population-based studies (54,336 patients) found that the presence of carotid bulb plaque on ultrasonography in comparison with common carotid IMT had a significantly higher diagnostic accuracy for the prediction of future myocardial infarction.[114] IMT measurement in the carotid bulb was found to be a significantly stronger predictor of cardiovascular events than IMT measurements in the common carotid artery; however, the presence of carotid plaque was a significantly stronger predictor than IMT measurement at either site.[114]

Considering that atherosclerosis is a chronic, systemic inflammatory process and that plaque develops multifocally and simultaneously, it would stand to reason that similar vulnerable plaque features might be found in plaques in various arterial beds. Zhao and colleagues[115] evaluated the association between coronary plaque characteristics on CT angiography and carotid plaque morphology on vessel wall MR imaging in 123 suspected CAD patients who underwent both examinations. Coronary plaques were identified as calcified, mixed, and noncalcified, and carotid plaques were evaluated for the presence of IPH, lipid-rich necrotic core, and calcification. There was a significant correlation between the presence of a mixed coronary plaque and carotid IPH (OR 1.5, P<.05). In addition, the mixed coronary plaque had the highest likelihood of predicting carotid IPH (area under the curve = 0.74). This result led the investigators to conclude that mixed calcified and noncalcified coronary plaques may indicate the presence of vulnerable carotid plaques, given their association with carotid IPH. In a separate

article, Zhao and colleagues[116] indicated that 98.2% and 28.6% of patients with less than 50% coronary artery stenosis had carotid atherosclerotic disease with a lipid-rich necrotic core and IPH, respectively. Underhill and colleagues[117] compared carotid plaque morphologic characteristics between 97 patients with obstructive CAD (≥50% stenosis on coronary angiogram) and 94 with normal coronary angiograms (controls). In male CAD patients compared with male controls, there was a significantly smaller lumen area (P<.001 and P = .006, respectively) and smaller total vessel area (P<.001 and P = .04, respectively) in the distal carotid bulb and internal carotid artery. For the distal bulb, there was also a significantly larger mean wall thickness (P = .002). There was no significant difference in plaque characteristics for females at any arterial segment, and no significant difference in the common carotid arteries for males. The presence of extracranial carotid artery atherosclerosis was significantly associated with incidence and progression of coronary artery calcification in a prospective cohort study of 5445 subjects.[118]

Extracranial carotid arteries are amenable to cross-sectional imaging, in particular MR imaging, considering their large size, linear anatomy, superficial location, and relative immobility; this is in contradistinction to the coronary arteries, which are very difficult to image because of their small size, cardiac and respiratory motion, and tortuous courses. For these reasons and considering the propensity of coronary plaques to outwardly remodel, thus limiting the ability to estimate plaque burden on luminal imaging, cross-sectional carotid plaque composition evaluation using MR imaging or ultrasonography may be a useful way to predict the presence and risk of CAD noninvasively.

LIMITATIONS OF MR IMAGING OF THE CAROTID ARTERIES

The clinical applicability of MR imaging of plaque must be considered in light of several limitations of this modality. The resolution of MR imaging is limited by the available signal of the tissue of interest. Dedicated carotid surface coils and higher-field MR imaging scanners, however, can provide a substantially improved signal. MR imaging examinations are typically more expensive, and MR imaging has limited accessibility in comparison with other cross-sectional imaging modalities, and for these reasons MR imaging likely cannot serve as a first-line screening tool for asymptomatic carotid atherosclerotic disease. MR imaging suffers from longer scan times, and for this reason is susceptible to motion artifacts.[119] Safety concerns also must be considered with MR imaging scanners, especially contraindications to magnetic-field exposure. Such concerns include metallic foreign bodies in the orbit or near vital structures, cochlear implants, and pacemakers. Local heating with skin burns can occur from certain medicine patches, tattoos, or permanent cosmetics. More commonly, claustrophobia poses a relative contraindication, although most patients are able to tolerate the examination with sedation or by using an open or wide-bore system. There has been recent concern with administration of gadolinium-based MR imaging contrast agents and evidence of intracranial tissue deposition, although the long-term significance of this is still unknown.[120–123]

SUMMARY

MR imaging has emerged as a tool capable of uncovering and characterizing atherosclerotic plaque before it has a hemodynamic effect on the lumen, allowing a means to study plaque characteristics associated with risk for rupture. Identifying and characterizing lesions that have gone unrecognized by angiography forces clinicians reconsider the guidelines for managing low-grade carotid stenosis. At present, MR imaging offers a tool that can identify the culprit lesion, a particular challenge with low-grade disease, creating management decisions not previously faced. Considering that atherosclerosis is a systemic disease, MR imaging can allow determination of the presence of disease within other parts of the cardiovascular system. Ultimately, understanding the nature of atherosclerosis formation in the extracranial carotid artery may allow clinicians to identify the vulnerable patient in whom systemic intervention could be initiated to prevent cardiovascular events.

REFERENCES

1. Standish BA, Spears J, Marotta TR, et al. Vascular wall imaging of vulnerable atherosclerotic carotid plaques: current state of the art and potential future of endovascular optical coherence tomography. AJNR Am J Neuroradiol 2012;33:1642–50.
2. Randomised trial of endarterectomy for recently symptomatic carotid stenosis: final results of the MRC European Carotid Surgery Trial (ECST). Lancet 1998;351:1379–87.
3. North American Symptomatic Carotid Endarterectomy Trial Collaborators. Beneficial effect of carotid endarterectomy in symptomatic patients with high-grade carotid stenosis. N Engl J Med 1991;325:445–53.
4. Rothwell PM, Eliasziw M, Gutnikov SA, et al. Analysis of pooled data from the randomised controlled trials of endarterectomy for symptomatic carotid stenosis. Lancet 2003;361:107–16.
5. Falk E, Shah PK, Fuster V. Coronary plaque disruption. Circulation 1995;92:657–71.
6. Fuster V, Badimon L, Badimon JJ, et al. The pathogenesis of coronary artery disease and the acute coronary syndromes (1). N Engl J Med 1992;326:242–50.
7. Fuster V, Badimon L, Badimon JJ, et al. The pathogenesis of coronary artery disease and the acute coronary syndromes (2). N Engl J Med 1992;326:310–8.
8. Grubb RL Jr, Derdeyn CP, Fritsch SM, et al. Importance of hemodynamic factors in the prognosis of symptomatic carotid occlusion. JAMA 1998;280:1055–60.
9. Powers WJ. Cerebral hemodynamics in ischemic cerebrovascular disease. Ann Neurol 1991;29:231–40.
10. Lovett JK, Gallagher PJ, Hands LJ, et al. Histological correlates of carotid plaque surface morphology on lumen contrast imaging. Circulation 2004;110:2190–7.
11. Redgrave JN, Lovett JK, Gallagher PJ, et al. Histological assessment of 526 symptomatic carotid plaques in relation to the nature and timing of ischemic symptoms: the Oxford plaque study. Circulation 2006;113:2320–8.
12. Spagnoli LG, Mauriello A, Sangiorgi G, et al. Extracranial thrombotically active carotid plaque as a risk factor for ischemic stroke. JAMA 2004;292:1845–52.
13. Barnett HJ, Taylor DW, Eliasziw M, et al. Benefit of carotid endarterectomy in patients with symptomatic moderate or severe stenosis. North American Symptomatic Carotid Endarterectomy Trial Collaborators. N Engl J Med 1998;339:1415–25.
14. Rothwell PM, Gutnikov SA, Warlow CP, et al. Reanalysis of the final results of the European Carotid Surgery Trial. Stroke 2003;34:514–23.
15. Wasserman BA, Wityk RJ, Trout HH 3rd, et al. Low-grade carotid stenosis: looking beyond the lumen with MRI. Stroke 2005;36:2504–13.
16. Fritz VU, Levien LJ. Therapy for isolated, low and high grade symptomatic carotid artery stenosis. Ann Vasc Surg 1988;2:367–72.
17. O'Leary DH, Polak JF, Kronmal RA, et al. Distribution and correlates of sonographically detected carotid artery disease in the Cardiovascular Health Study. The CHS Collaborative Research Group. Stroke 1992;23:1752–60.
18. Amarenco P, Bogousslavsky J, Callahan A 3rd, et al. High-dose atorvastatin after stroke or transient ischemic attack. N Engl J Med 2006;355:549–59.

19. Sillesen H, Amarenco P, Hennerici MG, et al. Atorvastatin reduces the risk of cardiovascular events in patients with carotid atherosclerosis: a secondary analysis of the Stroke Prevention by Aggressive Reduction in Cholesterol Levels (SPARCL) trial. Stroke 2008;39:3297–302.

20. Heart Protection Study Collaborative Group. MRC/BHF Heart Protection Study of cholesterol lowering with simvastatin in 20,536 high-risk individuals: a randomised placebo-controlled trial. Lancet 2002; 360:7–22.

21. Hegland O, Dickstein K, Larsen JP. Effect of simvastatin in preventing progression of carotid artery stenosis. Am J Cardiol 2001;87:643–5. A610.

22. Amarenco P, Labreuche J, Lavallee P, et al. Statins in stroke prevention and carotid atherosclerosis: systematic review and up-to-date meta-analysis. Stroke 2004;35:2902–9.

23. Ambrose JA, Tannenbaum MA, Alexopoulos D, et al. Angiographic progression of coronary artery disease and the development of myocardial infarction. J Am Coll Cardiol 1988;12:56–62.

24. Fuster V, Stein B, Ambrose JA, et al. Atherosclerotic plaque rupture and thrombosis. Evolving concepts. Circulation 1990;82:II47–59.

25. Little WC, Constantinescu M, Applegate RJ, et al. Can coronary angiography predict the site of a subsequent myocardial infarction in patients with mild-to-moderate coronary artery disease? Circulation 1988;78:1157–66.

26. Libby P. The interface of atherosclerosis and thrombosis: basic mechanisms. Vasc Med 1998;3:225–9.

27. Lovett JK, Gallagher PJ, Rothwell PM. Reproducibility of histological assessment of carotid plaque: implications for studies of carotid imaging. Cerebrovasc Dis 2004;18:117–23.

28. Libby P. Inflammation in atherosclerosis. Nature 2002;420:868–74.

29. Virmani R, Ladich ER, Burke AP, et al. Histopathology of carotid atherosclerotic disease. Neurosurgery 2006;59:S219–27 [discussion: S3–13].

30. Fayad ZA, Mani V, Woodward M, et al. Safety and efficacy of dalcetrapib on atherosclerotic disease using novel non-invasive multimodality imaging (dal-PLAQUE): a randomised clinical trial. Lancet 2011;378:1547–59.

31. Lei-xing X, Jing-jing G, Jing-xue N, et al. Combined application of 18F-fluorodeoxyglucose positron emission tomography/computed tomography and magnetic resonance imaging in early diagnosis of vulnerable carotid atherosclerotic plaques. J Int Med Res 2014;42:213–23.

32. Mani V, Woodward M, Samber D, et al. Predictors of change in carotid atherosclerotic plaque inflammation and burden as measured by 18-FDG-PET and MRI, respectively, in the dal-PLAQUE study. Int J Cardiovasc Imaging 2014;30:571–82.

33. Silvera SS, Aidi HE, Rudd JH, et al. Multimodality imaging of atherosclerotic plaque activity and composition using FDG-PET/CT and MRI in carotid and femoral arteries. Atherosclerosis 2009;207: 139–43.

34. Glagov S, Weisenberg E, Zarins CK, et al. Compensatory enlargement of human atherosclerotic coronary arteries. N Engl J Med 1987;316: 1371–5.

35. Benes V, Netuka D, Mandys V, et al. Comparison between degree of carotid stenosis observed at angiography and in histological examination. Acta Neurochir 2004;146:671–7.

36. Fishbein MC, Siegel RJ. How big are coronary atherosclerotic plaques that rupture? Circulation 1996;94:2662–6.

37. Inzitari D, Eliasziw M, Gates P, et al. The causes and risk of stroke in patients with asymptomatic internal-carotid-artery stenosis. North American Symptomatic Carotid Endarterectomy Trial Collaborators. N Engl J Med 2000;342:1693–700.

38. Dennis M, Bamford J, Sandercock P, et al. Prognosis of transient ischemic attacks in the Oxfordshire Community Stroke Project. Stroke 1990;21: 848–53.

39. Freilinger TM, Schindler A, Schmidt C, et al. Prevalence of nonstenosing, complicated atherosclerotic plaques in cryptogenic stroke. JACC Cardiovasc Imaging 2012;5:397–405.

40. Cheung HM, Moody AR, Singh N, et al. Late stage complicated atheroma in low-grade stenotic carotid disease: MR imaging depiction—prevalence and risk factors. Radiology 2011;260:841–7.

41. Altaf N, Daniels L, Morgan PS, et al. Detection of intraplaque hemorrhage by magnetic resonance imaging in symptomatic patients with mild to moderate carotid stenosis predicts recurrent neurological events. J Vasc Surg 2008;47:337–42.

42. Yoshida K, Sadamasa N, Narumi O, et al. Symptomatic low-grade carotid stenosis with intraplaque hemorrhage and expansive arterial remodeling is associated with a high relapse rate refractory to medical treatment. Neurosurgery 2012;70: 1143–50 [discussion: 1150–1].

43. Weinstein R. Noninvasive carotid duplex ultrasound imaging for the evaluation and management of carotid atherosclerotic disease. Hematol Oncol Clin North Am 1992;6:1131–9.

44. Qiao Y, Etesami M, Astor BC, et al. Carotid plaque neovascularization and hemorrhage detected by MR imaging are associated with recent cerebrovascular ischemic events. AJNR Am J Neuroradiol 2012;33:755–60.

45. Bayer-Karpinska A, Schwarz F, Wollenweber FA, et al. The carotid plaque imaging in acute stroke (CAPIAS) study: protocol and initial baseline data. BMC Neurol 2013;13:201.

46. Eliasziw M, Streifler JY, Fox AJ, et al. Significance of plaque ulceration in symptomatic patients with high-grade carotid stenosis. North American Symptomatic Carotid Endarterectomy Trial. Stroke 1994;25:304–8.

47. Kuk M, Wannarong T, Beletsky V, et al. Volume of carotid artery ulceration as a predictor of cardiovascular events. Stroke 2014;45:1437–41.

48. Madani A, Beletsky V, Tamayo A, et al. High-risk asymptomatic carotid stenosis: ulceration on 3D ultrasound vs TCD microemboli. Neurology 2011; 77:744–50.

49. Rothwell PM, Gibson R, Warlow CP. Interrelation between plaque surface morphology and degree of stenosis on carotid angiograms and the risk of ischemic stroke in patients with symptomatic carotid stenosis. On behalf of the European Carotid Surgery Trialists' Collaborative Group. Stroke 2000;31:615–21.

50. Streifler JY, Eliasziw M, Fox AJ, et al. Angiographic detection of carotid plaque ulceration. Comparison with surgical observations in a multicenter study. North American Symptomatic Carotid Endarterectomy Trial. Stroke 1994;25:1130–2.

51. Etesami M, Hoi Y, Steinman DA, et al. Comparison of carotid plaque ulcer detection using contrast-enhanced and time-of-flight MRA techniques. AJNR Am J Neuroradiol 2013;34:177–84.

52. Zhao H, Wang J, Liu X, et al. Assessment of carotid artery atherosclerotic disease by using three-dimensional fast black-blood MR imaging: comparison with DSA. Radiology 2015;274:508–16.

53. Virmani R, Kolodgie FD, Burke AP, et al. Lessons from sudden coronary death: a comprehensive morphological classification scheme for atherosclerotic lesions. Arterioscler Thromb Vasc Biol 2000;20:1262–75.

54. Davies MJ. Anatomic features in victims of sudden coronary death. Coronary artery pathology. Circulation 1992;85:I19–24.

55. Barger AC, Beeuwkes R 3rd, Lainey LL, et al. Hypothesis: vasa vasorum and neovascularization of human coronary arteries. A possible role in the pathophysiology of atherosclerosis. N Engl J Med 1984;310:175–7.

56. Carr S, Farb A, Pearce WH, et al. Atherosclerotic plaque rupture in symptomatic carotid artery stenosis. J Vasc Surg 1996;23:755–65 [discussion: 765–6].

57. McCarthy MJ, Loftus IM, Thompson MM, et al. Vascular surgical society of great britain and ireland: angiogenesis and the atherosclerotic carotid plaque: association between symptomatology and plaque morphology. Br J Surg 1999;86:707–8.

58. Burke AP, Kolodgie FD, Farb A, et al. Healed plaque ruptures and sudden coronary death: evidence that subclinical rupture has a role in plaque progression. Circulation 2001;103:934–40.

59. Mann J, Davies MJ. Mechanisms of progression in native coronary artery disease: role of healed plaque disruption. Heart 1999;82:265–8.

60. Farb A, Burke AP, Tang AL, et al. Coronary plaque erosion without rupture into a lipid core. A frequent cause of coronary thrombosis in sudden coronary death. Circulation 1996;93:1354–63.

61. Gronholdt ML, Wiebe BM, Laursen H, et al. Lipid-rich carotid artery plaques appear echolucent on ultrasound B-mode images and may be associated with intraplaque haemorrhage. Eur J Vasc Endovasc Surg 1997;14:439–45.

62. Schminke U, Motsch L, Hilker L, et al. Three-dimensional ultrasound observation of carotid artery plaque ulceration. Stroke 2000;31:1651–5.

63. de Weert TT, Cretier S, Groen HC, et al. Atherosclerotic plaque surface morphology in the carotid bifurcation assessed with multidetector computed tomography angiography. Stroke 2009;40:1334–40.

64. Wintermark M, Jawadi SS, Rapp JH, et al. High-resolution CT imaging of carotid artery atherosclerotic plaques. AJNR Am J Neuroradiol 2008;29: 875–82.

65. Saba L, Argiolas GM, Siotto P, et al. Carotid artery plaque characterization using CT multienergy imaging. AJNR Am J Neuroradiol 2013;34:855–9.

66. Saba L, Lai ML, Montisci R, et al. Association between carotid plaque enhancement shown by multidetector CT angiography and histologically validated microvessel density. Eur Radiol 2012; 22:2237–45.

67. Saba L, Piga M, Raz E, et al. Carotid artery plaque classification: does contrast enhancement play a significant role? AJNR Am J Neuroradiol 2012;33: 1814–7.

68. Grimm JM, Schindler A, Schwarz F, et al. Computed tomography angiography vs 3 T black-blood cardiovascular magnetic resonance for identification of symptomatic carotid plaques. J Cardiovasc Magn Reson 2014;16:84.

69. Clarke SE, Hammond RR, Mitchell JR, et al. Quantitative assessment of carotid plaque composition using multicontrast MRI and registered histology. Magn Reson Med 2003;50:1199–208.

70. Cai JM, Hatsukami TS, Ferguson MS, et al. Classification of human carotid atherosclerotic lesions with in vivo multicontrast magnetic resonance imaging. Circulation 2002;106:1368–73.

71. Cappendijk VC, Cleutjens KB, Kessels AG, et al. Assessment of human atherosclerotic carotid plaque components with multisequence MR imaging: initial experience. Radiology 2005;234: 487–92.

72. Puppini G, Furlan F, Cirota N, et al. Characterisation of carotid atherosclerotic plaque: comparison between magnetic resonance imaging and histology. Radiol Med 2006;111:921–30.

73. Saam T, Ferguson MS, Yarnykh VL, et al. Quantitative evaluation of carotid plaque composition by in vivo MRI. Arterioscler Thromb Vasc Biol 2005;25:234–9.

74. Albuquerque LC, Narvaes LB, Maciel AA, et al. Intraplaque hemorrhage assessed by high-resolution magnetic resonance imaging and C-reactive protein in carotid atherosclerosis. J Vasc Surg 2007;46:1130–7.

75. Hatsukami TS, Ross R, Polissar NL, et al. Visualization of fibrous cap thickness and rupture in human atherosclerotic carotid plaque in vivo with high-resolution magnetic resonance imaging. Circulation 2000;102:959–64.

76. Mitsumori LM, Hatsukami TS, Ferguson MS, et al. In vivo accuracy of multisequence MR imaging for identifying unstable fibrous caps in advanced human carotid plaques. J Magn Reson Imaging 2003;17:410–20.

77. Trivedi RA, U-King-Im JM, Graves MJ, et al. MRI-derived measurements of fibrous-cap and lipid-core thickness: the potential for identifying vulnerable carotid plaques in vivo. Neuroradiology 2004;46:738–43.

78. Wasserman BA, Casal SG, Astor BC, et al. Wash-in kinetics for gadolinium-enhanced magnetic resonance imaging of carotid atheroma. J Magn Reson Imaging 2005;21:91–5.

79. Wasserman BA, Smith WI, Trout HH 3rd, et al. Carotid artery atherosclerosis: in vivo morphologic characterization with gadolinium-enhanced double-oblique MR imaging initial results. Radiology 2002;223:566–73.

80. Kerwin W, Hooker A, Spilker M, et al. Quantitative magnetic resonance imaging analysis of neovasculature volume in carotid atherosclerotic plaque. Circulation 2003;107:851–6.

81. McCarthy MJ, Loftus IM, Thompson MM, et al. Angiogenesis and the atherosclerotic carotid plaque: an association between symptomatology and plaque morphology. J Vasc Surg 1999;30:261–8.

82. Altaf N, MacSweeney ST, Gladman J, et al. Carotid intraplaque hemorrhage predicts recurrent symptoms in patients with high-grade carotid stenosis. Stroke 2007;38:1633–5.

83. Singh N, Moody AR, Gladstone DJ, et al. Moderate carotid artery stenosis: MR imaging-depicted intraplaque hemorrhage predicts risk of cerebrovascular ischemic events in asymptomatic men. Radiology 2009;252:502–8.

84. Sun J, Underhill HR, Hippe DS, et al. Sustained acceleration in carotid atherosclerotic plaque progression with intraplaque hemorrhage: a long-term time course study. JACC Cardiovasc Imaging 2012;5:798–804.

85. Takaya N, Yuan C, Chu B, et al. Presence of intraplaque hemorrhage stimulates progression of carotid atherosclerotic plaques: a high-resolution magnetic resonance imaging study. Circulation 2005;111:2768–75.

86. Takaya N, Yuan C, Chu B, et al. Association between carotid plaque characteristics and subsequent ischemic cerebrovascular events: a prospective assessment with MRI—initial results. Stroke 2006;37:818–23.

87. Underhill HR, Yuan C, Yarnykh VL, et al. Arterial remodeling in [corrected] subclinical carotid artery disease. JACC Cardiovasc Imaging 2009;2:1381–9.

88. Kwee RM, van Oostenbrugge RJ, Mess WH, et al. MRI of carotid atherosclerosis to identify TIA and stroke patients who are at risk of a recurrence. J Magn Reson Imaging 2013;37:1189–94.

89. Gossl M, Versari D, Hildebrandt HA, et al. Segmental heterogeneity of vasa vasorum neovascularization in human coronary atherosclerosis. JACC Cardiovasc Imaging 2010;3:32–40.

90. Nagy E, Eaton JW, Jeney V, et al. Red cells, hemoglobin, heme, iron, and atherogenesis. Arterioscler Thromb Vasc Biol 2010;30:1347–53.

91. Sluimer JC, Kolodgie FD, Bijnens AP, et al. Thin-walled microvessels in human coronary atherosclerotic plaques show incomplete endothelial junctions relevance of compromised structural integrity for intraplaque microvascular leakage. J Am Coll Cardiol 2009;53:1517–27.

92. Sun J, Song Y, Chen H, et al. Adventitial perfusion and intraplaque hemorrhage: a dynamic contrast-enhanced MRI study in the carotid artery. Stroke 2013;44:1031–6.

93. Virmani R, Kolodgie FD, Burke AP, et al. Atherosclerotic plaque progression and vulnerability to rupture: angiogenesis as a source of intraplaque hemorrhage. Arterioscler Thromb Vasc Biol 2005;25:2054–61.

94. Stary HC, Chandler AB, Dinsmore RE, et al. A definition of advanced types of atherosclerotic lesions and a histological classification of atherosclerosis. A report from the Committee on Vascular Lesions of the Council on Arteriosclerosis, American Heart Association. Circulation 1995;92:1355–74.

95. Yuan C, Zhang SX, Polissar NL, et al. Identification of fibrous cap rupture with magnetic resonance imaging is highly associated with recent transient ischemic attack or stroke. Circulation 2002;105:181–5.

96. Millon A, Mathevet JL, Boussel L, et al. High-resolution magnetic resonance imaging of carotid atherosclerosis identifies vulnerable carotid plaques. J Vasc Surg 2013;57:1046–51.e2.

97. Underhill HR, Yuan C, Yarnykh VL, et al. Predictors of surface disruption with MR imaging in

asymptomatic carotid artery stenosis. AJNR Am J Neuroradiol 2010;31:487–93.

98. Shimizu Y, Kitagawa K, Nagai Y, et al. Carotid atherosclerosis as a risk factor for complex aortic lesions in patients with ischemic cerebrovascular disease. Circ J 2003;67:597–600.

99. Harloff A, Simon J, Brendecke S, et al. Complex plaques in the proximal descending aorta: an underestimated embolic source of stroke. Stroke 2010;41:1145–50.

100. Wang J, Bornert P, Zhao H, et al. Simultaneous noncontrast angiography and intraplaque hemorrhage (SNAP) imaging for carotid atherosclerotic disease evaluation. Magn Reson Med 2013;69: 337–45.

101. Saam T, Underhill HR, Chu B, et al. Prevalence of American Heart Association type VI carotid atherosclerotic lesions identified by magnetic resonance imaging for different levels of stenosis as measured by duplex ultrasound. J Am Coll Cardiol 2008;51: 1014–21.

102. Dong L, Underhill HR, Yu W, et al. Geometric and compositional appearance of atheroma in an angiographically normal carotid artery in patients with atherosclerosis. AJNR Am J Neuroradiol 2010;31:311–6.

103. Ota H, Reeves MJ, Zhu DC, et al. Sex differences of high-risk carotid atherosclerotic plaque with less than 50% stenosis in asymptomatic patients: an in vivo 3T MRI study. AJNR Am J Neuroradiol 2013;34:1049–55. S1041.

104. Zhao X, Underhill HR, Zhao Q, et al. Discriminating carotid atherosclerotic lesion severity by luminal stenosis and plaque burden: a comparison utilizing high-resolution magnetic resonance imaging at 3.0 Tesla. Stroke 2011;42:347–53.

105. Naghavi M, Libby P, Falk E, et al. From vulnerable plaque to vulnerable patient: a call for new definitions and risk assessment strategies: part I. Circulation 2003;108:1664–72.

106. Graner M, Varpula M, Kahri J, et al. Association of carotid intima-media thickness with angiographic severity and extent of coronary artery disease. Am J Cardiol 2006;97:624–9.

107. Kablak-Ziembicka A, Tracz W, Przewlocki T, et al. Association of increased carotid intima-media thickness with the extent of coronary artery disease. Heart 2004;90:1286–90.

108. Lekakis JP, Papamichael CM, Cimponeriu AT, et al. Atherosclerotic changes of extracoronary arteries are associated with the extent of coronary atherosclerosis. Am J Cardiol 2000;85: 949–52.

109. Den Ruijter HM, Peters SA, Anderson TJ, et al. Common carotid intima-media thickness measurements in cardiovascular risk prediction: a meta-analysis. JAMA 2012;308:796–803.

110. Helfand M, Buckley DI, Freeman M, et al. Emerging risk factors for coronary heart disease: a summary of systematic reviews conducted for the U.S. Preventive Services Task Force. Ann Intern Med 2009;151:496–507.

111. van den Oord SC, Sijbrands EJ, ten Kate GL, et al. Carotid intima-media thickness for cardiovascular risk assessment: systematic review and meta-analysis. Atherosclerosis 2013; 228:1–11.

112. Touboul PJ, Hennerici MG, Meairs S, et al. Mannheim carotid intima-media thickness consensus (2004-2006). An update on behalf of the Advisory Board of the 3rd and 4th Watching the Risk Symposium, 13th and 15th European Stroke Conferences, Mannheim, Germany, 2004, and Brussels, Belgium, 2006. Cerebrovasc Dis 2007;23:75–80.

113. O'Leary DH, Bots ML. Imaging of atherosclerosis: carotid intima-media thickness. Eur Heart J 2010; 31:1682–9.

114. Inaba Y, Chen JA, Bergmann SR. Carotid plaque, compared with carotid intima-media thickness, more accurately predicts coronary artery disease events: a meta-analysis. Atherosclerosis 2012; 220:128–33.

115. Zhao Q, Zhao X, Cai Z, et al. Correlation of coronary plaque phenotype and carotid atherosclerotic plaque composition. Am J Med Sci 2011;342:480–5.

116. Zhao X, Zhao Q, Chu B, et al. Prevalence of compositional features in subclinical carotid atherosclerosis determined by high-resolution magnetic resonance imaging in chinese patients with coronary artery disease. Stroke 2010;41: 1157–62.

117. Underhill HR, Yuan C, Terry JG, et al. Differences in carotid arterial morphology and composition between individuals with and without obstructive coronary artery disease: a cardiovascular magnetic resonance study. J Cardiovasc Magn Reson 2008;10:31.

118. Polak JF, Tracy R, Harrington A, et al. Carotid artery plaque and progression of coronary artery calcium: the multi-ethnic study of atherosclerosis. J Am Soc Echocardiogr 2013;26: 548–55.

119. Andre JB, Bresnahan BW, Mossa-Basha M, et al. Towards quantifying the prevalence, severity, and cost associated with patient motion during clinical MR examinations. J Am Coll Radiol 2015;12(7): 689–95.

120. Kanda T, Osawa M, Oba H, et al. High signal intensity in dentate nucleus on unenhanced T1-weighted MR images: association with linear versus macrocyclic gadolinium chelate administration. Radiology 2015;275:803–9.

121. McDonald RJ, McDonald JS, Kallmes DF, et al. Intracranial gadolinium deposition after contrast-enhanced MR imaging. Radiology 2015; 275:772–82.

122. Radbruch A, Weberling LD, Kieslich PJ, et al. Gadolinium retention in the dentate nucleus and globus pallidus is dependent on the class of contrast agent. Radiology 2015;275: 783–91.

123. Ramalho J, Castillo M, AlObaidy M, et al. High signal intensity in globus pallidus and dentate nucleus on unenhanced T1-weighted MR images: evaluation of two linear gadolinium-based contrast agents. Radiology 2015;276(3):836–44.

Unusual Cerebral Emboli

Nader Zakhari, MD, FRCPC[a,b], Mauricio Castillo, MD[c],
Carlos Torres, MD, FRCPC[d,e],*

KEYWORDS

- Cerebral embolism • Fat embolism • Air embolism • Septic emboli • Paradoxic embolism
- Myxoma

KEY POINTS

- A multiplicity of acute small infarcts in different vascular territories is a common manifestation of cerebral embolism.
- Diffuse white matter blooming foci on T2* MR imaging are considered a pathognomonic imaging pattern of cerebral fat embolism in the setting of bone fractures.
- Calcified cerebral embolism carries a high risk of recurrent embolic events in almost one-half of the patients.
- Using thin-slice thickness and window settings adjustment may improve visualization of cerebral air emboli on noncontrast computed tomography.
- Microbleeds are the most common asymptomatic manifestation of cerebral septic embolism in infective endocarditis.

INTRODUCTION

The heart and the carotid arteries are the most common sites of origin of embolic disease to the brain. These emboli consist mainly of red blood cells, platelets, and fibrin.[1] However, there are other less common cerebral emboli with different composition, including air, fat, calcium, and tumor cells. Some of these emboli could have a different site of origin, including the venous system. Although infarcts can be the final result of any type of embolism, here are described the ancillary and sometimes unique imaging features of less common types of cerebral emboli that may allow for a specific diagnosis to be made or at least suspected in many patients.

General Features of Cerebral Emboli

Emboli travel distally through progressively narrower arteries before lodging where the blood vessel becomes too small for further progression, especially at branching points.[2] Chung and colleagues[3] have shown that large emboli strongly favor the middle cerebral artery (MCA), while smaller emboli are carried proportionally to flow volume in the MCA and anterior cerebral artery (ACA) territories.

Emboli lodging in the proximal intracranial arteries result in territorial cortical infarcts, whereas smaller emboli lodging distally in terminal cortical branches result in small wedge-shaped peripheral infarcts centered at the gray-white matter

Disclosure: The authors have nothing to disclose.
[a] Department of Radiology, University of Ottawa, Ottawa, Ontario, Canada; [b] Department of Medical Imaging, The Ottawa Hospital, 1053 Carling Avenue, Ottawa, Ontario K1Y 4E9, Canada; [c] Division of Neuroradiology, Department of Radiology, University of North Carolina School of Medicine, Chapel Hill, Room 3326 Old Infirmary Building, Manning Drive, Chapel Hill, NC 27599-7510, USA; [d] Neuroradiology, Department of Radiology, University of Ottawa, Ottawa, Ontario, Canada; [e] Department of Medical Imaging, Ottawa Hospital Research Institute (OHRI), The Ottawa Hospital, Civic Campus, 1053 Carling Avenue, Ottawa, Ontario K1Y 4E9, Canada
* Corresponding author. Department of Medical Imaging, Ottawa Hospital Research Institute (OHRI), The Ottawa Hospital, Civic Campus, 1053 Carling Avenue, Ottawa, Ontario K1Y 4E9, Canada.
E-mail address: catorres@toh.on.ca

Neuroimag Clin N Am 26 (2016) 147–163
http://dx.doi.org/10.1016/j.nic.2015.09.013
1052-5149/16/$ – see front matter © 2016 Elsevier Inc. All rights reserved.

interface.[4] Uncommonly, embolic lacunar infarcts may occur in conditions causing massive showers of emboli. Overall, emboli are more likely to travel toward the leptomeningeal arteries rather than to the small perforators due to the smaller caliber and sharp angles of the perforators as they arise from parent vessels.[5]

A multiplicity of acute small infarcts in different vascular territories suggests emboli[4] and is best appreciated on the diffusion-weighted imaging (DWI)[6] (**Fig. 1**). However, multiple acute infarcts can also be seen with watershed infarcts, vasculitis, hypercoagulable

states, and in presence of anatomic variants connecting the anterior and posterior circulations (eg, fetal posterior cerebral artery [PCA] and persistent trigeminal artery) or connecting both hemispheres (eg, azygos A2 supplying the ACA territories bilaterally).[5–7] Of note, multiple acute infarcts exclusively affecting the posterior circulation are, in most cases, related to large-artery atherosclerosis.[5]

Hemorrhagic transformation is a common feature of embolic infarcts and is best seen on susceptibility blood-sensitive MR imaging sequences as petechial hemorrhage as opposed to the larger

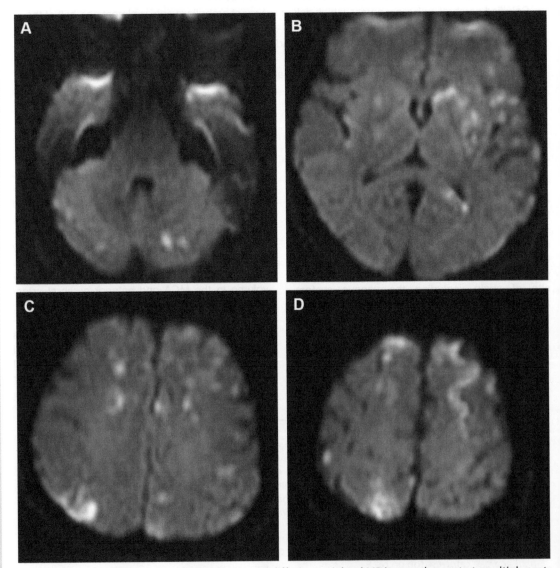

Fig. 1. Typical pattern of embolic infarcts: (*A–D*) Axial diffusion-weighted MR images demonstrate multiple acute small infarcts in different vascular territories in the supratentorial and infratentorial compartments bilaterally.

parenchymal hematomas that develop more commonly in territorial infarcts such as those involving the MCA.[2]

Cerebral Fat Embolism

Cerebral fat embolism (CFE) is a consequence of fractures, especially those involving the lower extremity long bones and the pelvis, orthopedic procedures, as well as nontraumatic conditions including bone infarcts in sickle cell disease and acute hemorrhagic pancreatitis. It presents as a triad of pulmonary and neurologic dysfunction and petechial rash.[8] The neurologic presentation varies from asymptomatic to subclinical to headache, confusion, and coma. The onset varies from a few hours up to 48 hours after trauma with a mean of 29 hours.[4,8,9] Clinically apparent fat embolism occurs in 0.5% to 3.5% of isolated long bone fractures[8,10] and in 5% to 10% of polytrauma patients.[8] Subclinical fat embolism is thought to occur in all cases of lower extremity and pelvic fractures.[8] The incidence of CFE is 0.9% to 2.2% of patients with a long bone fracture.[9,11]

CFE is thought to result from the exposure of medullary fat to damaged blood vessels with fat mechanically forced into the venous system.[12,13] An alternative theory suggests that stored fat is mobilized into the plasma due to increased levels of catecholamines and plasma lipase, resulting in fat droplets throughout the entire circulation.[12] Fat emboli cross the pulmonary circulation and reach the intracranial circulation even without an intracardiac shunt being present.[10]

Intracranially, fat emboli lodge in and mechanically occlude capillaries, producing ischemia and cytotoxic edema. However, the fat globules are deformable and tend to break up into smaller ones, which recycle through the pulmonary circulation. Hence, occlusions tend to be temporary, and changes may be reversible.[10,11,13] Cytotoxic edema may also result from the release of toxic metabolites (oleic acid and triglyceride triolein).[11] The release of toxic metabolites also results in opening of the blood-brain barrier (BBB), causing vasogenic edema and enhancement on contrast studies.[10,11]

Imaging Findings

The "star field" appearance (Fig. 2) is the most common imaging pattern found, and yet it remains nonspecific.[11,14] It is seen on DWI early in the acute phase as multiple foci of high signal scattered throughout the brain predominantly in the border zones and deep gray nuclei bilaterally.

These foci are thought to represent cytotoxic edema in acute cerebral infarcts.[11,14–16] As the occlusions are temporary, the findings can be reversible, leading to better outcome compared with other cerebral embolic events.[11] A second pattern seen on DWI, usually in the subacute phase, is the confluent bilateral symmetric periventricular and subcortical white matter cytotoxic edema and diffusion restriction.[11] This pattern portrays a worse prognosis.

T2* sequences may reveal innumerable foci of blooming low signal in the white matter[11,13,17] (Fig. 3). This pattern is best appreciated on susceptibility-weighted images (SWI)[17,18] and is to be pathognomonic of CFE.[11] The diffuse microhemorrhages can be secondary to microscopic hemorrhagic infarcts and vessel wall rupture due to embolism[13] or leakage of red blood cells because of abnormal BBB.[11] Alternatively, Suh and colleagues[18] suggested decreased blood flow secondary to embolism, leading to local increased deoxyhemoglobin levels as an underlying explanation for the extensive abnormalities seen on SWI.

White-matter T2/FLAIR (fluid attenuation inversion recovery sequence) hyperintense foci with no diffusion restriction can be seen, can reflect vasogenic edema, and may show contrast enhancement.[10,11] T2 abnormalities appear later than the DWI changes and are nonspecific.[14] However, the number of white matter lesions on T2-weighted images correlates with the patient's Glasgow coma scale score.[9] Magnetic resonance (MR) spectroscopy shows the presence of lipid peaks within the lesions, a finding related to the nature of the emboli or associated necrosis.[19,20]

CALCIFIED CEREBRAL EMBOLI

Calcified cerebral embolism is an uncommon cause of stroke[21] that has been recently estimated to occur in 3% of patients assessed for stroke and carries with it a high risk of recurrent embolic events in almost one-half of the patients.[22] Calcified emboli can occur spontaneously or secondary to surgery and catheterization. The sources of these emboli are the heart (especially calcified valves and calcified thrombus), the aortic arch, and neck arteries, including the carotid as well as the brachiocephalic and vertebral arteries. The most common sources are, however, a calcified aortic valve and carotid atherosclerosis.[21–26]

On computed tomography (CT), calcified emboli are small (2–3 mm) round or ovoid hyperdensities (162 HU)[22] (Figs. 4 and 5). The "salted pretzel"

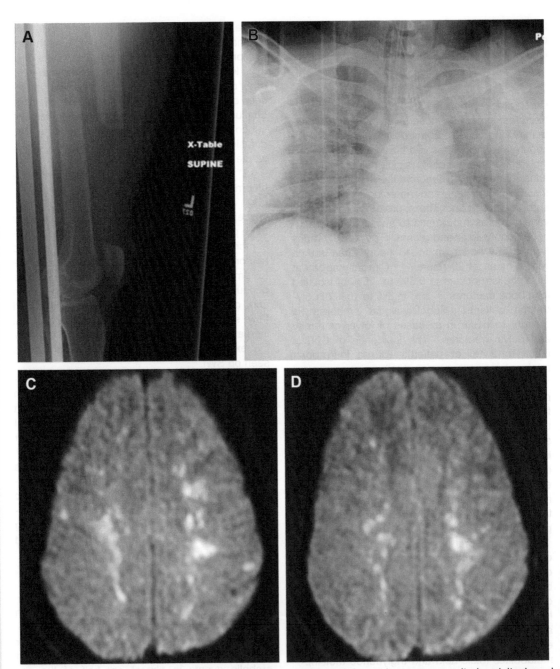

Fig. 2. "Star field" appearance of CFE: (*A*) Lateral radiograph of the left femur demonstrates a displaced diaphyseal fracture. (*B*) Anteroposterior (AP) radiograph of the chest shows patchy bilateral airspace disease. (*C, D*) Axial diffusion-weighted MR images show multiple bilateral scattered foci of high signal, which on the apparent diffusion coefficient (ADC) maps (not shown) demonstrated restricted diffusion, predominantly in the deep border zones.

sign describes a near pathognomonic unenhanced CT appearance of multiple calcified peripheral emboli in arteries along the pial surface of the brain, like salt on a pretzel.[23] Differential considerations include arterial wall calcification, which appears more linear than calcified emboli,[22] and other causes of superficial calcifications, including congenital infections, tuberous sclerosis, and prior intrathecal administration of pantopaque contrast media.[23]

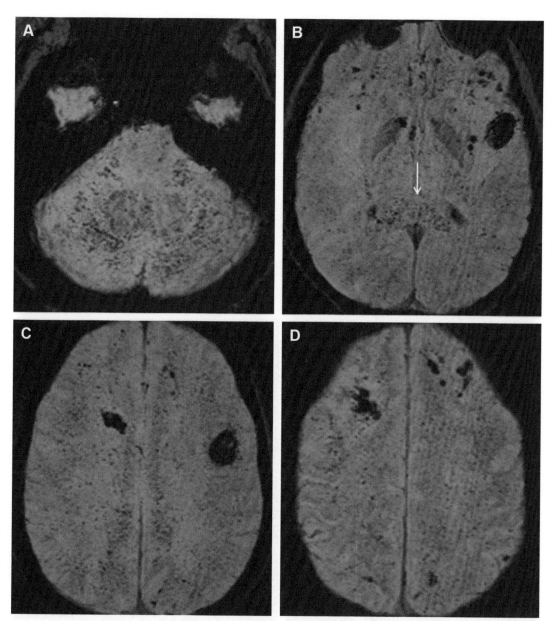

Fig. 3. Diffuse microhemorrhage in CFE: (*A–D*) Axial SWI MR images demonstrate innumerable tiny white matter blooming foci in the supratentorial and infratentorial compartments and through the splenium of the corpus callosum (*arrow* in *B*). Larger blooming areas in the frontal lobes are due to associated hemorrhagic contusions and diffuse axonal injury.

CEREBRAL AIR EMBOLISM

Introduction of air into the arterial or venous circulations is mostly iatrogenic and can occur in a variety of procedures including percutaneous lung biopsy, craniotomy with patient in the sitting position, cardiac surgery with cardiopulmonary bypass, atrioesophageal fistula after left atrial ablation,[27] angiography, and intravascular catheters, among others.[28–30] Less common noniatrogenic causes of air embolism include penetrating thoracic and cranial trauma and decompression sickness.[31] Accidental ingestion of hydrogen peroxide, an industrial bleaching agent, has also been reported to cause arterial or venous gas

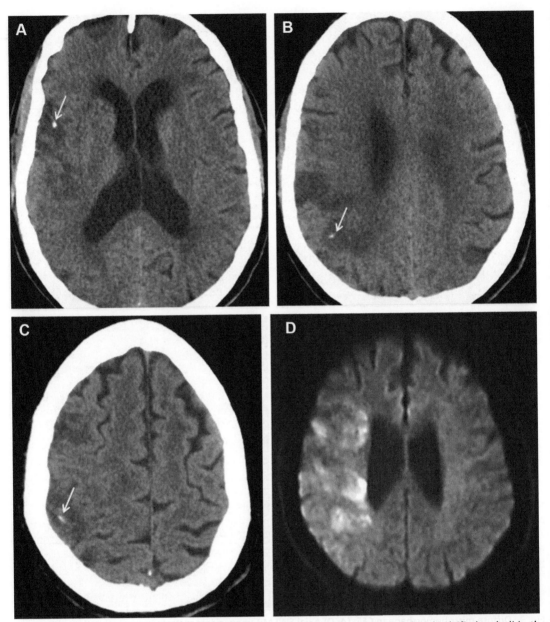

Fig. 4. Distal MCA calcific emboli: (A–C) Axial NCCT images demonstrate small peripheral calcified emboli in the distal right MCA branches (arrows) with adjacent acute embolic infarcts. (D) Diffusion-weighted MR image confirms the acute infarcts in the right MCA territory.

embolism as it decomposes into oxygen and water after absorption.[32]

During percutaneous lung biopsy, arterial air embolism may result from placement of the needle tip in a pulmonary vein or creation of a transient bronchovenous fistula with air bubbles traveling to the left cardiac chambers and the aorta[33,34] (Fig. 6). It has been shown that as little as 2 to 3 mL of air introduced in the pulmonary veins

can be fatal.[33] On the other hand, venous embolism may reach the arterial circulation through an intracardiac shunt or by overwhelming the pulmonary filtering mechanism.[28,30] It has been suggested that venous air may ascend retrograde to the cerebral veins in the upright position, leading to impairment of the venous outflow.[28] Cerebral arterial air emboli cause damage by mechanically blocking small arteries or eliciting an

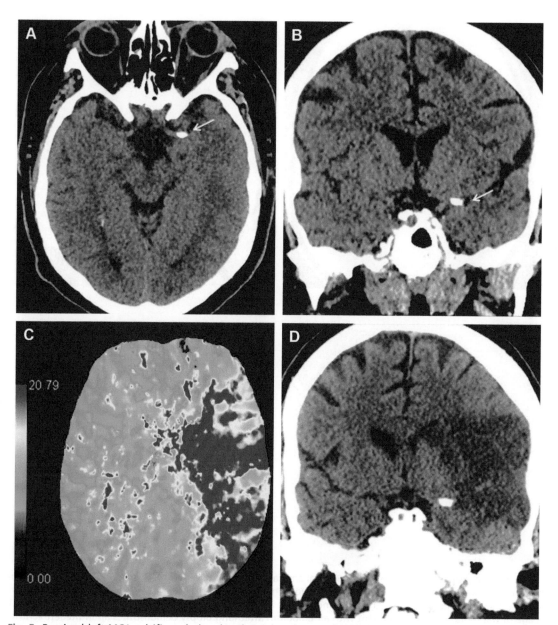

Fig. 5. Proximal left MCA calcific embolus: (*A, B*) Axial and coronal NCCT images at presentation demonstrate calcified embolus from calcified carotid plaque (not shown) lodged in the proximal left MCA M1 segment (*arrows*). Note the ovoid shape of the embolus as opposed to the usual linear appearance of MCA atherosclerotic calcifications. (*C*) CT perfusion time-to-peak (TTP) image demonstrates secondary prolongation of the TTP in the left MCA territory. (*D*) Twenty-four-hour follow-up coronal NCCT image demonstrates established acute infarction in the left MCA territory.

inflammatory response that results in endothelial damage.[28,30,34]

The clinical presentation is sudden and depends on the amount of air introduced and final destination of the gas emboli.[30,34] The only effective treatment available for arterial air embolism is hyperbaric oxygen treatment, which improves

oxygenation of ischemic tissues and resolves the mechanical vascular occlusion by accelerating nitrogen resorption and decreasing the size of the embolized bubbles.[33]

Cerebral air embolism (CAE) has a predilection for the supratentorial compartment and especially the right cerebral hemisphere (see **Fig. 6**), which

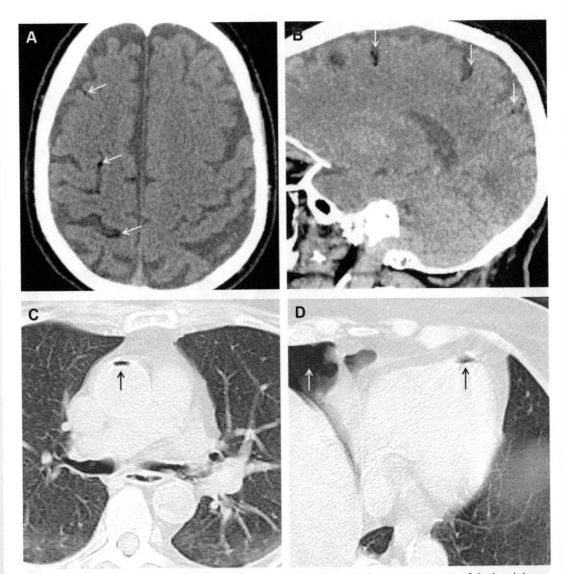

Fig. 6. Air embolism after lung biopsy: (*A, B*) Axial and sagittal 2-mm-thickness NCCT images of the head demonstrate rounded and curvilinear hypodensities in the right cerebral cortical sulci in keeping with air emboli (*arrows*). (*C*) Axial CT image of the thorax demonstrates air in the ascending aorta (*black arrow*). (*D*) Axial CT image of the thorax in another patient with air embolism after lung biopsy demonstrates air in the left ventricular apex (*black arrow*). Note incidental right-sided pneumothorax (*white arrow in D*).

may be explained by the fact that the brachiocephalic trunk is the first major branch of the aorta.[31,35,36] The patient's position has been suggested to affect the distribution of air emboli with the erect position causing emboli located mostly in the parietal and occipital lobes.[36] Posterior circulation emboli have been reported in the prone position due to preferential flow to the right vertebral artery.[35]

Noncontrast CT (NCCT) can directly visualize air emboli as small rounded or curvilinear hypodensities close to the cortical sulci (see **Fig. 6; Fig. 7**), representing air within cortical blood vessels, which are then resorbed into the general circulation.[27,31,36] Potential causes of false negative studies resulting in decreased sensitivity of NCCT include nonvisualization of small amounts of air, which can be clinically significant, resorption of gas emboli before scanning, and misinterpretation of gas attenuation values as fat.[28,31] Using thin-slice thickness (5 mm or smaller)[31] and demonstrating the air attenuation value by using

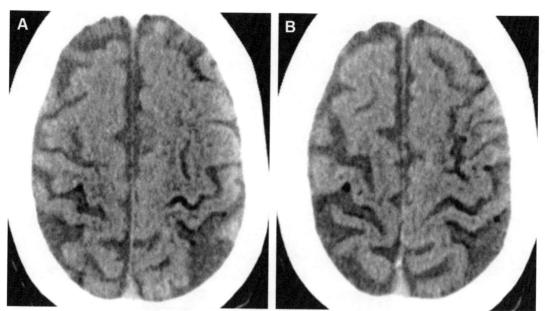

Fig. 7. CAE: (*A, B*) Axial CT images of the head in another patient demonstrate multiple curvilinear hypodensities bilaterally in the frontoparietal cortical sulci in keeping with extensive air emboli.

lung window settings and comparing with the air in the paranasal sinuses[36] can increase certainty on NCCT. Cerebral gas emboli can also be visualized on gradient echo MR sequences as hypointense foci due to susceptibility artifacts caused by air.[31,37]

SEPTIC EMBOLI

Embolization of infected cardiac vegetations in patients with infective endocarditis (IE) is associated with a high rate (up to 40%) of symptomatic neurologic complications with greater than 50% risk of recurrence.[38,39] In up to 47% of patients, it is the presenting symptom of IE.[40] Subclinical asymptomatic cerebral lesions in the acute phase of IE are even more common (71.5% in one study).[38] The risk of embolic events increases with *Staphylococcus aureus* as the causative organism, mitral valve involvement, and vegetations larger than 3 cm in size.[41]

Septic emboli may produce embolic infarcts, cerebral hemorrhages, or less likely, mycotic aneurysms and cerebral abscesses. Infarcts share the multiplicity and distribution of other emboli and thus are nonspecific. Infarcts of different ages are commonly coexistent even with a single clinical event.[38,42] Cerebral microbleeds (**Fig. 8**) are the most common abnormality seen in asymptomatic patients and have been shown to be significantly associated with IE, more frequently

as compared with age-matched controls; the strength of association increases with increasing number of microbleeds. Microhemorrhages seen on T2*-weighted imaging in IE tend to be cortical in location, larger and more heterogeneous compared with hypertension or amyloid-associated microbleeds seen in the elderly.[38,43]

The incidence of infectious (mycotic) aneurysms varies from 1% to 10% in patients with IE.[44] They develop due to infection and destruction of the vessel wall from the lumen or due to embolization of the vasa vasorum.[45] Infectious aneurysms tend to be multiple (up to 28%), fusiform in shape, and located in peripheral branches, most commonly of the MCA (55%)[45,46] (**Fig. 9**). Proximal infectious aneurysms (**Fig. 10**) occur in approximately one-third of cases and are difficult to differentiate from the more common berry aneurysms.[44,45] Multiplicity, presence of adjacent arterial stenoses, or occlusions and rapid morphologic changes favor infectious aneurysms over other types.[44] Infectious aneurysms may appear as foci of susceptibility artifacts on T2*-weighted imaging.[38] Infectious aneurysms carry a higher mortality than berry aneurysms and are managed with antimicrobial treatment as well as endovascular therapy or surgery.[46] The response to antibiotic therapy alone was shown to be highly variable with possible regression and resolution, rupture, or even de novo aneurysm formation[44] (see **Fig. 10**).

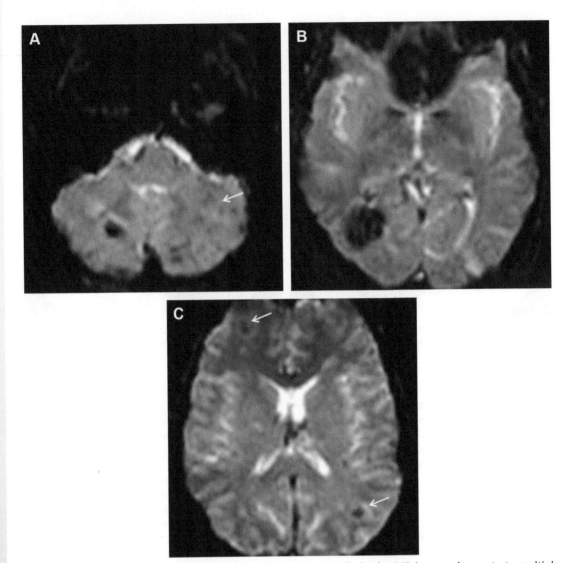

Fig. 8. Septic emboli with hemorrhage: (A–C) Axial gradient recalled echo MR images demonstrate multiple variable-sized supratentorial and infratentorial areas of blooming in keeping with hemorrhage in a patient with mitral-tricuspid IE and septic emboli (microbleeds are shown by *arrows*).

EMBOLISM FROM CARDIAC MYXOMA

Cardiac myxoma is the most common primary cardiac tumor in adults (83%); it is most commonly located in the left atrium (83%–88%) and is most frequent from the third to the sixth decades of life, with a 2:1 female predominance.[47] Systemic embolization is a known complication of this tumor and occurs in up to 50% of patients.[47–49] Embolization occurs due to surface thrombi or, less commonly, erosion and fragmentation of the tumor itself (tumor particles).[47,48] The cerebral arteries are affected in at

least 50% of cases,[48] and neurologic complications can be the initial and only clinical manifestations of this tumor.[50] Embolic stroke is the most common neurologic complication of cardiac myxoma[47,50] and is estimated to represent 0.5% of all strokes.[49] It affects most commonly the MCA territories.[49] Involvement of multiple vascular territories was seen in less than one-third of patients in one study.[47]

Myxomatous tumor emboli may result in cerebral aneurysm formation (Fig. 11) and metastatic space-occupying lesions. The preferred theory for aneurysm formation is that of transendothelial

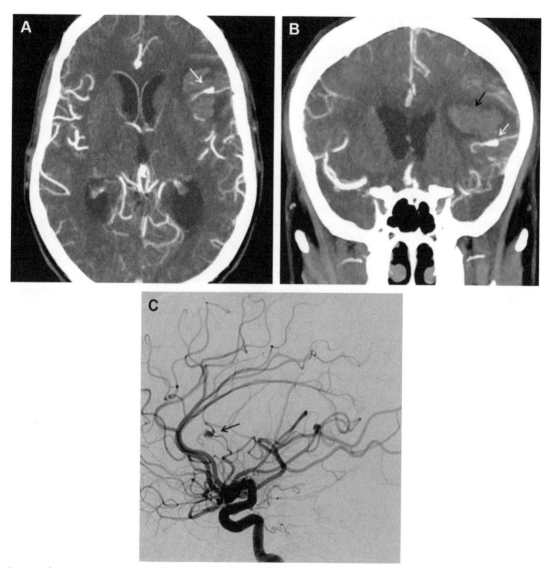

Fig. 9. Infectious left MCA aneurysm: (*A, B*) Axial and coronal maximum intensity projection (MIP) CTA images demonstrate fusiform peripheral left MCA aneurysm (*white arrows*) in a patient with methicillin-resistant *S aureus* mitral valve IE and left frontal intraparenchymal hematoma from aneurysm rupture (*black arrow* in *B*). (*C*) Conventional cerebral angiogram (lateral projection of left internal carotid artery [ICA] injection) demonstrates the fusiform infectious aneurysm (*arrow*).

invasion of the arterial wall by tumor cells with subintimal growth and disruption of the wall architecture leading to weakening and subsequent aneurysm formation.[47,48] Myxomatous aneurysms tend to be fusiform in shape and peripheral in location and may be multiple and similar to infectious aneurysms.[47,51] Sabolek and colleagues[51] found that most (74%) myxomatous aneurysms involved the MCAs. Contrast enhancement inside the aneurysm on MR imaging has been described, possibly related to slow flow or tumor within the aneurysm wall.[49] Intracranial hemorrhage can occur due to aneurysm rupture.[48] Finally, metastatic myxoma is rare, and intracranial metastasis is even less common.[47]

PARADOXICAL EMBOLISM

Paradoxical embolism (PDE) should be suspected in patients with embolic stroke in the absence of

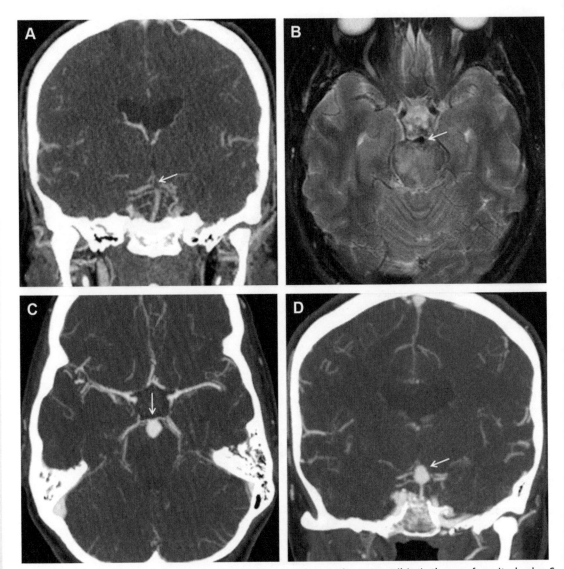

Fig. 10. Rapidly developing infectious basilar tip aneurysm in a patient on antibiotic therapy for mitral valve *S aureus* IE: (*A*) Coronal CTA MIP image at presentation demonstrates no obvious abnormality in the region of the basilar tip (*arrow*). (*B*) Axial T2-weighted MR image 2 days later demonstrates abnormal signal in the pons with diffusion restriction (not shown) in keeping with acute infarction and unremarkable basilar tip flow void (*arrow*). (*C, D*) Axial and coronal CTA MIP images (performed <24 hours after the MR imaging due to deterioration of the patient's clinical condition) demonstrate a new 1-cm basilar tip infectious aneurysm (*arrow*).

cardiac or proximal arterial sources. It requires the presence of systemic embolization, venous thrombosis, abnormal communication between the arterial and venous circulations, and a pressure gradient favoring a right-to-left shunt. The abnormal communication can be intracardiac or extracardiac (eg, pulmonary arteriovenous malformation).[52,53] The defect is most commonly a patent foramen ovale (PFO).[52,54] The right-to-left pressure gradient can be transient and physiologic (during Valsalva or coughing), and the most common source of PDE is venous thrombosis in the legs.[52]

A "definite diagnosis of PDE" can only be made by showing a thrombus that crosses an intracardiac defect at autopsy or at imaging in

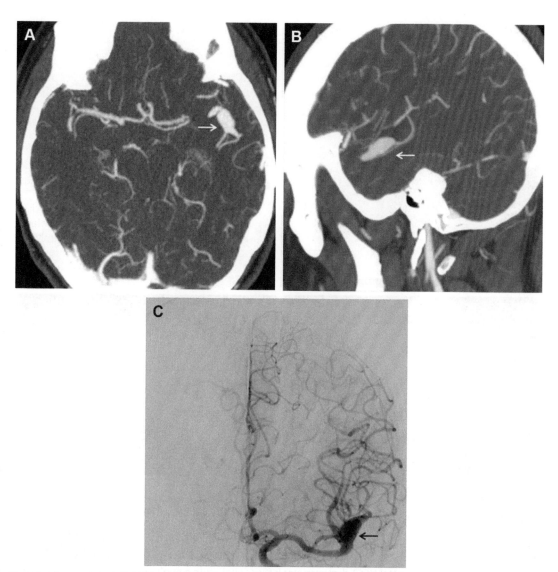

Fig. 11. Myxomatous left MCA aneurysm: (*A, B*) Axial and sagittal MIP CTA images demonstrate fusiform aneurysm of the left MCA (M2 segment, *arrows*) in a patient with known cardiac myxoma (not shown). (*C*) Conventional cerebral angiogram (AP projection of left ICA injection) demonstrates the fusiform myxomatous aneurysm (*arrow*).

the context of systemic embolization. A "presumptive diagnosis of PDE" can be made with a high level of confidence in the presence of an intracardiac communication, systemic embolization, and venous thrombosis.[52,55] The presence of systemic embolization and a PFO is considered "possible PDE."[52,56] PDE is one of the putative mechanisms of cryptogenic stroke, with some studies showing increased prevalence of pelvic DVT in patients with cryptogenic stroke as well as a high incidence of lower limb DVT

in patients with cryptogenic stroke and PFO.[55,57,58] Attention to ancillary findings on CT examinations performed for stroke assessment (eg, presence of pulmonary embolism) may provide a clue to the diagnosis (**Fig. 12**).

EMBOLIZATION SECONDARY TO ATRIOESOPHAGEAL FISTULA

Atrioesophageal fistula (AEF) is a rare (0.04%) and devastating complication of left atrial

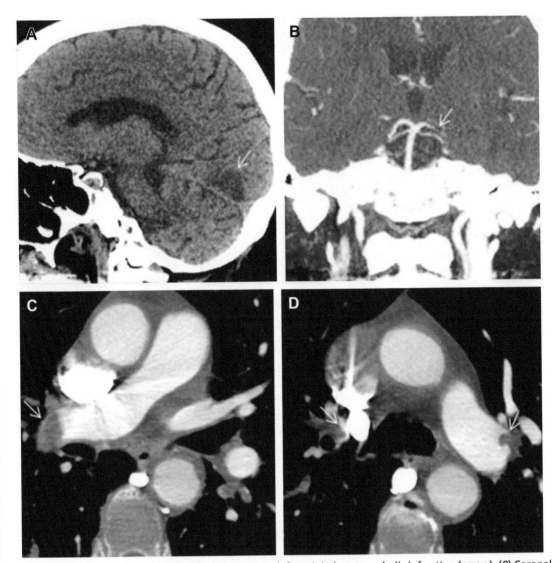

Fig. 12. Presumed PDE: (*A*) Sagittal NCCT demonstrates left occipital acute embolic infarction (*arrow*). (*B*) Coronal MIP CTA demonstrates filling defect in the left PCA (P1 segment, *arrow*). (*C, D*) Axial images from the same CTA demonstrate emboli in the pulmonary arteries and their branches (*arrows*).

ablation for treatment of atrial fibrillation.[59,60] After cardiac tamponade, it is the second most common cause of mortality (16%) in these patients.[59,60] The presentation is usually delayed, 1 to 6 weeks after the procedure, and is nonspecific.[59,61,62] Postprandial transient ischemic attack associated with fever has been described as one of the leading clinical manifestations.[62]

AEF may give rise to variable types of emboli, including food particles and air extending into the left atrium from the esophagus or thrombus formation within the left atrium (Fig. 13). These emboli may manifest as embolic infarcts, air embolism, meningitis, or abscesses[63] (see Fig. 13). These findings in a patient with recent atrial ablation should raise the suspicion of an underlying AEF and lead to urgent assessment and intervention.[59,63]

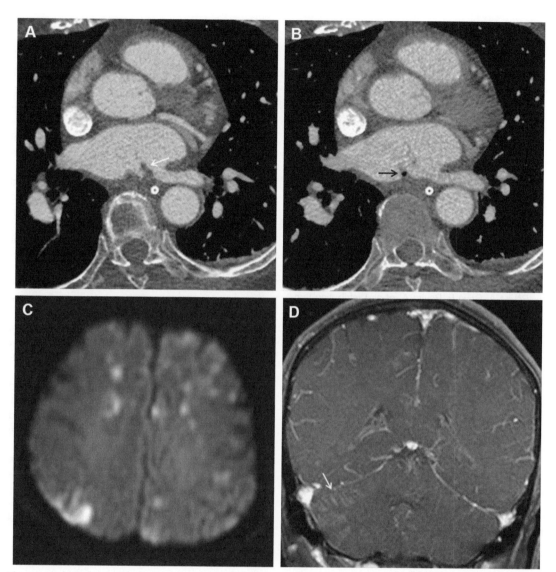

Fig. 13. Embolism secondary to atrioesophageal fistula 5 weeks after left atrial ablation: (*A, B*) Axial contrast-enhanced CT images of the thorax demonstrate filling defect (*white arrow* in *A*) and gas bubble (*black arrow* in *B*) in the left atrium adjacent to the esophagus with a nasogastric tube seen in place. (*C*) Axial diffusion-weighted MR image demonstrates multiple embolic infarcts. (*D*) Coronal T1-weighted MR image after contrast administration shows associated supratentorial (not shown) and infratentorial leptomeningeal enhancement (*arrow*) in keeping with meningitis.

SUMMARY

A wide variety of unusual cerebral emboli exists. Some may represent the earliest manifestation of the underlying condition (eg, myxoma, IE, cardiac shunt), can carry a high risk of recurrence (calcified and septic emboli), or could be amenable to a specific treatment (hyperbaric oxygen for air embolism). The diagnosis of unusual cerebral embolism could be made by attention to specific clinical scenarios, direct emboli visualization (eg, air and calcific emboli), specific imaging patterns (eg, diffuse white matter microhemorrhage in fat embolism and "salted pretzel" sign in calcified emboli), and ancillary findings on neurologic studies (eg, pulmonary embolism on head and neck CT angiography [CTA] in PDE). The radiologist's ability to identify these findings and to suggest the correct diagnosis may significantly impact patients' management and outcome.

REFERENCES

1. Niesten JM, van der Schaaf IC, van Dam L, et al. Histopathologic composition of cerebral thrombi of acute stroke patients is correlated with stroke subtype and thrombus attenuation. PLoS One 2014; 9(2):e88882.
2. Koroshetz WJ, González RG. Causes of ischemic stroke. In: González RG, Schwamm LH, Schaefer PW, et al, editors. Acute ischemic stroke. Imaging and intervention. 2nd edition. Berlin; New York: Springer; 2011. p. 27–40.
3. Chung EM, Hague JP, Chanrion MA, et al. Embolus trajectory through a physical replica of the major cerebral arteries. Stroke 2010;41(4):647–52.
4. Osborn AG. Acute cerebral ischemia—infarction. In: Osborn AG, editor. Osborn's brain: imaging, pathology, and anatomy. Salt Lake City (UT): Amirsys; 2013. p. 180–91.
5. Rovira A, Grivé E, Rovira A, et al. Distribution territories and causative mechanisms of ischemic stroke. Eur Radiol 2005;15(3):416–26.
6. Roh JK, Kang DW, Lee SH, et al. Significance of acute multiple brain infarction on diffusion-weighted imaging. Stroke 2000;31(3):688–94.
7. Cho AH, Kim JS, Jeon SB, et al. Mechanism of multiple infarcts in multiple cerebral circulations on diffusion-weighted imaging. J Neurol 2007;254(7): 924–30.
8. Johnson MJ, Lucas GL. Fat embolism syndrome. Orthopedics 1996;19:41–7.
9. Takahashi M, Suzuki R, Osakabe Y, et al. Magnetic resonance imaging findings in cerebral fat embolism: correlation with clinical manifestations. J Trauma 1999;46(2):324–7.
10. Simon AD, Ulmer JL, Strottmann JM. Contrast-enhanced MR imaging of cerebral fat embolism: case report and review of the literature. AJNR Am J Neuroradiol 2003;24:97–101.
11. Kuo KH, Pan YJ, Lai YJ, et al. Dynamic MR imaging patterns of cerebral fat embolism: a systematic review with illustrative cases. AJNR Am J Neuroradiol 2014;35(6):1052–7.
12. Bardana D, Rudan J, Cervenko F, et al. Fat embolism syndrome in a patient demonstrating only neurologic symptoms. Can J Surg 1998;41: 398–402.
13. Gibbs WN, Opatowsky MJ, Burton EC. AIRP best cases in radiologic-pathologic correlation: cerebral fat embolism syndrome in sickle cell β-thalassemia. Radiographics 2012;32(5):1301–6.
14. Parizel PM, Demey HE, Veeckmans G, et al. Early diagnosis of cerebral fat embolism syndrome by diffusion-weighted MRI (starfield pattern). Stroke 2001;32(12):2942–4.
15. Decaminada N, Thaler M, Holler R, et al. Brain fat embolism. A report of two cases and a brief review of neuroimaging findings. Neuroradiol J 2012;25: 193–9.
16. Ryu CW, Lee DH, Kim TK, et al. Cerebral fat embolism: diffusion-weighted magnetic resonance imaging findings. Acta Radiol 2005;46(5):528–33.
17. Lee J. Gradient-echo MRI in defining the severity of cerebral fat embolism. J Clin Neurol 2008;4(4): 164–6.
18. Suh SI, Seol HY, Seo WK, et al. Cerebral fat embolism: susceptibility-weighted magnetic resonance imaging. Arch Neurol 2009;66:1170.
19. Kokatnur L, Rudrappa M, Khasawneh KR. Cerebral fat embolism: use of MR spectroscopy for accurate diagnosis. Ann Indian Acad Neurol 2015;18(2): 252–5.
20. Guillevin R, Vallée JN, Demeret S, et al. Cerebral fat embolism: usefulness of magnetic resonance spectroscopy. Ann Neurol 2005;57(3):434–9.
21. Gearry RB, Sharr JP, Avery SF. Spontaneous calcific cerebral embolus. Australas Radiol 2005; 49(2):154–6.
22. Walker BS, Shah LM, Osborn AG. Calcified cerebral emboli, a "do not miss" imaging diagnosis: 22 new cases and review of the literature. AJNR Am J Neuroradiol 2014;35(8):1515–9.
23. Christian BA, Kirzeder DJ, Boyd J, et al. Showered calcific emboli to the brain, the 'salted pretzel' sign, originating from the ipsilateral internal carotid artery causing acute cerebral infarction. Stroke 2009;40(5):e319–21.
24. Moustafa RR, Antoun NM, Coulden RA, et al. Stroke attributable to a calcific embolus from the brachiocephalic trunk. Stroke 2006;37(1):e6–8.
25. Kavanagh EC, Fenton DM, Heran MK, et al. Calcified cerebral emboli. AJNR Am J Neuroradiol 2006;27(9):1996–9.
26. Doiron A, Blais C, Bonneau D. Spontaneous cerebral embolus from a calcified aortic valve. AJR Am J Roentgenol 1996;167(4):955–6.
27. Lempel JK, Jozwik B, Manfredi C, et al. Cerebral air embolism: a result of atrioesophageal fistula. AJNR Am J Neuroradiol 2012;33(3):E40–1.
28. Murphy A, Torres C, Lum C, et al. Whole brain CT perfusion after cerebral air embolism. Can J Neurol Sci 2011;38(3):522–5.
29. Heckmann JG, Lang CJ, Kindler K, et al. Neurologic manifestations of cerebral air embolism as a complication of central venous catheterization. Crit Care Med 2000;28:1621–5.
30. Muth CM, Shank ES. Gas embolism. N Engl J Med 2000;342:476–82.
31. Weiss KL, Macura KJ, Ahmed A. Cerebral air embolism: acute imaging. J Stroke Cerebrovasc Dis 1998; 7(3):222–6.
32. Ijichi T, Itoh T, Sakai R, et al. Multiple brain gas embolism after ingestion of concentrated hydrogen peroxide. Neurology 1997;48(1):277–9.

33. Hare SS, Gupta A, Goncalves AT, et al. Systemic arterial air embolism after percutaneous lung biopsy. Clin Radiol 2011;66(7):589–96.

34. Kau T, Rabitsch E, Celedin S, et al. When coughing can cause stroke—a case-based update on cerebral air embolism complicating biopsy of the lung. Cardiovasc Intervent Radiol 2008;31(5):848–53.

35. Suzuki K, Ueda M, Muraga K, et al. An unusual cerebral air embolism developing within the posterior circulation territory after a needle lung biopsy. Intern Med 2013;52(1):115–7.

36. Jensen ME, Lipper MH. CT in iatrogenic cerebral air embolism. AJNR Am J Neuroradiol 1986;7(5):823–7.

37. Jeon SB, Kang DW. Neurological picture. Cerebral air emboli on T2-weighted gradient-echo magnetic resonance imaging. J Neurol Neurosurg Psychiatry 2007;78(8):871.

38. Hess A, Klein I, Iung B, et al. Brain MRI findings in neurologically asymptomatic patients with infective endocarditis. AJNR Am J Neuroradiol 2013;34(8): 1579–84.

39. Ruttmann E, Willeit J, Ulmer H, et al. Neurological outcome of septic cardioembolic stroke after infective endocarditis. Stroke 2006;37(8):2094–9.

40. Heiro M, Nikoskelainen J, Engblom E, et al. Neurologic manifestations of infective endocarditis: a 17-year experience in a teaching hospital in Finland. Arch Intern Med 2000;160:2781–7.

41. García-Cabrera E, Fernández-Hidalgo N, Almirante B, et al. Neurological complications of infective endocarditis: risk factors, outcome, and impact of cardiac surgery: a multicenter observational study. Circulation 2013;127(23):2272–84.

42. Singhal AB, Topcuoglu MA, Buonanno FS. Acute ischemic stroke patterns in infective and nonbacterial thrombotic endocarditis: a diffusion-weighted magnetic resonance imaging study. Stroke 2002; 33(5):1267–73.

43. Klein I, Iung B, Labreuche J, et al. Cerebral microbleeds are frequent in infective endocarditis: a case-control study. Stroke 2009;40(11):3461–5.

44. Chapot R, Houdart E, Saint-Maurice JP, et al. Endovascular treatment of cerebral mycotic aneurysms. Radiology 2002;222(2):389–96.

45. Corr P, Wright M, Handler LC. Endocarditis-related cerebral aneurysms: radiologic changes with treatment. AJNR Am J Neuroradiol 1995;16(4):745–8.

46. Kannoth S, Thomas SV. Intracranial microbial aneurysm (infectious aneurysm): current options for diagnosis and management. Neurocrit Care 2009;11(1): 120–9.

47. Lee VH, Connolly HM, Brown RD Jr. Central nervous system manifestations of cardiac myxoma. Arch Neurol 2007;64(8):1115–20.

48. Herbst M, Wattjes MP, Urbach H, et al. Cerebral embolism from left atrial myxoma leading to cerebral and retinal aneurysms: a case report. AJNR Am J Neuroradiol 2005;26(3):666–9.

49. Nucifora PG, Dillon WP. MR diagnosis of myxomatous aneurysms: report of two cases. AJNR Am J Neuroradiol 2001;22(7):1349–52.

50. Zheng Z, Guo G, Xu L, et al. Left atrial myxoma with versus without cerebral embolism: length of symptoms, morphologic characteristics, and outcomes. Tex Heart Inst J 2014;41(6):592–5.

51. Sabolek M, Bachus-Banaschak K, Bachus R, et al. Multiple cerebral aneurysms as delayed complication of left cardiac myxoma: a case report and review. Acta Neurol Scand 2005;111(6):345–50.

52. Saremi F, Emmanuel N, Wu PF, et al. Paradoxical embolism: role of imaging in diagnosis and treatment planning. Radiographics 2014;34(6): 1571–92.

53. Desai SP, Rees C, Jinkins JR. Paradoxical cerebral emboli associated with pulmonary arteriovenous shunts: report of three cases. AJNR Am J Neuroradiol 1991;12:355–9.

54. Loscalzo J. Paradoxical embolism: clinical presentation, diagnostic strategies, and therapeutic options. Am Heart J 1986;112:141–5.

55. Stöllberger C, Slany J, Schuster I, et al. The prevalence of deep venous thrombosis in patients with suspected paradoxical embolism. Ann Intern Med 1993;119(6):461–5.

56. Travis JA, Fuller SB, Ligush J Jr, et al. Diagnosis and treatment of paradoxical embolus. J Vasc Surg 2001;34:860–5.

57. Liberman AL, Prabhakaran S. Cryptogenic stroke: how to define it? How to treat it? Curr Cardiol Rep 2013;15:423.

58. Cramer SC, Rordorf G, Maki JH, et al. Increased pelvic vein thrombi in cryptogenic stroke: results of the Paradoxical Emboli from Large Veins in Ischemic Stroke (PELVIS) study. Stroke 2004; 35(1):46–50.

59. Nair GM, Nery PB, Redpath CJ, et al. Atrioesophageal fistula in the era of atrial fibrillation ablation: a review. Can J Cardiol 2014;30:388–95.

60. Dagres N, Anastasiou-Nana M. Prevention of atrial-esophageal fistula after catheter ablation of atrial fibrillation. Curr Opin Cardiol 2011;26:1–5.

61. Hazell W, Heaven D, Kazemi A, et al. Atrio-oesophageal fistula: an emergent complication of radiofrequency ablation. Emerg Med Australas 2009;21: 329–32.

62. Stöllberger C, Pulgram T, Finsterer J. Neurological consequences of atrioesophageal fistula after radiofrequency ablation in atrial fibrillation. Arch Neurol 2009;66:884–7.

63. Finsterer J, Stöllberger C, Pulgram T. Neurological manifestations of atrio-esophageal fistulas from left atrial ablation. Eur J Neurol 2011;18:1212–9.

Plaque Imaging to Decide on Optimal Treatment
Medical Versus Carotid Endarterectomy Versus Carotid Artery Stenting

Jie Sun, MD[a], Thomas S. Hatsukami, MD[b],*

KEYWORDS

- Carotid artery disease • Optimal medical therapy • Carotid endarterectomy • Carotid artery stenting
- MR imaging

KEY POINTS

- Advancements in optimal medical therapy, comprising antiplatelet agents, statin therapy, and aggressive risk factor control, have substantially reduced the risk of stroke in individuals with carotid artery disease.
- Compared with the current clinical standard of attributing risk based on carotid stenosis, plaque imaging may be better able to stratify the risk for stroke, and identify those most likely to benefit from carotid endarterectomy (CEA) and carotid artery stenting (CAS).
- Although CAS is considered as an alternative to CEA, it currently has higher rates of periprocedural stroke and clinically silent hemispheric infarction. Preliminary results suggest that vessel wall imaging of plaque morphology, composition, and activity may be beneficial in planning CAS procedures, and thereby reduce periprocedural stroke.
- While evidence is increasing, larger outcome studies and randomized clinical trials are needed to confirm the value of carotid plaque imaging in deciding between optimal medical therapy, carotid endarterectomy, and CAS.

CURRENT CLINICAL CHALLENGES
Prevalence of Carotid Artery Disease

Carotid artery disease, a local manifestation of systemic atherosclerosis, is not an uncommon finding in clinical practice. Indeed, a recent study pooling individual participant data from 4 large population-based studies estimated that the prevalence of asymptomatic moderate carotid stenosis, defined as 50% or more based on duplex ultrasonography, was as high as 7.5% in the general population depending on subjects' age and sex.[1] Specifically, 2.3% of men and 2.0% women

in their 60s had carotid stenosis on ultrasonographic examination, which increased to 7.5% and 5.0% for individuals aged 80 years or older. In subgroups with cardiovascular risk factors or those with established coronary or peripheral artery disease, the prevalence of carotid stenosis is increased by severalfold compared with the general population.[2,3]

In addition, the prevalence of carotid artery disease that is significant, from a histopathologic point of view, may be underestimated. Nonstenotic or minimally stenotic carotid plaques can

Disclosure Statement: None (J. Sun); investigator-initiated research grants from Philips Healthcare (T.S. Hatsukami).
[a] Department of Radiology, University of Washington, 850 Republican Street, Seattle, WA 98109, USA;
[b] Department of Surgery, University of Washington, 850 Republican Street, Seattle, WA 98109, USA
* Corresponding author.
E-mail address: tomhat@u.washington.edu

1052-5149/16/$ – see front matter © 2016 Elsevier Inc. All rights reserved.

neuroimaging.theclinics.com

harbor substantial amounts of lipid and necrotic debris as a result of outward remodeling and the geometry of the carotid bulb. Furthermore, high-risk plaque features such as intraplaque hemorrhage (IPH), thin or ruptured fibrous cap, and plaque inflammation have been found in carotid plaques that are otherwise morphologically indistinct (Fig. 1).[4,5] In a 2008 study, 192 subjects underwent ultrasonography to quantify the degree of carotid stenosis, and MR imaging to identify the presence of complex plaques.[6] Complex plaques were defined as having IPH or luminal surface defect on multicontrast MR images and were more frequently found in plaques with higher grades of stenosis. Of note, however, complex plaques were detected in 21.7% of arteries with only 16% to 49% luminal stenosis. Increasingly, the advent of improved techniques for vessel wall imaging demonstrates that diagnostic imaging methods that only measure stenosis underestimate plaque burden, plaque complexity, and, hence, the true prevalence of histologically significant carotid artery disease.[4,5]

Clinical Outcomes with Medical Therapy Alone

Most carotid plaques have a relatively benign clinical course. However, once carotid artery disease becomes symptomatic, it often leads to disabling or devastating stroke without preceding signs. In the Asymptomatic Carotid Surgery Trial (ACST), half of the ipsilateral ischemic strokes in patients with asymptomatic carotid stenosis greater than 60% were disabling or fatal.[7] Carotid artery disease is a major source of ischemic stroke, accounting for approximately 15% of the 795,000 incident strokes that occur annually in the United States.[8] Less known is the role of nonstenotic but high-risk carotid plaques in cryptogenic strokes, of which a significant portion may be attributable to large-artery atherosclerosis,[9,10] as discussed elsewhere in this issue.

Medical therapy plays a pivotal role in the primary and secondary prevention of ischemic strokes ascribed to carotid artery disease. The benefit of aspirin has long been recognized, and

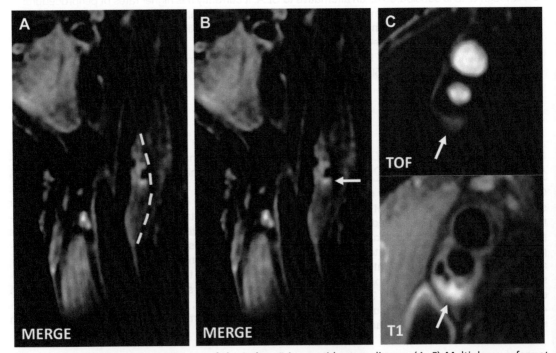

Fig. 1. Mild luminal stenosis as "the tip of the iceberg" in carotid artery disease. (A, B) Multiplanar reformat (MPR) of 3-dimensional volume data acquired using the motion-sensitized driven equilibrium prepared rapid gradient echo sequence (3D-MERGE)*, with centerlines in the common and internal carotid arteries. (A) A large plaque in a carotid artery with minimal luminal stenosis. The outer boundary of the plaque is delineated by the dotted yellow line. (B) Presence of intraplaque hemorrhage (white arrow) located near the outer boundary of the plaque. (C) Corresponding time-of-flight (TOF, upper) and T1-weighted (lower) images at the same level, confirming the presence of intraplaque hemorrhage. Plaque burden and complexity are disproportionate to the mild luminal narrowing. (* Balu N, Yarnykh VL, Chu B, et al. Carotid plaque assessment using fast 3D isotropic resolution black-blood MRI. Magn Reson Med 2011;63:627–37.)

it is currently listed as a class I recommendation in guidelines for the management of asymptomatic and symptomatic carotid artery disease. Multiple clinical trials have established the efficacy of 3-hydroxy-3-methylglutaryl coenzyme A reductase inhibitors (statins) in reducing the incidence of major cardiovascular events and stroke, which is proportional to individuals' baseline risk and absolute reduction in low-density lipoprotein cholesterol.[11] Annual event rates for recurrent strokes from all sources have decreased from 8.7% in the 1960s to 4.98% in the 2000s, in part attributed to more prevalent use of statins along with improved profiles in blood pressure, smoking, and antithrombotic agents.[12] In current guidelines, optimal medical therapy including aspirin and statin use, synergistic control of vascular risk factors, and lifestyle intervention forms the foundation of clinical management.[13,14]

Carotid Endarterectomy

Excision of the culprit carotid plaque can offer long-term benefits in selected patients. To ensure net benefit on an individual basis, the evaluation of operative risk and future stroke risk must be carefully compared (Fig. 2).

Symptomatic carotid artery disease

The North American Symptomatic Carotid Endarterectomy Trial compared carotid endarterectomy with medical therapy alone in patients with carotid artery disease and transient ischemic attack (TIA) or nondisabling stroke in the previous 180 days.[15] Carotid stenosis, as assessed on digital subtraction angiography, ranged from mild (<50%) to severe (≥70%). Net benefit was seen most robustly in the group with severe stenosis, whereas patients with mild stenosis did not have a significant reduction in 5-year rate of ipsilateral stroke.

Asymptomatic carotid artery disease

Earlier randomized trials demonstrated smaller but statistically significant benefit from CEA in asymptomatic patients with high-grade carotid stenosis, as shown in the Asymptomatic Carotid Atherosclerosis Study and the ACST study.[7,16]

However, the major clinical trials comparing CEA with medical therapy alone were conducted decades ago. Substantial advancements in medical therapy have been associated with progressive reduction in the risk for stroke. Most recent studies have reported an annual stroke rate of less than 1%. In 2009, Abbott[17] performed a systematic

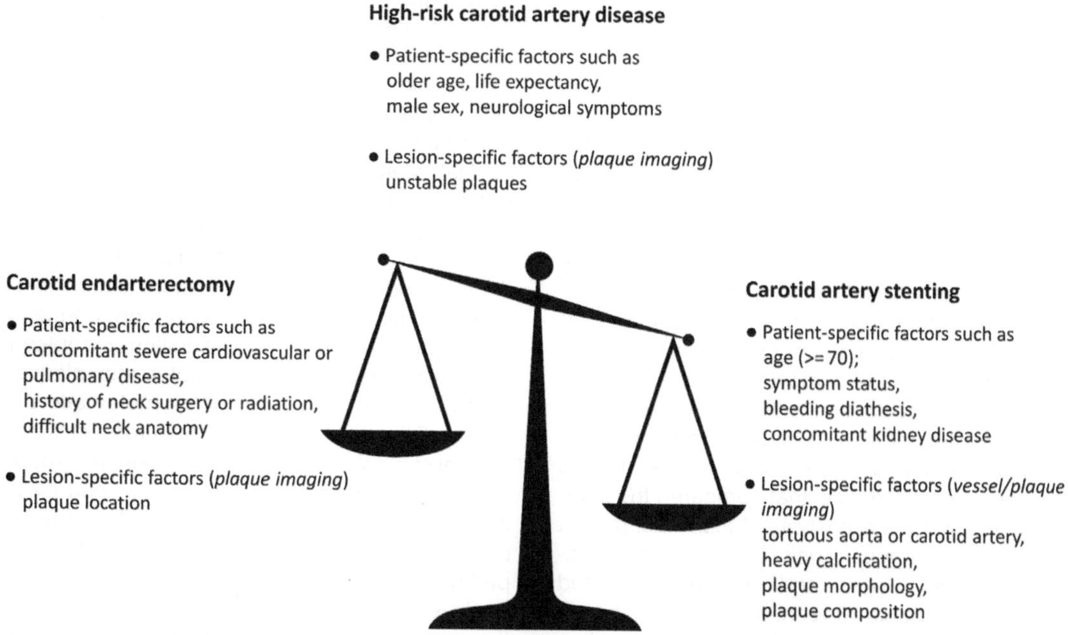

High-risk carotid artery disease

- Patient-specific factors such as older age, life expectancy, male sex, neurological symptoms

- Lesion-specific factors (*plaque imaging*) unstable plaques

Carotid endarterectomy

- Patient-specific factors such as concomitant severe cardiovascular or pulmonary disease, history of neck surgery or radiation, difficult neck anatomy

- Lesion-specific factors (*plaque imaging*) plaque location

Carotid artery stenting

- Patient-specific factors such as age (>= 70); symptom status, bleeding diathesis, concomitant kidney disease

- Lesion-specific factors (*vessel/plaque imaging*) tortuous aorta or carotid artery, heavy calcification, plaque morphology, plaque composition

Fig. 2. Weighing the future stroke and procedural risk in clinical decisions of carotid artery disease. Carotid revascularization should be reserved for those at a high risk for future ischemic stroke. If stroke risk is high, selection of CEA versus CAS is further based on both patient-specific and lesion-specific factors. In contrast to patient-specific factors, many lesion-specific factors require advanced vessel wall imaging and, unfortunately, are currently less used. Ultimately, large randomized clinical trials will be necessary to determine the exact contribution of plaque imaging in clinical decisions regarding optimal treatment.

review and analysis of published data on stroke risk associated with asymptomatic severe carotid stenosis. She found a progressive decrease in reported stroke rate with an average annual stroke risk estimated to be as low as those of the CEA arms in randomized trials performed before 2003. As the decision to proceed with surgical intervention must balance periprocedural risk and long-term event-free benefit, the net gain from surgical intervention for asymptomatic carotid stenosis is unclear in comparison with current optimal medical therapy.

Stroke risk, even in symptomatic cerebrovascular disease, can be substantially reduced with aggressive medical therapy. Recent guidelines have introduced alternative antiplatelet therapies and have taken into account the potential benefit of dual-antiplatelet therapy in the early phase following onset of symptoms.[14] Furthermore, high-intensity statins are now recommended in patients with symptomatic carotid artery disease irrespective of patients' lipid level.[18] In a 2013 observational study, which pooled individual patient data from multiple centers internationally, Merwick and colleagues[19] found that statin pretreatment was associated with lower 90-day stroke risk in patients with TIA and carotid stenosis, thereby highlighting the importance of acute statin treatment in preventing early strokes.

Is Carotid Artery Stenting a Viable Substitute for Carotid Endarterectomy?

In patients with high surgical risk, such as those with concomitant severe cardiovascular or pulmonary disease, previous history of neck surgery, or cervical radiation therapy, carotid artery stenting (CAS) offers a viable alternative to CEA (see **Fig. 2**). The SAPPHIRE (Stenting and Angioplasty with Protection in Patients with High Risk for Endarterectomy) trial showed that CAS was noninferior to CEA for the primary composite end point of death, stroke, and myocardial infarction within 30 days, and death and ipsilateral stroke within 1 year (16.3% vs 20.0%).[20] Controversy remains for patients with average surgical risk despite several randomized trials that compared the 2 approaches. In a meta-analysis of individual patient data from 3 European trials on symptomatic carotid stenosis, Bonati and colleagues[21] noted that CAS in patients 70 years or older had a higher perioperative risk of stroke or death when compared with carotid endarterectomy (8.9% vs 5.8% within 120 days). The CREST (Carotid Revascularization Endarterectomy versus Stenting Trial) is the largest trial used to compare CAS with CEA in both symptomatic and asymptomatic

carotid stenosis.[22] No significant difference was found in the estimated 4-year rates of the composite end point including stroke, myocardial infarction, and death during the periprocedural period and ipsilateral stroke within 4 years (7.2% vs 6.8%). However, during the periprocedural period stroke occurred more frequently in the CAS arm, whereas myocardial infarction occurred more frequently in the CEA arm.

Based on these data, CAS is indicated in guidelines as an alternative to CEA for patients with an average or low risk of complications associated with endovascular intervention. However, older age (≥70 years) is considered as a factor that may drive the equilibrium toward CEA. Furthermore, several lesion-specific conditions that increase the probability of embolization from CAS have been associated with increased periprocedural events, such as a tortuous aorta, angulation of carotid bifurcation, and heavily calcified carotid plaques. Identification of these factors before CAS would contribute to improved outcomes.

INFORMED CLINICAL DECISION MAKING WITH CAROTID PLAQUE IMAGING
The Heterogeneous Carotid Plaque

Much of our understanding of carotid plaque morphology and composition comes from histopathologic examination of CEA specimens. Histologic studies of CEA specimens have led to the appreciation that carotid atherosclerotic plaques are complex structures with considerable morphologic variation, and that plaque rupture and/or thrombosis, rather than restriction in flow from luminal stenosis, is the likely cause of most ischemic strokes. A 1996 study by Carr and colleagues,[23] which included CEA specimens from 25 symptomatic and 19 asymptomatic patients, found that fibrous cap rupture, cap thinning, and cap inflammation were seen more frequently in symptomatic patients. In addition, intraplaque fibrin was present in all symptomatic plaques, compared with only 68% of asymptomatic plaques. Other morphologic features including luminal stenosis did not differ between the groups. Studies by Spagnoli and colleagues[24] and Fisher and colleagues[25] also confirmed the fundamental role of plaque rupture and/or thrombosis in the pathogenesis of ischemic strokes. Furthermore, an inverse relationship was observed between the presence of these histologic features and time since symptom onset.

These studies have provided important insights into disease mechanisms and have shifted attention from stenosis to plaque structure and composition. Luminal narrowing may increase the risk of plaque rupture. However, an imaging focus limited to quantifying stenosis will fail to capture crucial aspects of plaque biology that determine the risk for plaque rupture, including lipid core size, thin fibrous cap, IPH, and inflammation.

In the past 2 decades, significant advancements have been made in imaging carotid plaques. Echolucent areas on ultrasonography indicate deposition of lipid and the possible presence of IPH.[26] More recently, multicontrast MR imaging has emerged as an accurate and reliable method to allow quantitative assessment of major plaque components, including calcification and lipid core.[27–32] Importantly, MR imaging has shown a unique capability for reliable detection of IPH, which seems to be a key feature of vulnerable plaques.[33–36] Through the use of contrast agents, ultrasonography, MR imaging, and PET have all demonstrated the capability of imaging neovasculature and inflammatory cell infiltration.[37–43] Given the highly selected population of patients undergoing carotid endarterectomy, studies of surgical specimens provide a limited window onto the pathogenesis of high-risk carotid atherosclerosis. Advanced imaging techniques can provide the tools necessary to study the natural history of carotid disease in broader populations. Furthermore, by revealing the interaction between plaque phenotypes and treatment on clinical outcomes, imaging presents new opportunities for the development of novel therapeutic strategies.

Optimal Medical Therapy: Is It Truly Optimal?

The current recommended regimen of medical therapy rests on the cumulative experience from many large-scale randomized controlled trials. However, it is evident that residual risk for ischemic events persists, likely because of variations in individual patient characteristics. The varied response to pharmacologic therapy attributed to differences in genetic, environmental, demographic, and associated clinical conditions is well documented. Less known is whether different plaque phenotypes may likewise respond differently to the same treatment.

In an observational study of 16% to 49% carotid stenosis, Underhill and colleagues[44] used MR imaging to monitor carotid plaque progression in relation to baseline clinical and imaging characteristics. Statin therapy was associated with plaque regression, but its effect was offset by the presence of IPH. A 2013 study leveraged the control arm of a contemporary clinical trial and found that despite optimal medical therapy, carotid plaques with and without IPH showed distinctively different progression patterns (**Fig. 3**).[45] Plaques

without IPH had a significant reduction in lipid core size and no apparent change in stenosis during the study period, whereas plaques with IPH became more stenotic owing to an expansion in overall plaque and lipid core size. A 2012 longitudinal study using serial imaging data over 4.5 years suggested that statin therapy does not prevent IPH development, and that once it develops the path of plaque progression continues unabated.[36]

From these preliminary observations, it is plausible that the presence of IPH may explain at least a portion of the residual stroke risk in the statin era. It remains to be seen whether carotid plaques with IPH would best respond to novel pharmacologic therapy or require revascularization. Large-scale, imaging-based clinical trials are needed to further investigate the etiology and nature of the residual risk experienced by some individuals. Furthermore, such studies are needed to better define pathophysiologic mechanisms to improve medical management strategies.

Carotid Revascularization: Whom to Treat?

Increasing evidence suggests that a subgroup of patients with rupture-prone carotid atherosclerosis are at greater risk for stroke and may benefit from carotid revascularization. Conversely, studies suggest that a subgroup of symptomatic patients, but with stable carotid plaque morphology, may be equally well managed with medical therapy alone.

Echolucent plaques on B-mode ultrasonography,[26] IPH and thin/ruptured fibrous cap on MR imaging,[46–48] and microembolic signals on transcranial Doppler[49] have been associated with an increased risk for future stroke in prospective studies. MR imaging detection of IPH seems to be associated with a greater than 10-fold increased risk of ischemic neurologic events in symptomatic patients.[47] Conversely, absence of IPH is associated with a favorable outcome, with an estimated annual stroke risk of only 0.6% even among recently symptomatic patients with 50% to 99% carotid stenosis.[46] These new imaging markers have the potential to provide more accurate prognostic information in clinical decision making. However, the best imaging target or combination of plaque features that will help clinicians guide management remains to be determined.

Carotid Artery Stenting: Imaging-aided Surgery Planning

Plaques with larger necrotic cores and IPH are likely more fragile and thrombogenic, creating a potential source for perioperative embolization. In addition, lack of preprocedural information of

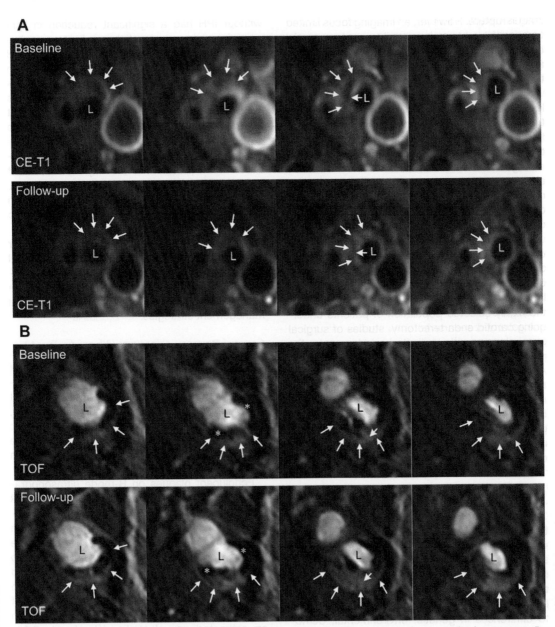

Fig. 3. Carotid plaque regression (A) and progression (B) under current standard-of-care medical treatment. For each plaque, 4 consecutive slices covering its major portion are compared between baseline and follow-up scans. (A) A plaque without IPH. Contrast-enhanced T1-weighted (CE-T1) images delineate lipid core as nonenhanced areas, and demonstrates regression of the core accompanied by decrease in total vessel area but no apparent lumen change. (B) A plaque with IPH. Time-of-flight (TOF) images show IPH as hyperintense areas, which expanded at follow-up. (*Modified from* Sun J, Balu, N, Hippe DS, et al. Subclinical carotid atherosclerosis: short-term natural history of lipid-rich necrotic core—a multicenter study with MR imaging. Radiology 2013;268:65–6; with permission.)

plaque morphology in an expansively remodeled carotid artery may result in residual edge disease and suboptimal stent placement, which has been implicated as a cause of early thrombosis in coronary stenting.[50]

To date, many studies examining the association between plaque information on noninvasive imaging and clinical outcomes of stenting have been in the coronary arteries[51] while data on carotid stenting remain scarce. In a single-center study of 112 patients undergoing CAS, Yoshimura and colleagues[52] tested the hypothesis that carotid plaques with IPH are at high risk for cerebral embolism during CAS. Preoperative time-of-flight images detected IPH in 34% of the patients. The comparison between preoperative and postoperative diffusion-weighted imaging of the brain found new ipsilateral ischemic infarcts in 65.8% of patients with carotid IPH versus 35.1% of those without. However, a study by Yoon and colleagues[53] in 91 subjects did not find a difference between the IPH group and the non-IPH group (10% vs 6.25%) in 30-day rates of stroke, myocardial infarction, and death.

Without data from large registries or clinical trials, it remains unclear whether particular plaques may need alternative forms of emboli protection during CAS, such as proximal protection devices, or whether these specific lesions would be better managed with CEA. The magnitude of malapposition and residual edge disease is unknown, as plaque imaging is rarely performed after stenting. Carotid MR imaging is able to provide detailed information on exact plaque burden, 3-dimensional plaque morphology, plaque composition, and plaque activity. It seems well suited to be used in surgical planning of CAS and may contribute to improved periprocedural outcomes.

SUMMARY

The severity of luminal stenosis has long served as the primary imaging feature to stratify patients for different treatment options. Nonetheless, clinical management of carotid artery disease has seen dramatic changes in the past 2 decades, including more effective medical therapy and improved interventional techniques. There is a gap in knowledge on stroke risk and the operative risks of CEA and CAS in the age of contemporary therapy, which highlights (1) the ineffectiveness of luminal stenosis in identifying high-risk carotid artery disease under modern medical therapy; and (2) the clinical need for better imaging for presurgical planning to minimize periprocedural risk. Information on carotid plaque morphology, composition, and activity present a promising solution to both aspects. New technical developments in carotid plaque imaging show great promise in helping to guide the management of carotid artery disease. Contemporary comparative effectiveness studies that incorporate plaque imaging are urgently needed to firmly establish the role of vessel wall imaging for more individualized, selective therapy.

REFERENCES

1. de Weerd M, Greving JP, Hedblad B, et al. Prevalence of asymptomatic carotid artery stenosis in the general population: an individual participant data meta-analysis. Stroke 2010;41:1294–7.

2. Tanimoto S, Ikari Y, Tanabe K, et al. Prevalence of carotid artery stenosis in patients with coronary artery disease in Japanese population. Stroke 2005; 36:2094–8.

3. Ahmed B, Al-Khaffaf H. Prevalence of significant asymptomatic carotid artery disease in patients with peripheral vascular disease: a meta-analysis. Eur J Vasc Endovasc Surg 2009;37:262–71.

4. Dong L, Underhill HR, Yu W, et al. Geometric and compositional appearance of atheroma in an angiographically normal carotid artery in patients with atherosclerosis. AJNR Am J Neuroradiol 2010;31:311–6.

5. Babiarz LS, Astor B, Mohamed MA, et al. Comparison of gadolinium-enhanced cardiovascular magnetic resonance angiography with high-resolution black blood cardiovascular magnetic resonance for assessing carotid artery stenosis. J Cardiovasc Magn Reson 2007;9:63–70.

6. Saam T, Underhill HR, Chu BC, et al. Prevalence of American Heart Association type VI carotid atherosclerotic lesions identified by magnetic resonance imaging for different levels of stenosis as measured by duplex ultrasound. J Am Coll Cardiol 2008;51: 1014–21.

7. Halliday A, Mansfield A, Marro J, et al. Prevention of disabling and fatal strokes by successful carotid endarterectomy in patients without recent neurological symptoms: randomised controlled trial. Lancet 2004;363:1491–502.

8. Mozaffarian D, Benjamin EJ, Go AS, et al. Heart disease and stroke statistics—2015 update: a report from the American Heart Association. Circulation 2015;131:e29–322.

9. Freilinger TM, Schindler A, Schmidt C, et al. Prevalence of nonstenosing, complicated atherosclerotic plaques in cryptogenic stroke. JACC Cardiovasc Imaging 2012;5:397–405.

10. Bayer-Karpinska A, Schindler A, Saam T. Detection of vulnerable plaque in patients with cryptogenic stroke. Neuroimag Clin N Am 2016, in press.

11. Baigent C, Keech A, Kearney PM, et al. Efficacy and safety of cholesterol-lowering treatment: prospective meta-analysis of data from 90,056 participants in 14 randomised trials of statins. Lancet 2005;366:1267–78.

12. Hong KS, Yegiaian S, Lee M, et al. Declining stroke and vascular event recurrence rates in secondary prevention trials over the past 50 years and consequences for current trial design. Circulation 2011; 123:2111–9.

13. Meschia JF, Bushnell C, Boden-Albala B, et al. Guidelines for the primary prevention of stroke: a statement for healthcare professionals from the American Heart Association/American Stroke Association. Stroke 2014;45:3754–832.

14. Kernan WN, Ovbiagele B, Black HR, et al. Guidelines for the prevention of stroke in patients with

stroke and transient ischemic attack: a guideline for healthcare professionals from the American Heart Association/American Stroke Association. Stroke 2014;45:2160–236.

15. Barnett HJ, Taylor DW, Eliasziw M, et al. Benefit of carotid endarterectomy in patients with symptomatic moderate or severe stenosis. North American Symptomatic Carotid Endarterectomy Trial Collaborators. N Engl J Med 1998;339:1415–25.

16. Endarterectomy for asymptomatic carotid artery stenosis. Executive Committee for the Asymptomatic Carotid Atherosclerosis Study. JAMA 1995;273:1421–8.

17. Abbott AL. Medical (nonsurgical) intervention alone is now best for prevention of stroke associated with asymptomatic severe carotid stenosis: results of a systematic review and analysis. Stroke 2009;40:e573–83.

18. Stone NJ, Robinson JG, Lichtenstein AH, et al. 2013 ACC/AHA guideline on the treatment of blood cholesterol to reduce atherosclerotic cardiovascular risk in adults: a report of the American College of Cardiology/American Heart Association Task Force on Practice Guidelines. Circulation 2014;129:S1–45.

19. Merwick A, Albers GW, Arsava EM, et al. Reduction in early stroke risk in carotid stenosis with transient ischemic attack associated with statin treatment. Stroke 2013;44:2814–20.

20. Yadav JS, Wholey MH, Kuntz RE, et al. Protected carotid-artery stenting versus endarterectomy in high-risk patients. N Engl J Med 2004;351:1493–501.

21. Bonati LH, Dobson J, Algra A, et al. Short-term outcome after stenting versus endarterectomy for symptomatic carotid stenosis: a preplanned meta-analysis of individual patient data. Lancet 2010;376:1062–73.

22. Brott TG, Hobson RN, Howard G, et al. Stenting versus endarterectomy for treatment of carotid-artery stenosis. N Engl J Med 2010;363:11–23.

23. Carr S, Farb A, Pearce WH, et al. Atherosclerotic plaque rupture in symptomatic carotid artery stenosis. J Vasc Surg 1996;23:755–66.

24. Spagnoli LG, Mauriello A, Sangiorgi G, et al. Extracranial thrombotically active carotid plaque as a risk factor for ischemic stroke. JAMA 2004;292:1845–52.

25. Fisher M, Paganini-Hill A, Martin A, et al. Carotid plaque pathology: thrombosis, ulceration, and stroke pathogenesis. Stroke 2005;36:253–7.

26. Gronholdt ML, Nordestgaard BG, Schroeder TV, et al. Ultrasonic echolucent carotid plaques predict future strokes. Circulation 2001;104:68–73.

27. Cai JM, Hatsukami TS, Ferguson MS, et al. In vivo quantitative measurement of intact fibrous cap and lipid-rich necrotic core size in atherosclerotic carotid plaque: comparison of high-resolution, contrast-enhanced magnetic resonance imaging and histology. Circulation 2005;112:3437–44.

28. Saam T, Ferguson MS, Yarnykh VL, et al. Quantitative evaluation of carotid plaque composition by in vivo MRI. Arterioscler Thromb Vasc Biol 2005;25:234–9.

29. Wasserman BA, Smith WI, Trout HH, et al. Carotid artery atherosclerosis: in vivo morphologic characterization with gadolinium-enhanced double-oblique MR imaging—initial results. Radiology 2002;223:566–73.

30. Takaya N, Cai JM, Ferguson MS, et al. Intra- and interreader reproducibility of magnetic resonance imaging for quantifying the lipid-rich necrotic core is improved with gadolinium contrast enhancement. J Magn Reson Imaging 2006;24:203–10.

31. Trivedi RA, U-King-Im JM, Graves MJ, et al. MRI-derived measurements of fibrous-cap and lipid-core thickness: the potential for identifying vulnerable carotid plaques in vivo. Neuroradiology 2004;46:738–43.

32. Sun J, Zhao XQ, Balu N, et al. Carotid magnetic resonance imaging for monitoring atherosclerotic plaque progression: a multicenter reproducibility study. Int J Cardiovasc Imaging 2015;31:95–103.

33. Bitar R, Moody AR, Leung G, et al. In vivo 3D high-spatial-resolution MR imaging of intraplaque hemorrhage. Radiology 2008;249:259–67.

34. Ota H, Yarnykh VL, Ferguson MS, et al. Carotid intraplaque hemorrhage imaging at 3.0-T MR imaging: comparison of the diagnostic performance of three T1-weighted sequences. Radiology 2010;254:551–63.

35. Wang J, Bornert P, Zhao H, et al. Simultaneous non-contrast angiography and intraplaque hemorrhage (SNAP) imaging for carotid atherosclerotic disease evaluation. Magn Reson Med 2013;69:337–45.

36. Sun J, Underhill HR, Hippe DS, et al. Sustained acceleration in carotid atherosclerotic plaque progression with intraplaque hemorrhage: a long-term time course study. JACC Cardiovasc Imaging 2012;5:798–804.

37. Coli S, Magnoni M, Sangiorgi G, et al. Contrast-enhanced ultrasound imaging of intraplaque neovascularization in carotid arteries: correlation with histology and plaque echogenicity. J Am Coll Cardiol 2008;52:223–30.

38. Staub D, Schinkel AF, Coli B, et al. Contrast-enhanced ultrasound imaging of the vasa vasorum: from early atherosclerosis to the identification of unstable plaques. JACC Cardiovasc Imaging 2010;3:761–71.

39. Kerwin WS, O'Brien KD, Ferguson MS, et al. Inflammation in carotid atherosclerotic plaque: a dynamic contrast-enhanced MR imaging study. Radiology 2006;241:459–68.

40. Calcagno C, Cornily JC, Hyafil F, et al. Detection of neovessels in atherosclerotic plaques of rabbits using dynamic contrast enhanced MRI and ^{18}F-FDG PET. Arterioscler Thromb Vasc Biol 2008;28:1311–7.

41. Gaens ME, Backes WH, Rozel S, et al. Dynamic contrast-enhanced MR imaging of carotid atherosclerotic plaque: model selection, reproducibility, and validation. Radiology 2013;266:271–9.

42. Rudd JH, Warburton EA, Fryer TD, et al. Imaging atherosclerotic plaque inflammation with [^{18}F]-fluorodeoxyglucose positron emission tomography. Circulation 2002;105:2708–11.

43. Tawakol A, Migrino RQ, Bashian GG, et al. In vivo ^{18}F-fluorodeoxyglucose positron emission tomography imaging provides a noninvasive measure of carotid plaque inflammation in patients. J Am Coll Cardiol 2006;48:1818–24.

44. Underhill HR, Yuan C, Yarnykh VL, et al. Arterial remodeling in the subclinical carotid artery disease. JACC Cardiovasc Imaging 2009;2:1381–9.

45. Sun J, Balu N, Hippe DS, et al. Subclinical carotid atherosclerosis: short-term natural history of lipid-rich necrotic core—a multicenter study with MR imaging. Radiology 2013;268:61–8.

46. Saam T, Hetterich H, Hoffmann V, et al. Meta-analysis and systematic review of the predictive value of carotid plaque hemorrhage on cerebrovascular events by magnetic resonance imaging. J Am Coll Cardiol 2013;62:1081–91.

47. Hosseini AA, Kandiyil N, Macsweeney ST, et al. Carotid plaque hemorrhage on magnetic resonance imaging strongly predicts recurrent ischemia and stroke. Ann Neurol 2013;73:774–84.

48. Gupta A, Baradaran H, Schweitzer AD, et al. Carotid plaque MRI and stroke risk: a systematic review and meta-analysis. Stroke 2013;44:3071–7.

49. Markus HS, King A, Shipley M, et al. Asymptomatic embolisation for prediction of stroke in the Asymptomatic Carotid Emboli Study (ACES): a prospective observational study. Lancet Neurol 2010;9:663–71.

50. Nakano M, Yahagi K, Otsuka F, et al. Causes of early stent thrombosis in patients presenting with acute coronary syndrome: an ex vivo human autopsy study. J Am Coll Cardiol 2014;63:2510–20.

51. Watabe H, Sato A, Akiyama D, et al. Impact of coronary plaque composition on cardiac troponin elevation after percutaneous coronary intervention in stable angina pectoris: a computed tomography analysis. J Am Coll Cardiol 2012;59:1881–8.

52. Yoshimura S, Yamada K, Kawasaki M, et al. High-intensity signal on time-of-flight magnetic resonance angiography indicates carotid plaques at high risk for cerebral embolism during stenting. Stroke 2011;42:3132–7.

53. Yoon W, Kim SK, Park MS, et al. Safety of protected carotid artery stenting in patients with severe carotid artery stenosis and carotid intraplaque hemorrhage. AJNR Am J Neuroradiol 2012;33:1027–31.

Clinical Perspective of Carotid Plaque Imaging

Leo H. Bonati, MD[a],*, Paul J. Nederkoorn, MD, PhD[b]

KEYWORDS

- Carotid plaque • Imaging • Stroke • Endarterectomy • Stenting • Personalized medicine

KEY POINTS

- At present, patients with carotid disease are selected for invasive recanalization therapies mainly based on the degree of luminal narrowing and the presence or absence of recent ischemic symptoms.
- A more sophisticated risk model takes into account other clinical variables, such as age, sex, and timing and type of recent symptoms as well as presence of irregular or ulcerated plaque.
- A growing body of evidence shows that noninvasive imaging of the carotid plaque by various methods reliably identifies structural correlates of plaque vulnerability, which are associated with an increased risk of cerebrovascular events.
- These observations are in line with current understanding of the pathophysiology of atherosclerosis according to which plaque rupture and subsequent embolism, rather than reduction in flow in the stenotic vessel, are key mechanisms leading to stroke.
- Integration of plaque imaging at baseline in randomized controlled trials is needed to test the hypothesis that plaque imaging helps select patients who benefit from carotid revascularization. If this holds true, then plaque imaging should be incorporated in management guidelines.

INTRODUCTION

Stroke is the leading cause of acquired disability in adult life and represents the second most common cause of death after ischemic heart disease in developed nations.[1] Atherosclerotic disease of the carotid artery causes about 10% to 15% of ischemic strokes.[2,3] Carotid atherosclerosis in Caucasian populations is most commonly located at the carotid artery bifurcation, typically involving the distal common carotid and the proximal internal carotid artery, and to a lesser extent the proximal external carotid artery. Carotid artery atherosclerosis is more frequent in men than in women, and its prevalence increases with age. Ultrasound screening studies in Central and Northern European and North American populations have shown a prevalence of at least a moderate degree of asymptomatic carotid stenosis (narrowing the lumen by ≥50%) of 2.3% in 60 to 69 year old men, 6.0% in 70 to 79 year old men, and up to 7.5% in men 80 years and older; in women, the prevalence rates were 2.0%, 3.6%, and 5.0%, in the same age groups, respectively.[4] Severe carotid stenosis measuring 70% or greater was present in 0.8%, 2.1%, and 3.1% in the same age groups in men, and in 0.2%, 1.0%, and 0.9% in women.

Disclosures: L.H. Bonati has received funding from the Swiss National Science Foundation (PBBSB-116873, 32003B-156658) and the University of Basel. He has served on scientific advisory boards for Bayer. P.J. Nederkoorn received funding as local PI of the Plaque At RISK (PARISK) study, supported by the Center for Translational Molecular Medicine (CTMM; Grant 01C-202).

[a] Stroke Center, Departments of Neurology and Clinical Research, University Hospital Basel, Petersgraben 4, Basel CH-4031, Switzerland; [b] Department of Neurology, Academic Medical Center Amsterdam, Meibergdreef 9, Amsterdam 1105 AZ, The Netherlands
* Corresponding author.
E-mail address: bonatil@uhbs.ch

Neuroimag Clin N Am 26 (2016) 175–182
http://dx.doi.org/10.1016/j.nic.2015.09.012
1052-5149/16/$ – see front matter © 2016 Elsevier Inc. All rights reserved.

Despite the high prevalence of carotid disease in the community, only a small proportion of the individuals affected will ever develop a transient ischemic attack (TIA) or a stroke. Although several randomized controlled trials (RCTs) have demonstrated that carotid endarterectomy (CEA), and in selected patients, carotid artery stenting (CAS), lowers the risk of stroke in patients with symptomatic and asymptomatic carotid stenosis, the numbers of interventions (number needed to treat; NNT) necessary to prevent one stroke are rather high. The present article reviews the current treatment dilemmas faced in the management of carotid disease and highlights the potential of carotid plaque imaging in selecting patients who benefit from carotid revascularization, thus allowing for more personalized treatment decisions.

STROKE RISK AND THE EFFECT OF REVASCULARIZATION IN PATIENTS WITH CAROTID DISEASE
Symptomatic Carotid Stenosis

The bulk of evidence on stroke risk under medical therapy for symptomatic carotid stenosis stems from the medical treatment groups of RCTs, which evaluated the benefit of CEA versus medical therapy alone 2 to 3 decades ago. In a pooled analysis of the North American Symptomatic Carotid Endarterectomy Trial (NASCET),[5] the European Carotid Surgery Trial (ECST),[6] and a third, smaller trial (the Veterans Affairs trial, VA309[7]), including 6092 patients and 35,000 patient-years of follow-up, the cumulative risk of ipsilateral stroke in patients with recently symptomatic severe carotid stenosis (causing 70%–99% narrowing) randomly allocated to medical therapy was approximately 26% at 5 years after randomization.[8] This risk was reduced by an absolute difference of 16% in the group of patients randomized to undergo CEA. In patients with moderate, 50% to 69% stenosis, the 5-year risk of ipsilateral stroke was about 18% and reduced by only 4.6%.[5] The risk of periprocedural stroke or death (which by definition includes outcome events occurring up to 30 days after treatment) was 7.1% in this pooled analysis and did not vary significantly with the degree of stenosis.

Importantly though, 55% of patients in the NASCET trial were randomized more than 30 days after the qualifying event (TIA or minor stroke), and in ECST, this proportion was 65%. These RCT data therefore do not allow estimating stroke risk in the first days after initial symptoms, which may be much higher. In large prospective registries of patients presenting with TIA, up to 20% of those with large artery atherosclerosis as the underlying

cause had a stroke within 90 days of the TIA, with most events occurring in the first 7 to 14 days.[2,9]

On the other hand, one has to acknowledge that ECST recruited patients between 1981 and 1994, and NASCET between 1988 and 1996. Medical therapy in these trials mainly consisted of aspirin only. In the NASCET trial, only 14% of patients were taking lipid-lowering therapy at the time of randomization. It is reasonable to assume that with more widespread use of statins and more aggressive antiplatelet regimes, the risk of early recurrent stroke in symptomatic carotid stenosis is lower today than reported in these earlier trials and TIA cohorts.

Since the time these trials were done, CAS has emerged as an alternative, less-invasive option to treat carotid stenosis and was compared against CEA in several RCTs, which enrolled mostly patients with symptomatic carotid stenosis. On average, CAS was as effective as CEA in these trials in maintaining the artery patent and preventing recurrent stroke in the long term.[10–13] However, CAS was associated with a higher risk of periprocedural stroke than surgery.[14] Subgroup analyses revealed that this excess risk in procedure-related stroke in CAS is mainly limited to patients older than 70 years, whereas CAS and CEA seem to be equally safe in younger patients.[15] Nonetheless, the fundamental problem of identifying patients in whom the risk of stroke under modern medical therapy is still high enough to warrant carotid revascularization has remained.

Asymptomatic Carotid Stenosis

Two large randomized trials, the Asymptomatic Carotid Atherosclerosis Study (ACAS), which recruited 1662 patients between 1987 and 1993, and the Asymptomatic Carotid Surgery Trial (ACST), which recruited 3120 patients between 1993 and 2003, consistently demonstrated an 11% risk of ipsilateral stroke in patients with asymptomatic carotid stenosis of 60% or higher who were assigned to initial medical management.[16,17] This risk was reduced by 6% in ACAS and 4% in ACST in patients assigned to immediate endarterectomy. Of note, fewer than 10% of patients in ACST were on lipid-lowering therapy at the beginning of recruitment in 1993, and this proportion steadily increased to more than 80% at termination of follow-up in 2008.

A meta-regression analysis of data from medical arms of randomized trials and prospective cohorts suggested that the risk of ipsilateral stroke associated with asymptomatic carotid stenosis has declined over the past 20 years and may now be only 1% per year or lower,[18] most likely attributable to advances in medical therapy. Indeed, under modern medical management of atherosclerosis, only a minority of patients with asymptomatic carotid disease may currently benefit from invasive revascularization.

CHANGING MANAGEMENT PARADIGMS AND THE ROLE OF CAROTID PLAQUE IMAGING
Current Guidelines and Their Limitations

Current guidelines for treatment of carotid stenosis in the United States and in Europe are informed by the evidence of the RCTs cited above, and hence, recommendations are largely based on degree of luminal narrowing and presence of recent ocular or cerebral ischemic events in the dependent vascular territory[19–23]: CEA within 2 weeks of presenting symptoms is recommended in patients with symptomatic carotid stenosis of 50% or higher; carotid stenting is considered an alternative treatment in patients with symptomatic carotid disease below the age of 70. CEA can be considered in patients with asymptomatic stenosis of at least 60% and a life expectancy of 5 years or longer.

Although widely established in clinical practice, these guidelines have major limitations. Even at the time when the RCTs of CEA versus medical therapy for symptomatic carotid stenosis were performed (and medical therapy was not very effective), many operations had to be done to prevent one stroke. Translating absolute risk reductions observed in these trials into numbers needed to treat (NNT), 9 men and 36 women with moderate or severe (50%–99% degree) symptomatic carotid stenosis had to be operated on to prevent a single stroke in each sex group after 5 years (Fig. 1). With advances in medical therapy for

atherosclerosis, NNTs are likely to be even higher today. This demonstrates that there is a strong need to improve the selection of patients with carotid disease who are at risk of stroke and are likely to benefit from revascularization, in order to reduce the number of unnecessary procedures performed.

The Risk Modeling Approach

Clinical risk modeling allows further differentiation of stroke risk in patients with symptomatic carotid stenosis. A score was derived from data of patients with 0% to 69% stenosis and validated with data of patients with 70% to 99% stenosis in ECST to predict the amount of benefit from CEA in individual patients.[24] This score included both angiographic findings and clinical patient characteristics associated with the risk of ipsilateral stroke during long-term follow-up under medical therapy (degree of stenosis, plaque surface irregularity, cerebrovascular events in the past 2 months, and type of clinical events: cerebral vs ocular) as well as variables associated with an increased risk of periprocedural stroke or death when undergoing CEA (female sex, peripheral vascular disease, and systolic blood pressure >180 mm Hg). The model nicely predicted net benefit from CEA in terms of reduction in 5-year ipsilateral stroke (Fig. 2). The distribution of this risk score in the trial population (see number of patients below the plot in Fig. 2) also demonstrated that only a minority of patients, that is,

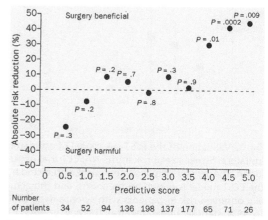

Fig. 2. Absolute reduction in 5-year risk of ipsilateral stroke or perioperative stroke or death through CEA in patients with symptomatic carotid stenosis. (*From* Rothwell PM, Warlow CP. Prediction of benefit from carotid endarterectomy in individual patients: a risk-modelling study. European Carotid Surgery Trialists' Collaborative Group. Lancet 1999;353(9170):2105–10; with permission.)

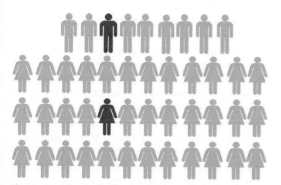

Fig. 1. Numbers of CEA procedures necessary to prevent a stroke in patients with symptomatic carotid stenosis. Visualization of the NNT for CEA to prevent one stroke after 5 years of follow-up: 9 men and 36 women with moderate or severe recently symptomatic carotid stenosis have to be operated to prevent a single stroke in each sex group.

those with a score of 4 or higher, clearly benefited from CEA. In a large proportion of patients, there was no clear benefit of surgery, and this proportion has likely increased since with availability of modern medical therapy.

The full data of the medical arm of ECST were later used to derive a model to estimate the 5-year ipsilateral stroke risk under medical therapy and were validated in the cohort of patients randomly assigned to medical treatment in NASCET (Fig. 3, Table 1).[25] The ECST model accurately predicted the risk of ipsilateral stroke among patients with symptomatic carotid stenosis in the medical group of the NASCET trial, while having no effect on the risk of periprocedural stroke or death in patients treated with endarterectomy. Thus, the ECST score represents a useful tool to select patients likely to benefit from revascularization.

The ongoing Second European Carotid Surgery Trial (ECST-2, ISRCTN97744893) has been designed to test the hypothesis that among patients with symptomatic or asymptomatic carotid stenosis and an expected 5-year risk of ipsilateral stroke of less than 15%, optimized medical therapy (OMT) is as efficient as OMT plus carotid revascularization combined. The trial uses a recalibrated version of the ECST-risk model, which takes into account the presumed lower risk of stroke under modern medical therapy, to select patients with symptomatic stenosis eligible for the trial. This recalibrated model can be accessed via http://s489637516.websitehome.co.uk/ECST2/CAR/index.html or downloaded as an app for iPhone/iPad and android devices free of charge. It also represents a useful tool to estimate stroke risk and benefit from revascularization in everyday clinical practice. Links can be found on the trial home page of www.ECST2.com.

Of note, the definition for irregular or ulcerated plaque was based on intra-arterial angiography, which was widely used at the time ECST and NASCET recruited patients, but which has in the meantime largely given way to noninvasive imaging, including duplex ultrasound and computed tomography (CT)- or magnetic resonance (MR)-based angiography. Presence of irregular or ulcerated plaque doubled the risk for ipsilateral stroke during follow-up (hazard ratio 2.03, 95% confidence interval 1.31–3.14; see Table 1). Criteria to define a plaque as irregular or ulcerated with noninvasive imaging are much less stringent.

Evolving Concepts in Carotid Imaging: The Vulnerable Plaque

The fact that the focus of carotid imaging has been limited to measuring degree of stenosis for a long time is partly explained by the historical concept of flow impairment as the main mechanism of cerebral ischemia. Limitation of intracranial flow requires a cross-sectional area of 4 to 5 mm^2 along a length of 3 mm; this area corresponds to less than 2 mm in the smallest 2-dimensional profile seen on an angiogram.[26] Up to this degree of luminal narrowing, any reduction in diameter is compensated for by an increase in blood flow velocity across the stenosis. Only a small minority of patients with carotid disease have such severely narrowed arteries, suggesting that other mechanisms may play a part in the strong association between stenosis severity and risk of recurrent stroke in medically treated patients.

That higher degree of stenosis is a risk factor for stroke in patients with recently symptomatic carotid stenosis may simply be explained by the fact that a larger burden of plaque is associated with a greater tendency to recurrent plaque rupture.[8] Interestingly though, the same relationship could not be consistently demonstrated in trials of CEA for patients with asymptomatic disease.[16,27]

Underlying the shift away from simply measuring degree of stenosis toward imaging of the carotid

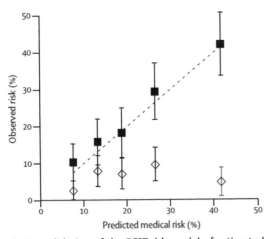

Fig. 3. Validation of the ECST-risk model of estimated ipsilateral 5-year stroke risk in the NASCET trial population. The 5-year risk of ipsilateral stroke predicted by the ECST model is shown on the x-axis, and the actually observed risk in patients with symptomatic 50% to 99% stenosis under medical therapy in NASCET (squares) is shown on the y-axis. In addition, the observed rate of periprocedural stroke or death in patients undergoing CEA is shown as diamonds. Error bars represent 95% confidence intervals. (*From* Rothwell PM, Mehta Z, Howard SC, et al. Treating individuals 3: from subgroups to individuals: general principles and the example of carotid endarterectomy. Lancet 2005;365:259; with permission.)

Table 1
Cox model for 5-year risk of ipsilateral ischemic stroke on medical treatment in patients with recently symptomatic carotid stenosis derived from European Carotid Surgery Trial

Risk Factor	Hazard Ratio (95% Confidence Interval)	P Value
Stenosis (per 10%)	1.18 (1.10–1.25)	<.0001
Near occlusion	0.49 (0.19–1.24)	.1309
Male sex	1.19 (0.81–1.75)	.3687
Age (per 10 y)	1.12 (0.89–1.39)	.3343
Time since last event (per 7 d)	0.96 (0.93–0.99)	.0039
Presenting event		
Ocular	1.000	.0067
Single TIA	1.41 (0.75–2.66)	—
Multiple TIAs	2.05 (1.16–3.60)	—
Minor stroke	1.82 (0.99–3.34)	—
Major stroke	2.54 (1.48–4.35)	—
Diabetes	1.35 (0.86–2.11)	.1881
Previous myocardial infarction	1.57 (1.01–2.45)	.0471
Peripheral vascular disease	1.18 (0.78–1.77)	.4368
Treated hypertension	1.24 (0.88–1.75)	.2137
Irregular/ulcerated plaque	2.03 (1.31–3.14)	.0015

Data from Eckstein HH, Ringleb P, Allenberg JR, et al. Results of the Stent-Protected Angioplasty versus Carotid Endarterectomy (SPACE) study to treat symptomatic stenoses at 2 years: a multinational, prospective, randomised trial. Lancet Neurol 2008;7:893–902.

plaque itself has been a change in the understanding of the pathophysiology of carotid atherosclerosis. Today, it is generally accepted that rather than impairment in blood flow, the predominant mechanism underlying cerebral ischemia associated with carotid stenosis is rupture of the atherosclerotic plaque with subsequent embolism of locally formed thrombus or plaque debris to the brain. This finding has fostered the concept of the vulnerable or unstable plaque, which is prone to rupture, as opposed to the stable plaque, which may remain inert over many years. A growing body of data supports that inflammation plays a key role in the pathophysiology of atherosclerosis and particularly in plaque rupture.[28–30] In the early phase of plaque formation, low-density lipoproteins accumulate in the vessel wall.[31] These lipoproteins undergo oxidation and thereby acquire pro-inflammatory biological functions unrelated to cholesterol homeostasis.[32] Oxidized lipoproteins activate endothelial cells by inducing expression of adhesion molecules, chemokines, and pro-inflammatory cytokines. They also help activate macrophages by triggering a variety of receptors of innate immune responses. Monocytes are attracted by chemokines and migrate into the plaque facilitated by expression of the vascular cell adhesion molecule-1 on endothelial cells.[33] Within the plaque, monocytes differentiate into macrophages, which take up oxidized lipoprotein particles and turn into so-called foam cells.[34] Foam cells secrete pro-inflammatory cytokines and a large array of proteases, including matrix metalloproteases, serine proteases, elastases, and cysteine proteases, that contribute to degradation of elastin and collagen in advanced lesions leading to destabilization of the plaque, thinning of its fibrous cap, and, ultimately, plaque rupture.[35,36] If the plaque surface ruptures, platelets are exposed to subendothelial collagen, von Willebrand factor, and local agonists such as adenosine diphosphate. Activated platelets bind to fibrinogen and secrete various pro-coagulatory and pro-inflammatory factors, which mediate the binding of leukocytes and enhance fibrin formation. A local thrombus may form on the plaque surface, leading to embolization and occlusion of arteries in the eye or the brain, manifesting as amaurosis fugax, TIA, or stroke.

Several plaque imaging modalities are available today that are capable of depicting key structural (or metabolic) correlates of plaque instability, including lipid-rich necrotic core, intraplaque hemorrhage (IPH), thinning or rupture of the fibrous cap, or plaque inflammation. These techniques and their ability to predict the risk of cerebrovascular events in patients with carotid disease are discussed in detail in the other articles in this issue.

Plaque imaging holds promise in greatly augmenting the capability to identify patients with carotid disease who are at high risk of stroke, and hence, most likely to benefit from invasive revascularization (even in the context of modern medical therapy), mainly because the information gathered is complementary to the data that currently inform the decision, such as degree of stenosis and clinical characteristics. A recent study in which the presence of IPH on plaque MRI was a much stronger predictor of recurrent stroke and TIA than was the degree of stenosis in patients with symptomatic carotid disease nicely illustrated this.[37]

A meta-analysis pooling data from studies reported the risk of the combined endpoint of TIA and stroke to be elevated by an odds ratio of 11.7 (95% confidence interval 5.2–26.5) with the presence of IPH on MRI among patients with symptomatic carotid stenosis and by 3.5 (2.6–4.7) in patients with asymptomatic stenosis.[38] As a limitation, most included studies combined recurrent stroke or TIA for reasons of increasing statistical power; therefore, no reliable estimates of increase in stroke risk based on the presence of IPH can be made at present. To obtain reliable estimates on prediction of stroke risk, pooling of individual patient-level data from these studies is required, and such efforts are currently being made. However, even if IPH was associated with a mere 5- or 6-fold increase in stroke risk in patients with symptomatic carotid stenosis (rather than the 12-fold increase in risk of stroke or TIA combined), it would by far be the marker contributing most strongly to the risk model (see **Table 1**).

Of note, plaque instability may not only impact the risk of recurrent stroke under medical therapy, but also impact the risk of procedure-related stroke in patients undergoing carotid revascularization. Data from the Carotid Revascularization Endarterectomy versus Stent Trial (CREST) trial, which randomly assigned 1321 patients with symptomatic carotid stenosis and 1181 patients with asymptomatic stenosis to CAS or CEA, support this. The risk of any stroke or death occurring between randomization and 30 days after treatment was 6.0% in the CAS group and 3.2% in the CEA group among patients with recent carotid-related symptoms, compared with 2.5% and 1.4%, respectively, in asymptomatic patients. The presence of recent symptoms can be regarded as a clinical marker of plaque instability, and it is evident that with both treatments, procedural risks were greater than if the plaque had been clinically stable (the definition of asymptomatic carotid stenosis in clinical trials is commonly absence of ischemic symptoms such as stroke, TIA, or ocular ischemia in the past 6 months).

The impact of imaging markers of plaque instability on treatment risks has also been demonstrated, particularly in patients undergoing CAS. An increased frequency of new ischemic brain lesions on cerebral MRI after stent procedures has been shown in patients with echolucent plaques on quantitative ultrasound,[39] high T1-signal intensity ratio on plaque MR imaging (as in IPH),[40,41] and hypodense plaque on CT.[42] The same associations could not be demonstrated for patients undergoing CEA.[39,41] These findings might indicate that plaque instability poses a greater risk of periprocedural embolic stroke in CAS than in CEA. During CAS, where blood flow toward the brain is usually maintained, debris of unstable plaques may be released during catheterization or stent insertion, causing embolism to the brain, and not all of these emboli may be captured by cerebral protection devices. In contrast, the carotid artery is clamped off during CEA protecting the brain from emboli more efficiently.

To evaluate whether plaque imaging not only helps identify patients at risk for stroke under medical therapy but also adds to established risk models (such as the ECST model) to select those who benefit from revascularization therapies requires an experimental setting in which the effect of revascularization can be reliably measured. This measurement is only possible in RCTs comparing revascularization versus current medical therapy. ECST-2, including patients with both symptomatic and asymptomatic carotid stenosis (see above), and the Carotid Revascularization and Medical Management for Asymptomatic Carotid Stenosis Trial (CREST-2, NCT02089217), which includes patients with asymptomatic disease, are 2 ongoing RCTs in which the usefulness of plaque imaging could be tested.

SUMMARY

Carotid plaque imaging has the potential to improve the identification of patients with atherosclerotic carotid disease who are at risk of stroke and who benefit from revascularization by CAS or CEA. Leading on from the growing number of prospective observational studies that demonstrated proof of concept that plaque imaging predicts the risk of cerebrovascular events, incorporation of plaque imaging into RCTs is now necessary to investigate to what magnitude the benefit from revascularization in terms of reducing long-term stroke risk can be predicted. A global model incorporating both clinical and plaque-imaging–based risk factor is likely to be superior to the current status quo, in which treatment decisions are largely based on symptom status and degree of stenosis alone.

REFERENCES

1. GBD 2013 Mortality and Causes of Death Collaborators. Global, regional, and national age-sex specific all-cause and cause-specific mortality for 240 causes of death, 1990-2013: a systematic analysis for the global burden of disease study 2013. Lancet 2015;385(9963):117–71.

2. Lovett JK, Coull AJ, Rothwell PM. Early risk of recurrence by subtype of ischemic stroke in population-based incidence studies. Neurology 2004;62:569–73.

3. Schneider AT, Kissela B, Woo D, et al. Ischemic stroke subtypes: a population-based study of incidence rates among blacks and whites. Stroke 2004;35:1552–6.

4. de Weerd M, Greving JP, Hedblad B, et al. Prevalence of asymptomatic carotid artery stenosis in the general population: an individual participant data meta-analysis. Stroke 2010;41:1294–7.

5. Barnett HJ, Taylor DW, Eliasziw M, et al. Benefit of carotid endarterectomy in patients with symptomatic moderate or severe stenosis. North American Symptomatic Carotid Endarterectomy Trial collaborators. N Engl J Med 1998;339:1415–25.

6. Randomised trial of endarterectomy for recently symptomatic carotid stenosis: final results of the MRC European Carotid Surgery Trial (ECST). Lancet 1998;351:1379–87.

7. Mayberg MR, Wilson SE, Yatsu F, et al. Carotid endarterectomy and prevention of cerebral ischemia in symptomatic carotid stenosis. Veterans Affairs cooperative studies program 309 trialist group. JAMA 1991;266:3289–94.

8. Rothwell PM, Eliasziw M, Gutnikov SA, et al. Analysis of pooled data from the randomised controlled trials of endarterectomy for symptomatic carotid stenosis. Lancet 2003;361:107–16.

9. Purroy F, Montaner J, Molina CA, et al. Patterns and predictors of early risk of recurrence after transient ischemic attack with respect to etiologic subtypes. Stroke 2007;38:3225–9.

10. Eckstein HH, Ringleb P, Allenberg JR, et al. Results of the stent-protected angioplasty versus carotid endarterectomy (space) study to treat symptomatic stenoses at 2 years: a multinational, prospective, randomised trial. Lancet Neurol 2008;7:893–902.

11. Mas JL, Arquizan C, Calvet D, et al. Long-term follow-up study of endarterectomy versus angioplasty in patients with symptomatic severe carotid stenosis trial. Stroke 2014;45:2750–6.

12. Bonati LH, Dobson J, Featherstone RL, et al. Long-term outcomes after stenting versus endarterectomy for treatment of symptomatic carotid stenosis: the International Carotid Stenting Study (ICSS) randomised trial. Lancet 2015;385:529–38.

13. Lal BK, Beach KW, Roubin GS, et al. Restenosis after carotid artery stenting and endarterectomy: a secondary analysis of crest, a randomised controlled trial. Lancet Neurol 2012;11:755–63.

14. Bonati LH, Lyrer P, Ederle J, et al. Percutaneous transluminal balloon angioplasty and stenting for carotid artery stenosis. Cochrane Database Syst Rev 2012;(9):CD000515.

15. Bonati LH, Dobson J, Algra A, et al. Short-term outcome after stenting versus endarterectomy for symptomatic carotid stenosis: a preplanned meta-analysis of individual patient data. Lancet 2010; 376:1062–73.

16. Endarterectomy for asymptomatic carotid artery stenosis. Executive committee for the asymptomatic carotid atherosclerosis study. JAMA 1995;273:1421–8.

17. Halliday A, Mansfield A, Marro J, et al. Prevention of disabling and fatal strokes by successful carotid endarterectomy in patients without recent neurological symptoms: randomised controlled trial. Lancet 2004;363:1491–502.

18. Abbott AL. Medical (nonsurgical) intervention alone is now best for prevention of stroke associated with asymptomatic severe carotid stenosis: results of a systematic review and analysis. Stroke 2009; 40:e573–83.

19. European Stroke O, Tendera M, Aboyans V, et al. ESC guidelines on the diagnosis and treatment of peripheral artery diseases: document covering atherosclerotic disease of extracranial carotid and vertebral, mesenteric, renal, upper and lower extremity arteries: the Task Force on the Diagnosis and Treatment of Peripheral Artery Diseases of the European Society of Cardiology (ESC). Eur Heart J 2011;32:2851–906.

20. Brott TG, Halperin JL, Abbara S, et al. 2011 ASA/ACCF/AHA/AANN/AANS/ACR/ASNR/CNS/SAIP/SCAI/SIR/SNIS/SVM/SVS guideline on the management of patients with extracranial carotid and vertebral artery disease. Stroke 2011;42:e464–540.

21. Eckstein HH, Kuhnl A, Dorfler A, et al. The diagnosis, treatment and follow-up of extracranial carotid stenosis. Dtsch Arztebl Int 2013;110:468–76.

22. Brown MM, Bonati LH, Söderman M, et al. Karolinksa stroke update consensus statement 2012: carotid endarterectomy vs. angioplasty and stenting. 2012. Available at: http://www.strokeupdate.org/Cons_Carotid_session_2012.aspx.

23. Kernan WN, Ovbiagele B, Black HR, et al. Guidelines for the prevention of stroke in patients with stroke and transient ischemic attack: a guideline for healthcare professionals from the American Heart Association/American Stroke Association. Stroke 2014;45:2160–236.

24. Rothwell PM, Warlow CP. Prediction of benefit from carotid endarterectomy in individual patients: a risk-modelling study. European Carotid Surgery Trialists' Collaborative Group. Lancet 1999;353:2105–10.

25. Rothwell PM, Mehta Z, Howard SC, et al. Treating individuals 3: from subgroups to individuals: general principles and the example of carotid endarterectomy. Lancet 2005;365:256–65.

26. Brice JG, Dowsett DJ, Lowe RD. Haemodynamic effects of carotid artery stenosis. Br Med J 1964;2:1363–6.

27. Halliday A, Harrison M, Hayter E, et al. 10-year stroke prevention after successful carotid endarterectomy for asymptomatic stenosis (ACST-1): a multicentre randomised trial. Lancet 2010;376:1074–84.

28. Ross R. Atherosclerosis–an inflammatory disease. N Engl J Med 1999;340:115–26.

29. Glass CK, Witztum JL. Atherosclerosis. The road ahead. Cell 2001;104:503–16.

30. Libby P, Ridker PM, Maseri A. Inflammation and atherosclerosis. Circulation 2002;105:1135–43.

31. Williams KJ, Tabas I. The response-to-retention hypothesis of early atherogenesis. Arterioscler Thromb Vasc Biol 1995;15:551–61.

32. Binder CJ, Chang MK, Shaw PX, et al. Innate and acquired immunity in atherogenesis. Nat Med 2002;8:1218–26.

33. Mestas J, Ley K. Monocyte-endothelial cell interactions in the development of atherosclerosis. Trends Cardiovasc Med 2008;18:228–32.

34. Johnson JL, Newby AC. Macrophage heterogeneity in atherosclerotic plaques. Curr Opin Lipidol 2009;20:370–8.

35. Shibata N, Glass CK. Regulation of macrophage function in inflammation and atherosclerosis. J Lipid Res 2009;50(Suppl):S277–81.

36. Dollery CM, Libby P. Atherosclerosis and proteinase activation. Cardiovasc Res 2006;69:625–35.

37. Hosseini AA, Kandiyil N, Macsweeney ST, et al. Carotid plaque hemorrhage on magnetic resonance imaging strongly predicts recurrent ischemia and stroke. Ann Neurol 2013;73:774–84.

38. Saam T, Hetterich H, Hoffmann V, et al. Meta-analysis and systematic review of the predictive value of carotid plaque hemorrhage on cerebrovascular events by magnetic resonance imaging. J Am Coll Cardiol 2013;62:1081–91.

39. Burow A, Lyrer PA, Nederkoorn PJ, et al. Echographic risk index and cerebral ischemic brain lesions in patients randomized to stenting versus endarterectomy for symptomatic carotid artery stenosis. Ultraschall Med 2014;35:267–72.

40. Akutsu N, Hosoda K, Fujita A, et al. A preliminary prediction model with MR plaque imaging to estimate risk for new ischemic brain lesions on diffusion-weighted imaging after endarterectomy or stenting in patients with carotid stenosis. AJNR Am J Neuroradiol 2012;33:1557–64.

41. Yamada K, Yoshimura S, Kawasaki M, et al. Embolic complications after carotid artery stenting or carotid endarterectomy are associated with tissue characteristics of carotid plaques evaluated by magnetic resonance imaging. Atherosclerosis 2011;215:399–404.

42. Uchiyama N, Misaki K, Mohri M, et al. Association between carotid plaque composition assessed by multidetector computed tomography and cerebral embolism after carotid stenting. Neuroradiology 2012;54:487–93.

Index

Note: Page numbers of article titles are in **boldface** type.

1052-5149/16/$ – see front matter © 2016 Elsevier Inc. All rights reserved.

neuroimaging.theclinics.com

Moving?

Make sure your subscription moves with you!

To notify us of your new address, find your **Clinics Account Number** (located on your mailing label above your name), and contact customer service at:

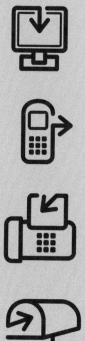

Email: journalscustomerservice-usa@elsevier.com

800-654-2452 (subscribers in the U.S. & Canada)
314-447-8871 (subscribers outside of the U.S. & Canada)

Fax number: 314-447-8029

Elsevier Health Sciences Division
Subscription Customer Service
3251 Riverport Lane
Maryland Heights, MO 63043

*To ensure uninterrupted delivery of your subscription, please notify us at least 4 weeks in advance of move.

ELSEVIER

Printed and bound by CPI Group (UK) Ltd, Croydon, CR0 4YY

03/10/2024

01040381-0020